**Prentice-Hall Series
in the Philosophy of Medicine**

Samuel Gorovitz,
Series Editor

Nursing

Th

Prentice-Hall, Inc., Englewood Cliffs, New Jersey 07632

Practice

Ethical Issues

ANDREW JAMETON

Institute for Health Policy Studies
Department of Mental Health and Community Nursing
University of California, San Francisco

with a foreword by
Ingeborg G. Mauksch
Lecturer-Consultant in Nursing

Library of Congress Cataloging in Publication Data

JAMETON, ANDREW.
  Nursing practice.

  (Prentice-Hall series in the philosophy of medicine)
  Includes bibliographies and index.
  1. Nursing ethics. I. Title. II. Series. [DNLM:
1. Ethics, Nursing. WY 85 J31n]
RT85.J35 1984   174'.2   83-17700
ISBN 0-13-627448-X

Editorial/production supervision: Elizabeth H. Athorn
Manufacturing buyer: Harry P. Baisley

Printed in the United States of America
10 9 8 7 6 5 4 3 2 1

ISBN 0-13-627448-X

Prentice-Hall-International, Inc., *London*
Prentice-Hall of Australia Pty. Limited, *Sydney*
Editora Prentice-Hall do Brasil, Ltda., *Rio de Janeiro*
Prentice-Hall Canada Inc., *Toronto*
Prentice-Hall of India Private Limited, *New Delhi*
Prentice-Hall of Japan, Inc., *Tokyo*
Prentice-Hall of Southeast Asia Pte. Ltd., *Singapore*
Whitehall Books Limited, *Wellington, New Zealand*

To Rachel

Contents

Nursing's Struggle for Autonomy 36

What Philosophers Do 58

PART TWO: CONVENTIONAL NURSING ETHICS PRINCIPLES AND PHILOSOPHICAL REFLECTION

Conventional Principles and Values 71

Competence: *Nurses Have an Obligation to Be Competent.* 80

Patient Good: *The Good of Patients Should Be the Nurse's Primary Concern.* **89**

Nonexploitation: *Nurses Should Not Use Their Positions to Exploit Patients.* **100**

Loyalty: *Nurses Should Be Loyal to Each Other.* **118**

10

Basic Moral Concepts and Theories **122**

11

Reason, Reflection, and Research in Ethics *152*

PART THREE: CASES AND PROBLEM AREAS IN NURSING PRACTICE

12

Talking with Clients *166*

13

Informed Consent *184*

14

Difficult Clients *201*

15
Death, Pain, and Suffering   *221*

16
Technology and Humanism: The Newborn Intensive Care Unit   *244*

17
Social and Political Responsibilities of Nurses   *261*

18
Making Hard Choices *278*

APPENDIX: SELECTED DOCUMENTS

Preface to the Series

It is a commonplace observation that there have been dramatic increases both in public and professional concern with questions of bioethics and in the role of philosophers in addressing those questions. Medical ethics is a well-established area of inquiry; not only does it include journals, widespread courses, professional specialists, and the other features of established fields, but philosophers now participate regularly in the deliberations of public agencies at both state and federal levels. Nonetheless, there is considerably more to the philosophy of medicine than medical ethics, and even within the area of medical ethics, there are many issues that have not been adequately explored.

The Prentice-Hall Series in the Philosophy of Medicine has been established in large measure in response to these two points. Some volumes in the series will explore philosophical aspects of medicine that are not primarily questions of ethics. They thereby contribute both to the subject matter of the philosophy of medicine and to an expanding appreciation of the breadth and diversity of the philosophy of medicine. Other volumes in the series will illuminate areas of ethical concern which, despite the recent prominence of medical ethics, have been inadequately considered.

Each volume is written by a philosopher, although none is written primarily for philosophers. Rather, the volumes are designed to bring the issues before an intelligent general readership, and they therefore presuppose no specific background in either the philosophical literature or the literature of the specific areas of medical practice or health policy on which they focus.

The problems considered in this series are of widespread public importance. We suffer from no delusions that philosophers hold the solutions; we do, however, share the conviction that these problems cannot be adequately addressed without an informed appreciation of their philosophical dimensions. We must always reach beyond philosophy in addressing problems in the world, but we should be wary of reaching without it. The volumes in this series are thus addressed to all those concerned with the practices and policies relating to medicine and health, and committed to considering such policies in a reflective and rational way.

SAMUEL GOROVITZ

Foreword

This book is very special. Not only does it deal sensitively with an important issue, but it also treats nursing practice with dignity and respect. Nurses have gradually learned to express respect for their domain and practice; but others, when writing or speaking about health and illness care, often still refer to nursing as if it were an afterthought, a lower case of health care practice, or a lesser form of medical care. This book addresses nursing as the significant health and illness care practice it now is.

Until recently, most nurses assumed that ethical decision making in the delivery of health and illness care was the sole province of the physician. Because physicians claimed ownership of patients and because nurses had a low sense of self-worth and little pride in their practice, they yielded significant accountability in the mistaken belief that that was as it should be. Today, nursing has come of age; this is reflected in its realization of the value of its practice and in its new insistence on autonomous ethical decision making, even when such decisions are in contrast to those made by other health care providers. They will find affirmation of this position in this volume.

The solutions of moral problems encountered in nursing practice are not arrived at readily. Competence in ethical decision making must be acquired through the study of ethics, the understanding of one's own values as they relate to basic morality and, finally, through a process of ethical reasoning which documents one's moral position. Only when this has been achieved and subsequently applied does the nurse behave as a truly accountable practitioner. This book provides a superb guide for the nurse in her endeavor to accomplish this! By providing a philosopher's perspective of nursing's state as a profession and as a meaningful practice, it assists the nurse in examining the components of her role, which is basic to her recognition of situations requiring ethical stances and moral making of decisions. The lucid discussion of professionalism, and professional relationships inherent in the practice of nursing, assists the nurse to grasp the enormousness of her complex practice role. The moral problems of health care in this society must be faced by nurses, as they assume their rightful place as principal, ethical decision makers in this domain. How to accomplish this is no easy task; yet the first section of the book offers guidance and ample material to achieve its mastery.

In his introduction to this entire series, Samuel Gorovitz indicates that philosophers, while not claiming to "corner the market" of ethical solutions, still have a basic significant contribution to make by supplying the "philosophical dimension." This book certainly amply supports this contention, as it guides the reader through a series of discussions of theories and basic morality. Furthermore, the concept of competence and the nurses' relationship to patients, to each other, and to other providers are discussed from a perspective of morality and within a context of reflection, both somewhat new dimensions to most nurses.

Jameton has opened a window for nurses to view a new, broad, and profound panorama of ethics and morality in their chosen field. The profession owes him a significant debt of gratitude.

INGEBORG G. MAUKSCH, PH.D., F.A.A.N.

Preface

Nursing is the morally central health care profession. Philosophies of nursing, not medicine, should determine the image of health care and its future directions. In its anxiety to control the institutions and technology of health care, medicine has allowed the central values of health care—health and compassion—to fall to the hands of nurses. Nurses thus supply the real inspiration and hope for progress in health care, and among health professionals, represent the least equivocal commitment to their clientele.

Nurses have struggled to find their rightful place in health care for over a century. Too many ethics texts, beginning with Isabel Hampton Robb's *Nursing Ethics: For Hospital and Private Use* (1900), have accepted the traditional subservience of nurses. This tradition makes the role of "ethics teacher" in nursing a delicate one: An element of presumption is inevitable in being a kibitzer on turf run roughshod by outsiders for a century. I have written a text supporting the increasing power of nurses. As a philosopher, I have offered what I believe to be the material most helpful in resolving ethical issues in nursing practice and have avoided egregious moralizing. I hope that nurses will let me know where this text is helpful, where it misinterprets nursing issues, and where more needs to be said.

In its recent decade of ferment, bioethics has directed the bulk of its analysis to the consciousness of physicians. But if not exactly a team effort, health care is the work of many occupations and professions. No issue in the ethics of health care can be understood well without appreciating the complex relationships that exist among practitioners. Moreover, the dominance of physicians over patients, so often criticized by bioethicists, cannot be studied properly without analyzing power among practitioners—an area too often dismissed by bioethicists as a matter of "etiquette." I hope this text will help redress that imbalance.

I have not tried to stake out a new field of study, "nursing ethics," independent of ethics in general. But I do not accept that the study of ethics in nursing is simply "applied ethics"—the application of philosophical principles to a new set of facts. There is a rich and complex relationship between the moral conventions of nursing practice and the philosophical imagination. Study of ethics in nursing raises serious questions about the aims of theory formation in ethics, the meaning of philosophical principles of ethics, the nature of philosophical solutions to ethical problems, and the modes of work necessary for progress in philosophical ethics. Philosophers not only bring their ideas to bear on nursing; they also have much to learn from nurses about what they should be thinking about in ethics.

This text is a general description and discussion of the clinical and philosophical ethics issues arising in nursing practice. It includes a balanced mixture of cases, methods for resolving nursing ethics problems, and clinical observations, but it is not intended as a clinical handbook, nor does it insist on one particular method for analyzing cases. Talking with many nurses about their work has shown me a great richness and diversity of concepts and concerns, too much to present fairly and still satisfy my sense of philosophical rigor. I regard many points in this text not as philosophical conclusions but as occasions on which to begin philosophical discussion.

I have included considerable empirical and descriptive material in this text. Some of the material is from my own fieldwork—interviews with nurses and observation in hospitals. (Unless otherwise indicated, cases and incidents are from my fieldwork, and names used in cases are fictional.) I have made heavy use of the historical, sociological, anthropological, psychological, and health policy research in health care. This is because I believe that only part of philosophical theorizing in ethics rests on analysis of broad principles; the other part requires detailed observation of daily life. Ideas are not solutions to ethical problems; new ways of life are.

The issues and material in this text are not limited to nursing practice alone: Nurses have long been vocal about human values in health care delivery as a whole. The text thus addresses broad issues in health care on which nurses have views, and mentions or discusses issues in pharmacy, health administration, social work, and especially medicine. As closely linked, gender-segregated professions, medicine and nursing have had many years to observe each other closely. As "the Other," to use Simone de Beauvoir's term, nursing has been far the better observer. Physicians dissatisfied with current practice and seeking more humane ways to provide care have much to learn from nurses. Wise residents rely on nurses for guidance in their clinical work. Indeed, this should cease to be an informal practice; medical schools should welcome nurses on their clinical faculty. Moreover, much of the case for the power of nursing can be found in the medical literature: Powerful critiques of medicine come from physicians on the basis of research that nurses would not be permitted by physicians to conduct.

If nurses assume the professional role appropriate to their knowledge and humane commitments, physicians and health administrators will have to adjust their modes of practice. But this process is part of more widespread adjustments men have to make to respect the rights of women and institutions have to make to respect the rights of those who work in them. The case for nursing is part of a larger struggle for the autonomy and equality of people generally. I hope that the study of ethics in nursing will encourage nurses, bioethicists, philosophers, physicians, and others to look to nursing for conceptions of human progress. The moral problems of health care will not be solved by philosophers alone, but by those involved in it, clients and clinicians alike.

In this text, I use the terms *client* and *patient* equivalently. *Medicine* and *medical practice* refer to the expertise and practice of physicians, not to health and health care.

Many people have contributed to completing this book, especially the many nurses who had powerful stories to tell about their experiences in patient care. I cannot name all those willing to talk with me about their work without violating the strictures of confidentiality. But I want to express my gratitude here to them and to many nurses and others whom I can name and who gave me information, provided access to clinical settings, criticized the manuscript, gave me ideas, and maintained support and inspiration: William Andereck, Mila Aroskar, Lynn Ashcraft, Aileen Atwood, Elsie Bandman, Jan Broek, Susan Chapman, Elaine Cichowski, Grace Damman, Grace Davis, Joan Dunkel, Suellyn Ellerbe, Andrew Feenberg, Marsha Fowler, Pat Franks, Steve Gabel, Sally Gadow, Lucy Ann Geiselman, Pamela Hefernan, Mary Clare Hornof, Beverly Hall, Phyllis Harding, Helen Heise, David Holman, Frank Jacobsen, Albert R. Jonsen, Kenneth Kipnis, Barbara Koenig, Carol Korenbrot, John Ladd, Karen Lebacqz, Mary Jo Lery, Lauren LeRoy, Ellen Lewin, Bernard Lo, Hal Luft, Sister Francesca Lumpp, Ruth Macklin, Kay Martz, Tarran McDaid, Diane Meier, Christine Mitchell, Lynda P. Nauright, Virginia Olesen, Maria O'Rourke, Henry Perkins, Donald Provence, Carolyn Rees, Leonard Rifas, Helen Ripple, Jonathon Showstack, Mark Siegler, Deborah Streeter, Maureen Stein, Dan Todes, Mary Topalis, Doris Wellenkamp, and Dan Wikler.

I particularly want to thank Laurence McCullough for his careful critique of the text, Ingeborg Mauksch for her commentary and support, Janet Jaskula for her commentary and clinical observations, Robin Linden for her careful proofreading and bibliographical research, Barbara Stoops for her excellent research and reading of the text, and Anne J. Davis for ideas and inspiration. The staff at the Institute for Health Policy Studies provided much support, and I especially want to thank Philip R. Lee, Eunice Chee, and Phyllis Fetto for marshaling resources, and Les Gates, Cathy Kulka, and Nancy Ramsay for help in preparing the manuscript. I want to thank Lee Glickstein and the staff at Blue Ox for word processing and Liz Athorn and staff at Prentice-Hall for getting the manuscript through its final stages. I received financial support from a variety of sources during the years I worked on the text and want to thank the Institute for Health Policy Studies, the National Endowment for the Humanities, the Henry J. Kaiser Family Foundation, the Commonwealth Fund, the Landsberg Bequest, the Josiah Macy, Jr., Foundation, and the Battelle Human Affairs Research Center.

I am grateful for the continuing attention to the text and emotional support of Christine Cassel, Michael McCally, Ruth Purtilo, and Leah Beckwith. I am grateful to Samuel Gorovitz for initiating this project and for his steady support throughout its production.

CHAPTER 1

Introduction:
Ethics, Nursing,
and the Crisis
in Health Care

Ethics has always been an integral part of nursing. Throughout the history of nursing one can find codes of ethics, statements of moral principles, expressions of high ideals, and discussions of moral issues. References to ethical issues in nursing the sick go back to ancient times, and ethical discussion and teaching are an important part of the development of nursing as a profession in the nineteenth and twentieth centuries.[1] Moreover, nursing is morally worthy work: Caring for and treating the sick, and comforting and protecting the suffering, are basic benefits of human culture. Traditionally, people express altruism and idealism by attending the sick.

In the 1970s ethics began to expand as a special field of study in nursing. This development was part of the expansion of interest in ethical issues in all the health professions. The aims, values, and principles of nursing, medicine, and the allied health professions were subjected to study not only by health professionals, but also by people outside health care, such as philosophers, ministers, sociologists, politicians, and lawyers. A new field of study, *bioethics,* grew up. It dealt with such subjects as informed consent, abortion, research on human subjects, compassionate treatment of the dying, new technology, the cost of care, and the right to health care.[2]

This rich and flourishing field did not spring up just by chance. It grew out of rapid changes, almost a sense of crisis, in the provision of health care. In the 1970s health care providers sensed basic value conflicts in conducting their work and became concerned about their ability to express their ideals in it. Because of their

[1]M. Adelaide Nutting and Lavinia L. Dock, *A History of Nursing,* vol. I (New York: G.P. Putnam's Sons, 1907), pp. 31, 43–45, 64–66, 104–7, 134, 138–43, 156. For nineteenth- and twentieth-century works, see Further Readings, chap. 1, and footnote 1, chap. 3.

[2]One of the first writers to use the term *bioethics* was Van Rensselaer Potter, in *Bioethics: Bridge to the Future* (Englewood Cliffs, N.J.: Prentice-Hall, Inc., 1971). See *Encyclopedia of Bioethics,* 1978 ed., s.v. "Bioethics," by K. Danner Clouser.

central and basic position in the care of patients, nurses vividly and directly encountered many of these problems. And for the same reason, the nursing profession now has an important opportunity to deal with these issues and to take the lead in resolving them.

In this chapter, I sketch how the crisis in health care gives rise to moral problems and how they are related to the issues of nursing practice. The book as a whole is a philosopher's approach to bioethical issues as they arise in and are shaped by nursing practice.

The Crisis in Health Care

The health care delivery system probably will not collapse tomorrow, and health professionals have worried for decades about its adequacy. So, *crisis* may be too strong a word to describe this period of rapid change in health care. Yet social changes in the last twenty years have made more acute the chronic frailties of health delivery, such as fiscal pressures, unequal distribution, problematic technology, undependable decision processes, and internal conflict.

The eruption of ethical questions is a symptom of crisis. Ethical questions arise alongside fundamental social, political, and scientific questions and reflect sharpened feelings of frustration, chaos, and loss of control. As providers and clients accommodate to change in health care, they reconsider basic assumptions about the ethics of practice. So in order to consider well, we should first identify some of the changes creating the occasion for bioethics.

The number and variety of health professionals, specialists, technicians, and other workers have increased dramatically since the turn of the century. In 1900, there were about 200,000 health workers, most of them physicians. By 1960 there were about 2,500,000 workers, half of them physicians,[3] and in 1976, the U.S. government estimated that there were about 5,080,500 to 5,118,400 people working in health care out of a work force of about 90,000,000 people.[4] Nursing grew from a tiny band of dedicated women to become the largest health profession, and nurses became strikingly varied in training, roles, competencies, and specializations. In 1980, there were 1,662,382 registered nurses (RNs) in the U.S., about 77 percent of them employed,[5] and 557,000 licensed practical nurses (LPNs) or licensed vocational nurses (LVNs).[6] Also employed were about 1,500,000 nursing aides, orderlies, and attendants. This compares with about 467,679 physicians, the

[3]"Allied Health Education and Accreditation," *Journal of the American Medical Association,* 244 (1980), 2838.

[4]National Center for Health Statistics, *Health Resources Statistics: Health Manpower and Health Facilities,* 1976–1977 ed., (Hyattsville, Md.: U.S. Department of Health, Education, and Welfare, 1979). Other major occupational groups in health care include clinical laboratory scientists, technologists, technicians, and aides; dentists; dental hygienists, assistants, and laboratory technicians; administrators; dietitians; nutritionists; dietary technicians; librarians; medical record clerks; food and drug inspectors; funeral directors; embalmers; pharmacists; radiological technicians; secretaries; office workers; social workers and assistants; emergency medical technicians; psychologists; home health aides; and midwives.

[5]"National Sample of Registered Nurses, November 1980" (U.S. Department of Health and Human Services, Division of Health Professions Analysis, 1982).

[6]Projection in "Second Report to the Congress, March 15, 1979 (Revised): Nurse Training Act of 1975" (Washington, D.C.: U.S. Department of Health, Education, and Welfare, 1975).

next largest group of health care workers.[7] Medicine fragmented into specialties and subspecialties, and the types of allied health professions number at least one hundred. Relationships among health professionals thus became increasingly complex.

Giant medical centers, university hospital complexes, multinational drug companies, insurance companies, chains of proprietary hospitals, health maintenance organizations, and the like changed health care delivery from an informal cottage industry into a centralized, corporate, and bureaucratic system. Growing corporate and governmental influence in the "medical-industrial complex"[8] created pressures for efficiency and cost cutting and began to challenge the health professions for control of health care decisions. Federal and state governments increasingly underwrote the costs of care. Public policies increased access to care and created an opportunity to distribute health care more justly. At the same time, government involvement increased prices, fostered centralization, and complicated regulation of health care delivery, and increasing fiscal limitations threatened the hope of providing equal access to quality care.

Broad social movements changed the expectations of patients and health professionals. The Civil Rights movement exposed racial and economic discrimination in health care delivery. The radicalism of the 1960s facilitated the moral examination of respected public institutions. Unions made increasing efforts to bargain over workplace health hazards. Feminism linked the oppression of nurses to discrimination against women as patients and employees generally. Labor unions and professional organizations competed to represent health workers. Crises in other areas of the U.S. economy—inflation, energy shortages, unemployment—placed the crisis in health care in a national and international social context.

Patient advocacy organizations developed to defend their interests and to educate their membership. These groups varied from organizations of kidney transplant and dialysis patients, diabetics, and the chronically ill to patients' groups in direct conflict with licensed practitioners, such as women's groups challenging traditional obstetric and gynecological practice and organizations defending the rights of psychiatric patients. Renewed professions, such as midwives and nurse practitioners, challenged traditional licensure practices, and patients supporting nonstandard therapies such as acupuncture challenged traditional modes of care. Such ideals as the right to health, the right to treatment, and patients' rights were deployed in legal and political actions pressing for change.

Rapid developments in health care technology increased the stakes involved in treatment decisions and professional qualifications. Opiates, a cup of tea, and purgatives gave way to respirators, dialysis machines, CAT-scanners, newborn intensive care units, coronary artery bypass surgery, chemotherapy, powerful antibiotics, major and minor tranquilizers, amniocentesis, and fetal surgery. These technologies changed the meaning and experience of illness for both practitioner and patient. Health care technology and an awareness of its problems were linked to nonmedical technological developments and their problems. For instance, inquiry into the ethics of human experimentation was linked to the concern about the effects of science aroused forcefully by development of nuclear weapons.

[7]Center for Health Policy Research, "Physician Distribution and Medical Licensure in the U.S." (Chicago: American Medical Association, 1980).

[8]Arnold S. Relman, "The New Medical-Industrial Complex," *The New England Journal of Medicine*, 303 (1980), 963–70; and Paul Starr, *The Social Transformation of American Medicine* (New York: Basic Books, Inc., Publishers, 1983).

Changes in demographic patterns of illness and death created pressure to reexamine traditional goals of health care and modes of delivery. Health care did not cope well with problems of prevention, chronic illness, and handicaps. Poverty on an international scale continued to pose problems of starvation, infection, and parasitic diseases. Poverty in the U.S. kept infant mortality rates high in many rural and inner-city areas. Meanwhile the perils of wealth, such as too much food and too little exercise, and of individual behavior, such as smoking and alcoholism, challenged health professionals. The health problems of social organization and technology—occupational hazards, chemical pollutants, automobile accidents, iatrogenic illness, stress, radiation—combined to raise questions about a health care delivery system focused on acute, individual interventions.

These changes created in many people a sense of crisis in health care, a sense that health care is faced with unpredictable changes and insoluble problems. Bioethics developed as a field of study partly because traditional values and principles of the health professions did not provide solutions to these new problems.

Ethics and Morals

Bioethics is the study of ethics as it relates to biology and the health professions. But, what is *ethics?* What is *morality?* When asked to characterize what sorts of issues are ethical or moral ones, people offer the following sorts of definitions:

1. Issues concerned with important social values or norms such as respect for life, personal independence, love, and the like
2. Issues arousing the conscience or such feelings as guilt, shame, self-esteem, courage, or hope
3. Issues we respond to with words like *ought, should, right, wrong, good, bad,* and so on
4. Issues that appear unusually complex, frustrating, unresolvable, or difficult in some indefinable way

Another way to define ethical and moral issues is to distinguish them from technical, "how-to," or scientific problems. These latter concerns are sometimes labeled the *descriptive* aspects of professional practice, and they are distinguished from its *normative* aspects, that is, its ethics and morality. For example, describing *how* to put a patient on kidney dialysis is a descriptive, scientific, or technical problem. Deciding whether we *ought* to do so is a normative or ethical problem. In ethics and morals, we evaluate and choose goals, set priorities among conflicting values, interpret and give meaning to our actions, make judgments about right and wrong courses of action, express ideals and aspirations, and establish minimal expectations of conduct.

People often ask what the difference is between *ethics* and *morals,* and appear to use the two terms to make a number of contrasts, though sometimes they also use them equivalently. Two of the more important contrasts that can be made are between *professional* and *personal,* and between *commitment* and *inquiry:*

1. *Professional* versus *personal:* In this contrast, *ethics* refers to publicly stated and formal sets of rules or values, such as professional codes of ethics. For example, the American Nurses' Association's "Code for Nurses" and the International

Council of Nurses' "Code for Nurses" (see Appendix) are statements of professional *ethics*. *Morals* refers to a set of values or principles to which one is *personally* committed. Moral values or principles may be formal or informal, explicit or implicit. Examples of personal moral principles are "Do unto others as you would have them do unto you," "Always act lovingly," "Look out for number one," and "Give others the benefit of the doubt."

2. *Commitment* versus *inquiry:* Here, *morals* refers to principles and values to which people are actually *committed,* that is, those they follow and defend in daily life. These may include both the professional and personal commitments mentioned above. *Ethics* refers to the systematic study of principles and values, in other words, the theories and research by means of which we question, study, inquire into, critique, and eventually change our morals.

In short, *ethics* is the more formal and theoretical term, *morals* the more informal and personal term. This text is primarily an inquiry into the professional ethics of nursing, but it touches on other aspects of ethics and morality as well. Nurses are legitimately concerned about bioethics, medical ethics, personal morality, and the ethics of public policy. This text sometimes uses the terms *ethics* and *morals* to make the two distinctions described above, but since these concepts overlap so extensively, there are many places in the text where either or both terms could be used. The general definitions given here should be adequate to begin our discussion, and these concepts will be enriched as the text develops.

Moral Problems in Nursing

The moral and ethical dimensions of the crisis in health care are poignantly reflected by individuals working in it. In order to make their work meaningful and to avoid burning out, nurses need their work to express their values and realize their expectations of proper patient care. Nurses experience stress and anger as they attempt to reconcile their ideals about health care with its uncertainties, inadequacies, and abuses. In *Reality Shock,* Marlene Kramer records some of the comments of nurses reacting to their first hospital jobs:

> Like wow! It's awful. I can't believe it; I never thought it would be like this. I knew it wouldn't be a picnic, but this is ridiculous.
>
> I'm somewhat disappointed because they don't care as much about patients as I had been led to believe. And nurses don't make the decisions my instructors always said they would . . .
>
> And then there's the sleep syndrome: when you go home all you want to do is sleep so you can get up and go to work the next day. Pretty soon all you are doing is sleeping and working.[9]

Although the stress that new nurses experience comes from a variety of sources,

[9]From Marlene Kramer, *Reality Shock: Why Nurses Leave Nursing* (St. Louis: The C.V. Mosby Company, 1974), p. 7.

many of these conflicts are experienced as ethical or moral problems,[10] and coming to terms with them requires ethical thinking.

Moral and ethical problems in the hospital can be sorted into three different types. *Moral uncertainty* arises when one is unsure what moral principles or values apply, or even what the moral problem is. For example, an elderly patient is somewhat neglected and his or her problem is given little attention. One feels dissatisfied with the patient's treatment, but the nature and cause of the inadequacy are hard to pinpoint.[11] *Moral dilemmas* arise when two (or more) clear moral principles apply, but they support mutually inconsistent courses of action. It seems terrible to give up either value, and yet the loss seems inescapable.[12] For example, the commitment to maintain life leads us to want to put a young child with kidney disease on dialysis, but the commitment to avoid suffering leads us to think that the child may be "better off dead." *Moral distress* arises when one knows the right thing to do, but institutional constraints make it nearly impossible to pursue the right course of action. For example, a hospital may routinely give all entering patients an unnecessary battery of blood tests. This costly practice imposes unnecessary risks on patients, and is therefore an unethical practice. But staff nurses employed by the hospital have neither the personal authority nor access to decision-making channels needed to change the practice. Moreover, it is personally risky for staff to criticize a practice that helps the hospital make ends meet.

Moral and ethical problems arise for nurses in relation to a wide variety of persons and institutions:

Patients
Other nurses
Supervisors and administrators
Physicians
Aides, orderlies, and attendants
Technicians, pharmacists, and other health care workers
Hospitals
Potential patients
Family and friends of patients

[10]Some of the problems that Kramer describes can be seen as ethical conflicts (for an example, see text p. 97). Sharol P. Jacobson, "Stressful Situations for Neonatal Intensive Care Nurses," *MCN: The American Journal of Maternal Child Nursing,* 3 (1978), 144–52, found that the leading type of stressful situation in the newborn intensive care nursery was philosophical and emotional conflict.

[11]Christine K. Cassel and Andrew L. Jameton, "Dementia in the Elderly: An Analysis of Medical Responsibility," *Annals of Internal Medicine,* 94 (1981), 802–7, analyzes the case of an elderly demented man whose case presents moral *uncertainties.*

[12]John Lemmon, "Moral Dilemmas," in *Contemporary Issues in Bioethics,* eds. Tom L. Beauchamp and LeRoy Walters (Encino, Calif.: Dickenson Publishing Co., Inc., 1978), classifies different types of dilemmas. The concept of a *dilemma* is closely related to the concept of a *contradiction* in European philosophy, but European philosophy sets these conflicts in a historical context: contradictions reveal the changing nature of reality and are resolved by social change through time. For an outline of the concept of contradiction, see Georges Politzer, *Elementary Principles of Philosophy* (New York: International Publishers Co., Inc., 1976), pp. 105–116. See also Anne J. Davis and Mila A. Aroskar, *Ethical Dilemmas and Nursing Practice* (Englewood Cliffs, N.J.: Prentice-Hall, Inc., 1978), pp. 6–8.

Professional associations and unions
Licensure boards
The law
Society[13]

The nature of nursing practice is an important factor in the genesis of ethical issues in the relationships listed above. It is an important source of values and principles to which nurses can appeal in dealing with moral problems as they arise, and it offers resources, personal support, and opportunities for action in solving these problems. It is important for students of nursing ethics to be familiar with the character and experience of nursing practice. No textbook can completely display, and no non-nurse can fully appreciate, the subtle and complex details of the experience of being a nurse, but in order to orient those unfamiliar with nursing, I attempt here a brief sketch of the nature and scope of nursing practice.

Nursing Practice

As the largest health care profession, nursing has grown rapidly since 1873, when the first three U.S. nursing schools modeled on Florence Nightingale's ideas were founded. In its century of development, nursing has become the most varied of the health professions. It has annexed tasks from medicine, entered newly developing institutions, specialized, generalized, expanded, and pioneered new conceptions of practice.

The broadest division in nursing is between *registered nurses* (RNs) and *licensed practical nurses* (LPNs), sometimes called *licensed vocational nurses* (LVNs). LPNs and LVNs generally have had about a year's training in a hospital school, although programs may vary from nine to twenty-four months. RNs may have any of a wide variety of educational backgrounds. *Diploma* nurses generally have been trained in hospital-based schools. *Associate Degree* nurses receive their education in two- or three-year community college programs. *Baccalaureate* nurses receive B.S. degrees after four- or five-year college educations. RNs increasingly have master's and doctoral degrees. In order to practice, all nurses must pass state examinations and be licensed by state boards of nursing practice.

The practice of LPNs and RNs can be distinguished in several ways. For the most part, LPNs are trained in basic nursing procedures and tasks, but they are not expected to be familiar with the theoretical and scientific background of these practices. RNs receive a broad education in biological, social, and psychological theories of health and disease and are expected to make use of these in practice. RNs generally have more autonomy in their practices than LPNs. Many RNs work as independent practitioners, but LPNs generally work under supervision. RNs typ-

---

[13]Some nursing ethics texts sort out the issues according to such categories as nurse-patient, nurse-doctor, and nurse-hospital. Good examples of this approach are Ruth B. Purtilo and Christine K. Cassel, *Ethical Dimensions in the Health Professions* (Philadelphia: W.B. Saunders Company, 1981); Martin Benjamin and Joy Curtis, *Ethics in Nursing* (New York: Oxford University Press, 1981); and James L. Muyskens, *Moral Problems in Nursing: A Philosophical Investigation* (Totowa, N.J.: Rowman and Littlefield, 1982).

ically supervise the work of LPNs in acute care settings, and LPNs do not often supervise RNs. LPNs can be found in subacute, chronic, and convalescent settings more often than RNs, who function more prominently in acute care settings.

RNs and LPNs often supervise and are assisted by auxiliary nursing personnel, such as *nursing aides, orderlies,* and *attendants.* These workers are generally trained on the job, generally do not think of themselves as professionals, and are less well paid. They do much basic patient care and have an important impact on the quality of care.

Another important type of nursing practice is that of the *nurse practitioner* (related concepts are *clinical nurse specialist* and *nurse clinician*). Nurse practitioners receive additional training beyond their RN education, sometimes in a master's degree program. They represent a developing role for nurses and work more independently than other nurses. They usually provide primary care for their patients and have an independent nurse-patient relationship. They sometimes function like attending physicians as clients of the hospital with admitting privileges, rather than as hospital employees. Nurse practitioners take patients' histories, perform comprehensive physical examinations, diagnose common acute illnesses and stable chronic health problems, order and interpret laboratory tests, and in some states, prescribe therapy including medication. Some work as specialists in critical care units; others provide primary care. Some are nurse-midwives; others practice specialties such as occupational health therapy or cancer chemotherapy. Historically, nurses have worked in independent settings, such as public health, midwifery, private duty, and geographically isolated areas, and in specialties such as anesthesia, but the certification and development of independent nursing is for the most part recent. Indeed, work settings sometimes influence what nurses do more than their certification and training. Some RNs and LPNs work independently, for instance, as midwives, while nurse practitioners may work in settings that offer them no more autonomy than hospital staff nursing.

Most nurses work in hospitals. Sixty to 65 percent work in acute care settings. Another 10 percent work in nursing homes. Nurses work in physicians' offices, registries, occupational health settings, public health agencies, blood banks, schools, clinics, and clients' homes. They also work in teaching, counseling, research, utilization review, supervision, administration, record keeping, court investigation, and a host of other jobs less directly related to primary clinical care. They specialize in a wide variety of areas, such as maternal and child health, medical and surgical nursing, psychiatric and mental health nursing, and community health. Some specialties parallel medical specialties such as pediatrics, geriatrics, and oncology. Others relate more closely to hospital units, such as intensive and coronary care.

Because most nurses work in hospital settings, this text focuses on ethical issues of staff nurses in the hospital. Readers should keep in mind that this is a gross oversimplification. The problems of hospital staff nurses do not represent the entire profession. Tasks and settings of nursing vary widely, and many nursing ethics issues are beyond the scope of this book.

In acute care hospitals, the nursing department is usually operated as a coherent unit and spends the largest portion of the hospital budget. It is directed by a nurse, who may also be a hospital administrator. Nursing supervisors mediate between the director and the head nurses, who are key figures in directing nursing care at the patient's bedside. The *head nurse* is usually an RN in charge of a ward, surgical recovery room, or critical care unit. The head nurse usually assigns nursing duties to both LPNs and RNs on the ward. The work may be organized by type of task, by assignment to patients, or in teams. The head nurse usually has responsibility for evaluating nursing work, keeping records and schedules, and performing a certain amount of patient care. The head nurse usually works on the day shift and a *charge nurse* performs head nurse functions on other shifts. Conferences at shift changes are essential to ongoing work.

LPNs and aides do much of the basic bedside work. They feed, bathe, dress, and undress patients. They take vital signs (temperature, pulse, blood pressure), observe signs and symptoms, dress wounds, give enemas, suction mucus, and tend catheters. They may make beds and clean rooms, although these are usually housekeeping functions. They sterilize equipment, assist patients in walking, and perform many other tasks. LPNs, but not aides, administer medications, give blood, and perform some oxygen procedures. RNs can perform all of these functions. They also formulate nursing treatment plans, keep records, and supervise other nurses. They administer potent and toxic medications, including heart stimulants, cancer chemotherapy, and intravenous (IV) therapy, for all manner of illnesses. They set up heart monitors, conduct patient rounds with or without physicians, and perform a variety of tests. In intensive care units, RNs are responsible for a variety of highly technological and specialized tasks.

Who does what varies from hospital to hospital and changes over time. Hospital nursing tasks can be roughly divided into what used to be called *independent nursing functions* and *dependent nursing functions*. Primary among *independent* functions are patient safety, comfort, and welfare in the hospital. Nurses create and implement nursing care plans directed to patients' overall psychological, social, and health needs. They observe patients closely and support them in dealing with the difficulties caused by disease. Nurses conduct patient education and advocate the needs and interests of patients. Nurses manage the nursing department, allocate hospital resources, and delegate housekeeping functions. Since nurses allocate care among many patients, they set priorities for patient care. These independent functions are coordinated with *dependent* functions. The primary dependent function is carrying out the medical treatment plan. Although the medical treatment plan could be considered part of the overall nursing care plan, hospitals traditionally expect the medical treatment plan to shape the nursing plan. Reporting significant observations, signs, and symptoms of patients to physicians is also a dependent function.

Although hospital practice still reflects the power relationship suggested by the term "dependent," many prefer to describe these dependent tasks as *overlapping* functions. Nurses carry out some of these under *standing orders*. These are orders written by physicians to be filled at the nurse's discretion. To facilitate nursing acquisition of traditional medical tasks, some nursing practice acts have created the concept of *standardized procedures*. By writing standardized procedures for carrying out tasks, a hospital committee can turn traditional medical functions over to nurses. Some independent nursing functions, such as patient teaching, are also overlapping functions.

Nursing differs from medicine in a number of ways. Nursing students receive education on global factors affecting patient health; they are not as focused as medical students on the biological sciences. Nursing schools integrate medical topics with material from sociology, anthropology, and psychology. Nurses have a stronger orientation toward health maintenance, disease prevention, patient education, and holistic modes of patient care. Physicians are sometimes said to focus on the *cure* functions, while nurses focus on the *care* functions, though each profession performs both of these interrelated functions.

Hospitals are dizzyingly complex. Nurses thus experience a variety of responsibilities and allegiances which create opportunities for conflict and power. According to the best health care practice, the nurse's primary responsibility is to the *client* or *patient*, but nurses also have important responsibilities to the *hospital*. They are hired and fired by the hospital, and their conditions of work are set by hospital policy, sometimes by negotiation with a labor representative. Nurses are expected to follow hospital procedures, report significant incidents and mishaps to supervisors, and, with physicians, organize work on wards and in such hospital departments as laboratory, pharmacy, respiratory therapy, x-ray, dietary, and so on. Although a hospital's main duty is in principle patient care, it may be poorly organized for it. Hospitals may be understaffed; procedures for patient protection may not be operational; cutting corners, substandard care, and even patient abuse may occur. Thus, conflicts between duties to patient and duties to employer arise for nurses in hospital settings.

These conflicts are complicated by the additional expectation that nurses have responsibilities to *physicians* to see that medical instructions are carried out. Nurses may be responsible both to in-house medical staff employed by the hospital and to attending physicians, who as clients of the hospital are present only to see their private patients. When there are conflicts among medical staff over proper patient care, the nurse may play an important role in determining the course of care. Hospitals expect nurses to make sure that physicians follow hospital policy and do not misuse facilities. Physicians expect nurses to implement hospital policies to serve their patients.

Nurses thus work within a *triangle* of responsibilities—to client, hospital, and physician. This triangle is embellished by the fact that nurses supervise other nurses and also have supervisory and peer relations with other departments in the hospital. In different hospitals, the mutual rights, responsibilities, and tasks are worked out in various ways. In some settings, close teamwork exists; work is conducted with grace and respect for everyone involved. In other settings, ancient and momentous struggles for power, accumulated bitterness, frustration, and despair dominate negotiations over these functions.

Like many professions, nursing gains unity by focusing on a prized and sacred activity—bedside care. Yet nursing has become so diverse that other concepts of care, for example, health education or hospital administration, threaten the profession with loss of definition. Many of the ethical conflicts nurses experience arise from unresolved questions about the nature, scope, and goals of nursing practice.

1. On one hand, nurses express strong ideals of health maintenance and patient education. On the other, most nurses work in hospitals—absolutely the worst place for conducting these activities.
2. On one hand, nurses have a strong tradition of humanizing health care through their personal relationships with patients. On the other, new technology invites nurses to gain prestige by acquiring more sophisticated medical skills and devoting less time to basic bedside care.
3. On one hand, equality with physicians in status and autonomy is necessary to end the gender-stereotyped history of clinical practice. On the other, physicians' roles tend to offer more power and prestige than most clinicians desire.

4. There are conflicts within the nursing profession. LPNs have a stronger claim to the prized ideal of bedside care than RNs.[14] Yet, RNs have a stronger claim to the concept of professionalism. Will nurses split more completely into two groups—the professional versus the technical nurse? Whose interests do these status distinctions serve?
5. Staff nurses have conflicts with administrative nurses along the traditional lines of worker versus manager. Can professional nursing organizations represent effectively the interests of both groups?
6. After years of struggle, nurses are gaining increased autonomy and better professional recognition. But this is occurring at a historical moment when the health professions are encountering the interests of investors, managers, and administrators in acquiring more control over the conduct and delivery of health care.[15] How will nurses establish and maintain the power to do their job well according to their own professional judgment?

Many questions like these, all of them difficult, lurk in the background of ethical questions, color them, and even create them. For example, the ethical question of what to tell dying patients revolves around interprofessional power conflicts surrounding patient education in the acute care setting. Ethical issues in discontinuing therapy for dying patients arise from conflicts over humanizing technology. Issues of power, autonomy, and unity affect all ethical issues that nurses face.

Nurses work in particularly difficult circumstances because of their central role in large health organizations, their close contact with patients, the dominance of the medical profession, and tensions in the directions and definition of nursing. For bioethics to continue growing as a field, and to discover solutions to problems in the health care crisis, active nursing participation and influence are needed.

The Approach of This Book

The next three chapters introduce the main elements needed to discuss issues of nursing ethics. Since the ethical tradition of first importance to nursing practice is that of the nursing profession, Chapter 2 treats the relationship of professionalism to ethics. Chapter 3 introduces the most problematic and pervasive issue of nursing ethics—the autonomy of nurses. Chapter 4 introduces the main features of philosophical ethics and describes the functions of philosophers and bioethicists in clinical settings. Chapter 4 also outlines a sample procedure for resolving moral questions in nursing practice.

[14]A major study found that LPNs and aides spend more time with individual patients than RNs. The study measured how many minutes out of each 20-minute period ward patients spent with staff. It found that on the average each ward patient spent .75 minutes with an RN and 2.39 minutes with LPNs, aides, and technicians. Ward patients saw medical house staff .58 minutes and an attending .01 minute. (The figures for semiprivate accommodations were: attendings .19, house staff .41, RNs .63, and others 1.78 minutes out of every 20.) Raymond S. Duff and August B. Hollingshead, *Sickness and Society* (New York: Harper & Row, Publishers, Inc., 1968), pp. 234, 236.

[15]For instance, the director of the Midwest Business Group on Health remarked: "Business wants to support the health-care system, but it wants to play a more influential role in deciding how the system operates." Quoted in Robert Cassidy, "How Tightly Will Big Business Control Your Practice?" *Medical Economics* (June 7, 1982), 254.

Part Two of the text unfolds four well-established professional and conventional principles of nursing practice. Chapter 5 discusses the ethical significance of widely held conventional principles, and Chapters 6 through 9 discuss in more detail each of these four main principles—competence, the patient's good, nonexploitation, and loyalty. The function of these chapters is both descriptive and evaluative; I describe how these principles are used and what they mean in concrete detail and briefly indicate their main strengths and weaknesses. But reflective ethical decision making in health care practice requires deeper and broader concepts and principles. And here we must turn to philosophical ethics. Chapter 10 introduces five important philosophical ethics concepts—respect for persons, justice, values, rights, and responsibility—and two ethical theories—formalism and utilitarianism. Chapter 11 discusses some of the differences between ethics and scientific thinking and major issues in ethical reasoning and research.

Part Three discusses several important problem areas in nursing practice. Chapter 12 is about disclosing information to clients, giving advice, describing side effects, and related topics. Chapter 13 is about informed consent mechanisms, patients' rights, and the issue of mental capacity to consent to therapy. Chapter 14 discusses difficult and disliked clients, such as those who abuse their health, those who do not follow clinical advice, and those who are dangerous to nurses. Chapter 15 is about death, pain, and suffering. It details considerations in discontinuing therapy and in using pain medication. Chapter 16 discusses the role of the nursing profession in humanizing health care technology, and it uses the newborn intensive care unit as an instance of this concern. Chapter 17 discusses the social and political responsibilities of nurses. It treats justice, the right to health care, and the problem of racism in health care delivery. Finally, Chapter 18 discusses two important areas of nursing choice and responsibility—coping with medical errors and going on strike. Other chapter topics could have been chosen, but I picked these because nurses often raise these issues, they seem important to practice, and they raise interesting philosophical issues. Discussion in Part Three is designed to provide helpful clinical considerations, to develop the conventional principles and philosophical concepts introduced in earlier chapters, and to identify problems for future discussion.

Part Three has an additional objective. Chapters 12 through 17 are partly intended as an extended argument to support the view that nursing is the "moral center" of health care practice, that is, that the values and principles most closely associated with nursing are the most significant to health care practice, and that clinical practice would pose fewer ethical dilemmas and benefit patients more if nurses directed health care practice more actively and received more recognition for their professional viewpoint.

In each of the problem areas of Part Three, I have attempted to sketch the main issues, and except for a few instances, I have steered away from final judgments and answers. This is for two reasons. First, this is a text by a philosopher, not a nurse. It would be presumptuous for an outsider to give prescriptions to the nursing profession. Instead, I have tried to display as best I can in a short space sample concepts, principles, and perspectives of philosophical ethics, and to open some doors to ethical reasoning and philosophical inquiry. Second, I believe that philosophical approaches to moral problems experienced in clinical settings can give only limited help to nurses. Social changes are needed in order to diminish the basic conflicts that give rise to many of the ethical issues nurses now face. Individual nurses and the nursing profession will need to make basic choices about what changes they would like to see.

Summary

Ethics has always been an integral part of nursing practice. The field of *bioethics,* the study of ethics in health care and biology, arises from the experience of nurses and other health professionals who face many moral and ethical problems in health care. Clinicians experience moral *uncertainty, dilemmas,* and *distress.* These problems are symptoms of a crisis of rapid change in the health care delivery system. Bioethics is part of the study of *ethics.* Ethics investigates what we should do in terms of basic values and principles. Competence in *ethics* can be distinguished from *technical* or scientific competence. *Ethics* and *morals* can also be loosely distinguished; *ethics* is the more formal and theoretical concept, *morals* is the more informal and personal concept.

To appreciate how ethical problems arise in nursing, it is important to understand the nature and variety of nursing practice and the institutional context in which nurses work. Nurses play a central and varied role in patient care and the management of health care delivery. Nurses practice many specialties, are educated at many different levels, hold a variety of academic degrees, and can perform many different jobs in patient care and administration. They face many ethical conflicts arising from the crisis in health care. These conflicts arise in relationship to clients, hospitals, physicians, nurses, and others. Nurses discover and resolve many ethical questions arising in clinical settings, and their choices in regard to ethical problems are important to the future development of health care.

The book is divided into three parts: introduction to professionalism, autonomy, and ethics; conventional and philosophical approaches to ethics; and cases and problem areas in clinical practice.

FURTHER READINGS

Nursing

ALFANO, GENROSE, "The Concept of Joint Practice," *Proceedings of the Third National Conference on Joint Practice.* Chicago: National Commission, 1979.

ANDERSON, PEGGY, *Nurse.* New York: St. Martin's Press, Inc., 1978.

BARHYDT, NANCY R., "Nursing," in *Health Care Delivery in the United States,* ed. Steven Jonas. New York: Springer Publishing Co., Inc., 1977, pp. 96–119.

CHASKA, NORMA L., ED., *The Nursing Profession: A Time to Speak.* New York: McGraw-Hill Book Company, 1983.

———, ED., *The Nursing Profession: Views through the Mist.* New York: McGraw-Hill Book Company, 1978.

CORWIN, RONALD G., AND MARVIN J. TAVES, "Nursing and Other Health Professions," in *Handbook of Medical Sociology,* ed. Howard Freeman, Sol Levine, and Leo G. Reeder, pp. 187–212. Englewood Cliffs, N.J.: Prentice-Hall, Inc., 1963.

DAVIS, ANNE J., AND JANELLE C. KRUEGER, EDS., *Patients, Nurses, Ethics.* New York: American Journal of Nursing, Educational Services Division, 1980.

DAVIS, FRED, ED., *The Nursing Profession: Five Sociological Essays.* New York: John Wiley & Sons, Inc., 1966.

DONNELLY, GLORIA FERRARO, ET AL., *The Nursing System: Issues, Ethics, and Politics.* New York: John Wiley & Sons, Inc., 1980.

FITZPATRICK, M. LOUISE, "Nursing," *Signs: Journal of Women in Culture and Society,* 2, 4 (Summer 1977), 818–34.

HARDEGREE, ELEANOR E., AND EDWINA A. McCONNELL, "RN's and NA's Working Together: Two Perspectives," *Nursing '80,* 10, 8 (August 1980), 89–93.

HENDERSON, VIRGINIA, "The Concept of Nursing," *Journal of Advanced Nursing,* 3 (1978), 113–30.

KALISCH, BEATRICE J., AND PHILIP A. KALISCH, *Politics of Nursing.* Philadelphia: J.B. Lippincott Company, 1982.

KELLY, LUCIE YOUNG, *Dimensions of Professional Nursing* (4th ed.). New York: Macmillan Publishing Co., Inc., 1981.

KINLEIN, LUCILLE M., *Independent Nursing Practice with Clients.* Philadelphia: J. B. Lippincott Company, 1977.

KOHNKE, MARY F. *Advocacy, Risk and Reality.* St. Louis: The C. V. Mosby Company, 1982.

———, ANN ZIMMERN, AND JOCELYN A. GREENIDGE, *Independent Nurse Practitioner.* Garden Grove, Calif.: Trainex Press, 1974.

LEE, ANTHONY, "Why Feelings Run High on the Professional/Technical Split," *R.N.,* 42, 3 (March 1979), 52–58.

MAUKSCH, INGEBORG G., "Critical Issues of the Nurse Practitioner Movement," *Nurse Practitioner,* 3, 6 (November/December 1978), 15.

OLESEN, VIRGINIA L., AND ELVI W. WHITTAKER, *The Silent Dialogue: A Study in the Social Psychology of Professional Socialization.* San Francisco: Jossey-Bass, Inc., Publishers, 1968.

PARTRIDGE, KAY B., "Nursing Values in a Changing Society," *Nursing Outlook* (June 1978), 356–60.

POPIEL, EDNA S., ED., *Social Issues and Trends in Nursing: Chataqua 77.* Thorofare, N.J.: Charles B. Slack, Inc., 1979.

RAMSAY, JANICE A., JOHN K. McKENZIE, AND DAVID G. FISH, "Physicians and Nurse Practitioners: Do They Provide Equivalent Health Care?" *American Journal of Public Health,* 72 (1982), 55–57.

REISSMAN, LEONARD, AND JOHN H. ROHRER, EDS., *Change and Dilemma in the Nursing Profession,* pp. 44–59. New York: G.P. Putnam's Sons, 1957.

ROWLAND, HOWARD S., ED., *The Nurse's Almanac.* Germantown, Md.: Aspen Systems Corporation, 1978.

ROY, SISTER CALLISTA, AND SISTER MARCIA OBLOY, "The Practitioner Movement—Toward a Science of Nursing," *American Journal of Nursing,* 78 (1978), 1698–1702.

SHEAHAN, SISTER DOROTHY, "The Game of the Name: Nurse Professional and Nurse Technician," *Nursing Outlook,* 20 (1972), 440–44.

STRAUSS, ANSELM L., ET AL., *Psychiatric Ideologies and Institutions,* "The Nurse at PPI," pp. 206–27. New York: The Free Press, 1964.

SULLIVAN, JUDITH A., "Research on Nurse Practitioners: Process behind the Outcome?" *American Journal of Public Health,* 72 (January 1982), 8–9.

TERKEL, STUDS, *Working,* "Carmelita Lester, Practical Nurse, Old People's Home;" "Cathleen Moran, Hospital Aide;" and "Ruth Lindstrom, Baby Nurse." New York: Avon Books, 1974.

WALKER, VIRGINIA H., *Nursing and Ritualistic Practice.* New York: Macmillan, Inc., 1967.

Bioethics: Texts and Collections

BANDMAN, ELSIE L., AND BERTRAM BANDMAN, EDS., *Bioethics and Human Rights: A Reader for Health Professionals.* Boston: Little, Brown & Company, 1978.

BEAUCHAMP, TOM L., AND JAMES F. CHILDRESS, *Principles of Biomedical Ethics*. New York: Oxford University Press, 1979.

BEAUCHAMP, TOM L., AND LEROY WALTERS, EDS. *Contemporary Issues in Bioethics* (2nd ed.). Belmont, Calif.: Wadsworth Publishing Co., Inc., 1982.

BRODY, HOWARD, *Ethical Decisions in Medicine* (2nd ed.). Boston: Little, Brown & Company, 1981.

ENCYCLOPEDIA OF BIOETHICS, 1978 ed.

FROMER, MARGOT JOAN, *Ethical Issues in Health Care*. St. Louis: The C.V. Mosby Company, 1981.

GOROVITZ, SAMUEL, ET AL., EDS. *Moral Problems in Medicine* (2nd ed.). Englewood Cliffs, N.J.: Prentice-Hall, Inc., 1983.

HUNT, ROBERT, AND JOHN ARRAS, EDS., *Ethical Issues in Modern Medicine* (2nd ed.). Palo Alto, Calif.: Mayfield Publishing Co., 1983.

MAPPES, THOMAS A., AND JANE S. ZEMBATY, EDS. *Biomedical Ethics*. New York: McGraw-Hill Book Company, 1981.

MUNSON, RONALD, ED., *Intervention and Reflection: Basic Issues in Medical Ethics*. Belmont, Calif.: Wadsworth Publishing Co., Inc., 1979.

PURTILO, RUTH B., AND CHRISTINE K. CASSEL, *Ethical Dimensions in the Health Professions*. Philadelphia: W.B. Saunders Company, 1981.

REISER, STANLEY JOEL, ARTHUR J. DYCK, AND WILLIAM J. CURRAN, EDS., *Ethics in Medicine: Historical Perspectives and Contemporary Concerns*. Cambridge: The MIT Press, 1977.

VEATCH, ROBERT M., *A Theory of Medical Ethics*. New York: Basic Books, Inc., Publishers, 1981.

————, *Case Studies in Medical Ethics*. Cambridge, Mass.: Harvard University Press, 1977.

Nursing Ethics: Texts and Collections

BENJAMIN, MARTIN, AND JOY CURTIS, *Ethics in Nursing*. New York: Oxford University Press, 1981.

CAMPBELL, A.V., *Moral Dilemmas in Medicine: A Coursebook in Ethics for Doctors and Nurses*. Edinburgh: Churchill Livingstone, 1972.

CARROLL, MARY ANN, AND RICHARD A. HUMPHREY, *Moral Problems in Nursing: Case Studies*. Washington, D.C.: University Press of America, 1979.

CATHOLIC HOSPITAL ASSOCIATION, *Ethical Issues in Nursing: A Proceedings*. St. Louis: Catholic Hospital Association, 1976.

CURTIN, LEAH, AND M. JOSEPHINE FLAHERTY, *Nursing Ethics: Theories and Pragmatics*. Bowie, Md.: Robert J. Brady Co., 1982.

DAVIS, ANNE J., AND MILA A. AROSKAR, *Ethical Dilemmas and Nursing Practice* (2nd ed.). Englewood Cliffs, N.J.: Prentice-Hall, Inc., 1983.

FENNER, KATHLEEN M., *Ethics and Law in Nursing: Professional Perspectives*. New York: D. Van Nostrand Company, 1980.

NATIONAL LEAGUE FOR NURSING, *Ethical Issues in Nursing and Nursing Education*. New York: National League for Nursing, 1980.

PATERSON, JOSEPHINE G., AND LORETTA T. ZDERDAD, *Humanistic Nursing*. New York: John Wiley & Sons, Inc., 1976.

ROSS, CARMEN F., *Personal and Vocational Relationships in Practical Nursing* (2nd ed.). Philadelphia: J.B. Lippincott Company, 1965.

SHELLEY, J., *Dilemma: A Nurse's Guide for Making Ethical Decisions*. Downers Grove, Ill.: Intervarsity Press, 1980.

SPICKER, STUART F., AND SALLY GADOW, EDS., *Nursing: Images and Ideals: Opening Dialogue with the Humanities*. New York: Springer Publishing Co., Inc., 1980.

STEELE, SHIRLEY M., AND VERA M. HARMON, *Values Clarification in Nursing* (2nd ed.). Englewood Cliffs, N.J.: Prentice-Hall, Inc., 1983.

TATE, BARBARA L., *The Nurse's Dilemma: Ethical Considerations in Nursing Practice.* Geneva: Florence Nightingale International Foundation, International Council of Nurses, 1977.

THOMPSON, JOYCE BEEBE, AND HENRY O. THOMPSON, *Ethics in Nursing.* New York: Macmillan, Inc., 1981.

Nursing Ethics: Articles

AROSKAR, MILA ANN, "Ethical Issues in Community Health Nursing," *Nursing Clinics of North America,* 14 (March 1979), 35–44.

———— ET AL., "The Most Pressing Ethical Problem Faced by Nurses in Practice," *Advanced Nursing Science,* 1, 3 (April 1979), 89–97.

BANDMAN, ELSIE L., "Why Ethics in Nursing Practice?" *Imprint,* 26, 5 (December 1979), 34.

BERGMAN, REBECCA, "Ethics—Concepts and Practice," *International Nursing Review,* 20 (1973), 140.

BUNZL, MARTIN, "A Note on Nursing Ethics in the USA," *Journal of Medical Ethics,* 1 (1975), 184–86.

CARPENTER, WILLIAM T., AND CAROL A. LANGSNER, "The Nurses' Role in Informed Consent," *Nursing Times,* 71 (1975), 1049–51.

CHRISTMAN, LUTHER, "Moral Dilemmas for Practitioners in a Changing Society," *Journal of Nursing Administration,* 3, 2 (March/April 1973), 15–17.

CHURCHILL, LARRY R., "Ethical Issues of a Profession in Transition," *American Journal of Nursing,* 77, 5 (May 1977), 873–75.

DAVIS, ANNE J., "Ethical Dilemmas and Nursing Practice," *Linacre Quarterly,* 44 (1977), 302–11.

————, "Ethics Rounds with Intensive Care Nurses," *Nursing Clinics of North America,* 14, 1 (March 1979), 45–55.

GADOW, SALLY, "Toward a New Philosophy of Nursing," *Nursing Law and Ethics,* 1, 8 (1980), 1.

JOHNSON, PRISCILLA, "The Gray Areas—Who Decides?" *American Journal of Nursing,* 77, 5 (1977), 856–58.

LEVINE, MYRA E., "Nursing Ethics and the Ethical Nurse," *American Journal of Nursing,* 77 (1977), 845–49.

MAHON, KATHLEEN A., AND SALLY J. EVERSON, "Moral Outrage—Nurses' Right or Responsibility: Ethics Rounds for Nurses," *Journal of Continuing Education in Nursing,* 10, 3 (1979), 4–7.

MOONEY, MARY MARGARET, "The Ethical Component of Nursing Theory," *Image,* 12, 1 (February 1980), 7–9.

NORRIS, CATHERINE M., "Delusions That Trap Nurses," *Canadian Nurse,* 69, 6 (June 1973), 37–40.

PELLEGRINO, EDMUND D., "Ethical Implications in Changing Practice," *American Journal of Nursing,* 64 (1964), 110–12.

QUAIFE, FRANCES M., "Ethics of Nursing," *American Journal of Nursing,* 4 (April 1904), 520–23.

ROMANELL, PATRICK, "Ethics, Moral Conflicts, and Choice," *American Journal of Nursing,* 77 (1977), 850–55.

ROSEN, ELLEN, AND CAROLYN DAROCY, "Ethical Issues in Nursing: Your Responses to JPN's Fourth Annual Survey," *Journal of Practical Nursing* (November/December 1981), 29–40.

ROSS, ANNIE H., "A Few Points of Ethics," *American Journal of Nursing,* 3 (1902), 41–42.

SHELP, EARL E., AND CLARA TERNES, "Moral Integrity for Nurses," *Nursing Law and Ethics*, 1, 9 (November 1980), 1.

SILVA, MARY CIPRIANO, "Science, Ethics, and Nursing," *American Journal of Nursing*, 74 (1974), 2004–7.

VEATCH, ROBERT M., "Nursing Ethics, Physician Ethics, and Medical Ethics," *Law, Medicine and Health Care* (October 1981), 17–19.

Bibliographies

AMERICAN NURSES' ASSOCIATION, *Ethics in Nursing: References and Resources*. Kansas City, Mo.: American Nurses' Association, 1979.

SOLLITTO, SHARMON, AND ROBERT M. VEATCH, *Bibliography of Society, Ethics and the Life Sciences*. Hastings-on-Hudson, N.Y.: The Hastings Center, series, 1973–.

WALTERS, LEROY, ED., *Bibliography of Bioethics*. Detroit: Gale Research Co., annual series, vol. 1, 1975.

CHAPTER 2

Professionalism

Concern for ethical standards and ideals is not unique to nursing. Virtually every group of working people that calls itself a profession practices with explicit and tacit assumptions about ethical standards and goals of practice. Virtually all publish codes of ethics and make statements of ideals and purposes. Associations of engineers, social workers, lawyers, teachers, physicians, accountants, real estate agents, airline flight attendants, and so on take public positions on the ethics of their membership.[1] What is it about the concept of being a professional that is so closely associated in many people's minds with ethics? The answer to this question lies in the concept of professionalism.

What a Profession Is

For many people, being a professional involves having a certain attitude toward one's work. Having a profession is something like having a *calling*. A calling is something one feels called upon to do, perhaps by God, by some deep need in one's being, or by the demands of historical circumstance. Like the role of priestess, a calling is central to one's life and gives it meaning. One is dedicated to creating something one sees as good and important. This good may be a widely recognized social or religious one, or it may represent a more private conception such as a cabinetmaker's pride in craft. Like those who feel called, professionals feel responsible for the quality of their work, identify with others who share their perspective, and feel that they are being paid in order to work instead of working in order to be paid. But seeing work as a profession usually demands less than seeing it as a calling. Professionals maintain more of a private life apart from their work and expect more concrete rewards for their devotion. People with a professional attitude

---

[1]Jane Clapp, *Professional Ethics and Insignia* (Metuchen, N.J.: Scarecrow Press, Inc., 1974).

18

are not found only within the professions; they can also be found among people who do technical work or manual labor.

But professionalism involves more than personal attitude. It has a social dimension shaped by one's relationships with co-workers and the organizations one joins. For example, the professional-client relationship usually requires a level of confidentiality that the clerk-customer relationship does not. Professional organizations gather with different aims and ideals than labor unions. Educational requirements, examinations, licensure, and registration distinguish professions from other occupational, labor, and business careers.

When people have tried to get to the core meaning of the word *professional* they have come up with many different definitions. Three common criteria for defining *professional* are adequate for understanding why professionals concern themselves so conspicuously with ethics.[2]

Maximal Competence

Professionals claim maximal competence in an activity of production or service. This means that they claim to provide a service better than any other group of people claiming to do the same. Professional groups establish their claim to competence in various ways. They may impose requirements on entry, such as extensive education, training, or a standard examination. They may require continuing education or repeated examinations for relicensure. They may claim that long association and familiarity with the details of certain tasks make them more competent at them than others. They may appeal to a theory of practice or a scientific foundation for their techniques. For example, the American Nurses' Association "Code for Nurses" states,

> Point 7: The nurse participates in activities that contribute to the ongoing development of the profession's body of knowledge. (ANA, 1976)

The ANA emphasizes the profession's association with nursing science.

> A unique body of verified knowledge provides both framework and direction for the profession in all of its activities and for the practitioner in the provision of nursing care. (Point 7.1, ANA, 1976)

Professions in transition or in conflict with other professions may become involved in disputes over the appropriateness of various theories or techniques, definitions of realms of competence, and related issues of appropriate education, credentials, and licensure. For example, in the late nineteenth century, the medical profession conducted an aggressive campaign against a wide variety of health care practices, such as patent medicines, homeopathic and chiropractic medicine, and midwifery. This helped to establish a standard conception of training and scientific

---

[2]Defining the professions is a favorite sociological enterprise. For a brief review and bibliography see *International Encyclopedia of the Social Sciences*, 1968 ed., s.v. "Professions," by Talcott Parsons. For a standard analysis, see Eliot Freidson, *The Profession of Medicine* (New York: Dodd, Mead, & Company, 1973), pp. 71–84. I use the brief definition of Kenneth Kipnis, "Professional Responsibility and the Responsibility of Professions," unpublished.

practice associated with the M.D. degree.[3] This campaign had the effect of defining who was and was not a physician at the same time that it defined a realm of medical competence.

The conflicts over health care practice in the mid–twentieth century have again opened questions about what counts as appropriate and maximal competence in caring for the sick. For example, clinical pharmacy is a new kind of pharmacy practice emphasizing consultation and hospital-based clinical work. Clinical pharmacists sometimes claim that since they know so much more about medications—their activity, indications, benefits, hazards, and interactions—than anyone else, they should have a major responsibility for prescribing medicines. Nurses educated in special types of medication, such as cancer chemotherapy, may be much more knowledgeable about them than physicians and claim maximal competence in that area. Nurses have also made a variety of claims to maximal and special competence in such areas as patient education and advocacy, integration of health services, primary care, and health maintenance.

Normally, an accepted profession has a generally agreed upon realm of maximal competence (such as nursing care) combined with borderline, overlapping, and disputed areas of competence. The claims that established professional groups make to maximal competence are sometimes hard to assess in an objective or neutral manner. There are two reasons for this. First, since the claim to competence is part of the concept of a profession, serious critiques of a profession's theory of practice threaten the self-concept and livelihood of its practitioners. Second, the practitioners of the discipline become the public authorities in the field, so that external critiques appear untrustworthy.

The criterion of competence will be crucially important to many of the ethical issues discussed in this text. The authority, trustworthiness, and responsibility of nurses and physicians to make recommendations and decisions with regard to patient care depend on their claims to be maximally competent in specific practice areas. Practitioners who overstep undisputed areas of competence risk charges of paternalism as well as incompetence. Moreover, the debate over nursing autonomy and authority in relationship to physicians, hospitals, and patients is closely linked with debate over definitions of nursing practice (see Chapter 3).

Significant Value

Professionals claim to practice work that has some significant social value. They link their competence to something important to most people: health, justice, education, land use, safety in air travel, and so on. They call attention to the dangers posed by unskilled practitioners in these socially valuable realms. Badly designed airplanes and bridges, clumsy surgeries, drug dosage errors, and malicious lawsuits capture public imagination and create support for identifiable groups of people that certify that their members will do their jobs well. Groups such as poets, craftspeople, and philosophers tend not to be seen as major professions, as their errors—obtuse imagery, careless leatherwork, and illusory metaphysics—pose less obvious public hazards.

---

[3]William G. Rothstein, *American Physicians in the Nineteenth Century: From Sects to Science* (Baltimore: Johns Hopkins University Press, 1972), pp. 9–10, 15–18.

Autonomy

Finally, professionals possess a high degree of autonomy in their work. *Autonomy* means *discretion, control, say-so, self-government,* or *independence* (see also p. 50). Professionals control various aspects of their work: details of how work is done, choice of goals toward which to work, choice of clientele, whether to work and with whom, and so on. The American Nurses' Association's "Code for Nurses" states, for example,

> Point 9: The nurse participates in the profession's efforts to establish and maintain conditions of employment conducive to high quality nursing care. (ANA, 1976)

Here, a professional nursing association claims a degree of control over conditions of employment. Professions vary widely in the amount and kinds of autonomy they experience. Moreover, the autonomy of the profession as a whole can be distinguished from the autonomy of its individual members.

Professions maintain their autonomy partly through their claim to maximal competence. So long as people believe that the professionals are the only ones who fully understand their work, it is very hard to supervise or criticize them. Professions also maintain their autonomy by means of *monopoly* over their work. In our competitive culture, people do not achieve autonomy simply by declaring it or believing in it. Professions maintain their control over their work partly by keeping people with other skills and other ideas from doing the same work. Only nurses may legally practice nursing. Licensure, educational requirements, certification of schools, and the like help nurses maintain control over nursing practice. This control is strengthened when nurses—rather than physicians and nonprofessionals—control the processes of licensure and certification. Autonomy is also maintained by a sense of unity and common interest among nurses. Ethical codes and traditions help to maintain this sense of unity.

Nursing as a Profession

Over the years, people have sometimes doubted nursing's standing as a profession. Like teaching, it is sometimes designated as a *semiprofession* to indicate its borderline standing. The grounds of doubt are not centered on whether nurses have professional attitudes or organizations. The doubts center on whether nurses meet the three criteria of professionalism. Many of these doubts can be traced to the backdrop of sexism against which nursing has had to assert itself.

First, some people have doubted whether nurses have a special area of competence. The charge has not been that nurses lack skill. Instead, it is claimed that nursing skills are not unique to nurses, or that these skills are an inborn and unteachable talent. The classic judgment on this issue comes from no less than Florence Nightingale: "You might as well register mothers as nurses. A good nurse must be a good woman."[4] More recent expressions of this attitude can still be found:

[4]M. Adelaide Nutting and Lavinia L. Dock, *A History of Nursing,* vol. II (New York: G.P. Putnam's Sons, 1907), p. 277.

Nursing has become professionalized to excess. . . . In my view the single most important improvement in patient care would be the availability of a person whose time would be spent in small-talk with the patients: somebody with a simple love for people and a liking for chit-chat.[5]

Nurses familiar with the skills and training required for patient care will scarcely credit these claims, and the claims can be dismissed as unreasonable. Attitudes like these, however, have been influential obstacles to payment and protection for nurses.

No one seriously doubts that nurses perform an important social good. However, people sometimes believe that nursing functions are less important social goods than the functions of physicians. This belief comes about because people often overlook the *care* function of health care and direct most of their attention to the *cure* function of health care. Since nurses are more closely associated in many people's minds with the care functions and physicians with the cure functions, nurses are sometimes seen as being less important than physicians in health care. Later in this text (Chapter 15) I will argue that the care functions are more important than the cure functions. This debate, however, is not to the point. Caring and curing are highly integrated tasks; nurses and physicians do both. Thus, there is no doubt that nursing care is a significant human good.

The criterion of autonomy is the main source of doubts about nursing as a profession. A close look at patterns of autonomy and subservience in nursing history indeed reveals a mixed picture, but one progressing toward greater autonomy. The discussion of nursing autonomy in the next chapter, together with the arguments for important nursing decision-making responsibilities discussed in Part Three, resolves the question in favor of increasing autonomy. Thus, nursing should be seen as a full profession in spite of some continuing resistance.

Characteristics of Professional Ethics

The three features of professionalism—a claim to competence, a socially valued goal, and autonomy—naturally lead professionals to a special concern with ethics. What distinguishes professionals' concern with ethics from our ordinary concern? For example, what makes confidentiality a special professional obligation different from the concern we would ordinarily have for tact or discretion in keeping secrets of friends? There are a number of differences, which together give an institutional structure to professional ethics and which make ethics basic to professions.

Unlike one's personal morality, one's professional ethics is not a fundamentally private concern. Ethical aspects of professional conduct are subject to *public scrutiny*. They may be legitimately observed, discussed, and judged by other professionals, clients, and the larger public. For example, it would be the legitimate concern of other nurses if one of the staff earnestly behaved in a racist way toward patients. Moreover, ethical aspects of professionals' work are subject to *review*. Professional groups and licensure boards can use ethics criteria for admission to

---

[5]Reprinted from Jose M. Segarra, "Medical Response to Layman's Perception of Illness," by permission of *The New England Journal of Medicine*, 296 (1977), 763.

membership in a profession and can use *sanctions* to punish violations of codes of practice. It is thus the *conduct* of a professional that is at issue, not what is held secret in one's heart. Professions are not so concerned with one's inner sympathy with the goals of the profession or with one's private motives. The well-meaning but incompetent practitioner endangers patients more than the competent but resentful clinician. This places professional ethics into sharp contrast with some major ethical traditions, such as Christianity, in which one's deeper feelings are at issue more than one's outward conduct.

Of course, intentions, feelings, and actions are not readily separable in the course of a lifetime. If one is in nursing entirely for status and security and has not an inkling of concern for people, then there is a good chance that those motives will show themselves in a course of action, for example, when it comes to admitting a mistake. There are also times when a nurse may be alone with a patient and no one else will know what transpires between the two. Or, if a group of people has two motives in patient care, as may happen with a research group doing clinical trials, it is possible for the research motive to show itself in uncaringly keeping a patient alive in order to complete a protocol. Or, if a profession has become corrupt and its conventions unacceptable in one's heart, this is also likely to surface in attempts to defend one's patients against other professionals, disillusionment, and "burnout," expressed by leaving a profession or by mechanical and cursory attention to one's work. Thus, although the focus of professional ethics is on outward conduct, one's private experiences and feelings enter the account at some point or other.

The ethics of a profession also represent a *tradition* carried by an identifiable and limited group of people. A professional group is not a community—which normally aggregates people into a place and which concerns itself with many aspects of their lives. Professionals are dispersed within a population, and their ethics concern primarily their work—not their personal relationships, births, and ceremonial occasions. Yet, the ethics of a professional group are like that of a community in that its traditional conventions reflect the experience, moral judgments, and explicit discussion of principles and goals of members over a period of time. They also reflect discussion and interaction with outsiders—patients, members of other professions, and the public.

Professional ethics thus functions something like *policy* in that it represents the resolution of debates over specific issues in the history of the profession.[6] For example, the sensitive area of nursing decision making in relationship to physicians has been a subject of debate and change in the codes of ethics of nursing professional organizations. The first ANA code of 1950 eliminated the references to nursing subservience found in earlier proposed codes, and the 1973 ICN code eliminated a statement of loyalty to physicians from its 1953 version. Or for example, a complex area of ethics, such as disclosure of information to cancer patients, may be aided by a careful statement of considerations and professional goals. A group of nurses may meet to develop a consensus and make recommendations, as did the Massachusetts Cancer Nurses' Group in its "Statement of Beliefs Related to Giving Cancer Patients Information" (see Appendix).

Ethical principles may be developed *formally,* as in the revision of a code of ethics. The American Nurses' Association has a standing ethics committee that bears the main organizational responsibility for the "Code for Nurses." A position

[6]Ivan Waddington, "The Development of Medical Ethics: A Sociological Analysis," *Medical History,* 19 (1975), 36–49.

on an ethical issue may also emerge *informally* within a profession. For example, in some hospitals nurses follow a practice of giving patients "no new information" that they have not already been told by their physician. This practice does not result from any written policy or meeting of those concerned. Instead, it is a practice that grew from the experiences of nurses.

To call attention to the special concern of professionals with ethics is not to claim that they are, or should be, "more ethical" than others, nor to say that they are better people than others (even though some professionals think that they are). It is to say that professionals are *accountable* to each other for the ethical conduct of their work. In other words, practitioners can be examined, assessed, and held responsible for the ethics of their practice. This accountability is limited in scope: It does not extend to judgments on the private morality of practitioners. It is nevertheless an important realm of study. Competence in the ethics of a profession stands alongside clinical skills to constitute basic competence in health care practice. It is part of the task of this book to give an account of *ethical competence* in nursing practice.

How the Concept of a Profession Shapes Its Ethics

Not just professionals but most people are concerned with ethical issues in the workplace. However, professionals approach these issues in a conscious, formal, and institutionalized way. For example, if nursing had taken a different form of organization, such as militant trade unionism, its expressions of ethical principles might well have taken a different form. Given that nursing is a profession, we can see why it is concerned with ethics in a conscious and institutionalized way.

AUTONOMY. The most obvious source of professional ethical traditions is the autonomy of professions. Autonomy is not total freedom. It is *self*-regulation as contrasted to regulation from outside or by others. To the degree that nurses regulate themselves, they need a set of rules or principles by which to do so.

MONOPOLY. Since autonomy of professions is protected in part by monopoly, one effect of nursing organizations is to *exclude* others from doing nursing. To the degree that nurses have control over the supply of people who can provide nursing services, the profession *incurs an obligation* to perform nursing care and to maintain standards. By encouraging cooperation and discouraging criticism among professionals, codes of ethics also help professions to maintain their monopoly power.[7]

CONCERN FOR PATIENTS. As part of their dedication to an important social good (the second criterion of a profession), nurses are expected to place the welfare of clients at the center of their professional concerns. Since demands are made on nurses from many sources, an explicit expression of ethical principles can protect this concern. A promise of confidentiality, for example, can protect nurses from demands upon them by others to reveal personal information that may be harmful to patients. The International Council of Nurses' "Code for Nurses" states,

The nurse holds in confidence personal information and uses judgment in sharing this information. (ICN, 1973)

[7]Jeffrey Berlant, "Medical Ethics and Professional Monopoly," *Annals of the American Association of Political and Social Sciences,* 437 (1978), 49–61.

The American Nurses' Association's code has a slightly stronger statement of this provision.

> Point 2: The nurse safeguards the client's right to privacy by judiciously protecting information of a confidential nature. (ANA, 1976)

Ethical principles can thus give clarity to the aims of nursing practice and help nurses keep patients' interests to the fore.

TRUST.   Since the nursing profession is not under the control of patients, and since patients are rarely knowledgeable about nursing, patients are dependent on and vulnerable to nurses. Patients must therefore place trust in nurses. A tradition of ethical principles helps ensure that patients are treated with respect and that trust will not be abused. By publishing principles in codes of ethics, nurses let patients and others know the terms of their *promises* to patients and some of the things for which patients can trust them.

BENEFITS.   It is sometimes argued that various professions *owe* duties to public welfare because they have received public benefits. Nurses, for example, benefit from public support for hospitals, nursing schools, scholarships, and so on. This debt can be paid by dedication to public service expressed by the ethical conventions of the profession. Since many nurses have doubted whether being a nurse is a benefit, however, this argument does not carry much weight. Nurses do not receive the rewards of money, power, and status of other professions to which this argument is directed.

THE NURSE-CLIENT RELATIONSHIP.   The ethical considerations involved in any important human relationship affect professional practice. Fairness, honesty, mutual autonomy, and respect need to be given specific expression in nursing practice in ways that reflect the realities of the nurse-client relationship.

PRACTICAL ARTS.   The knowledge and skills of nursing are not practiced merely for their own sake; they are always directed toward a good, such as the health of patients. So, we can call nursing a *practical art*. When we say that a skill represents a practical art, we emphasize that it is oriented to some valuable end or purpose. The end or purpose need not be distant in time from the act itself. It may be realized immediately as a result of the act. Giving a patient a massage gives the patient immediate satisfaction and relaxation. Giving a child a vaccination may later protect the child from polio. Both massages and vaccinations have their purposes and meaning primarily in connection with their intended results, although the result of one is immediate and of the other distant in time.

Sometimes nurses work just for the personal gains of job security, personal challenge, and income. Thus, personal benefits could be seen as the end or purpose of nursing work. Although it is legitimate to benefit from one's profession, this sort of purpose does not generate professional values and principles. The concept of professionalism integrates a skill with specific ends defining a particular profession, not just any end. Indeed, it is part of the function of professional ethics to warn practitioners against misusing their skills for extrinsic purposes.[8]

Since practical arts integrate skills with goals, reasoning about *means and*

---

[8]Goals can be *internal* or *external* to practices. For instance, the good of clients is an internal goal, and income is an external one. Skills in patient care enable nurses to achieve a goal intrinsic to nursing, and these skills can thus be called professional *virtues*. See Alasdair MacIntyre, *After Virtue* (Notre Dame, Ind.: University of Notre Dame Press, 1981), p. 178.

ends characterizes practical thinking. Thinking about means and ends in a professional context leads one inevitably to ethics. This transition from immediate practical concerns to ethics can be analyzed into four different levels.

First, at the most basic level, one needs to be able to choose the right means for the ends one has chosen. One needs to be able to tell when to address anxiety with communication and when Valium is the appropriate response. One needs to be able to choose the right needle size, to keep air out of dialysis lines, to approach distressing or disgusting situations with aplomb, to identify an abnormal heartbeat on a monitor, and so on. These kinds of choices represent the more technical side of competence.

Second, in order to do more than implement procedures, one needs to evaluate their various effects. The night nurse, for example, may need to balance the patient's need for quiet and comfort against the need to obtain vital signs. Or, for example, a nursing student objected because in her judgment a resident physician was prescribing an excessive dose of an antibiotic for an intestinal infection. The student was concerned that the patient might suffer side effects such as hearing loss or kidney damage. The resident replied with the maxim, "If you have no patient, you have no side effects." In this case, the aims "avoid death" and "avoid side effects" were being evaluated, and the physician was claiming that it was more important to guarantee that the patient live than to avoid side effects.[9]

Third, in order to make these evaluations well, one needs to *understand* the various goals of health care. One needs to understand what a good outcome is in order to appreciate how it can be achieved and to judge whether or not it has been achieved. Historically, this understanding has been divided into two rough divisions:

1. The *descriptive* aspects of understanding health care theory—the psychology of illness, physiology and stress, social processes in chronic disease, and so on
2. The *normative* aspects of health care theory—the concept of health, the significance of human suffering, the rights of patients, the dimensions of human compassion, the meaning of death, and so on

To practice competently, one must be able to integrate both descriptive and normative understanding of one's discipline. This integration is usually called "philosophy of nursing." Statements of philosophy or purpose often precede codes of ethics, bylaws, or statements of standards of professional organizations. For example, the American College of Nurse-Midwives asserts as part of its philosophy,

> Comprehensive maternity care, including education and emotional support as well as management of physical care throughout the childbearing years, is a major means for intercession into, and improvement and maintenance of, the health of the nation's families. Comprehensive maternity care is most effectively and efficiently delivered by interdependent health disciplines.
>
> Nurse midwifery is an interdependent health discipline focusing on the family and exhibiting responsibility for insuring that its practitioners are provided with excellence in preparation and that those practitioners demonstrate professional behavior in keeping with these stated beliefs.[10]

[9]In this case, the patient suffered the side effect of terminal and fatal kidney failure.

[10]American College of Nurse-Midwives, "Philosophy of the American College of Nurse-Midwives," April 22, 1972.

Fourth, competent thinking about the goals characterizing one's profession necessarily involves thinking about values and goals *extrinsic* to, or separate from, the profession. Health, compassion, protection, relief from illness, and so on are not the only goods to be considered in one's decisions. Although these are significant values, there are many other significant values in life which have to be considered in order to maintain a balanced perspective on nursing practice. For example, an elderly patient may consider the *independence* of living at home, however risky, a greater benefit than better physical *health* in more dependent circumstances. Costs must also be considered—time off from work to attend a clinic, money for medicines that might have gone for a child's coat, rent payments, or better food. Nursing skills are not so limitless as to address every value relevant to health and happiness. Any analysis of nursing goals must be conducted with a broad concern for human values in general.

I have sorted out these four levels of thinking to show how easily we move from a focus on daily tasks to broad moral values underlying them when these tasks are part of important practical arts like nursing. In reality, however, professional practice does not divide neatly into specific job skills and general moral principles. Professions *integrate* both of those in their practice. In this way, the practice of nursing acts as a solution to moral problems. Consider, for example, the moral problem of responding humanely to suffering caused by disease and death; nursing is one major solution our culture offers.

Practical thinking in nursing thus expresses both its technical and ethical aspects in every detail of work life. Nursing functions like a small social system. It exemplifies how societies generally integrate scientific and moral beliefs through practical arts and institutions.[11] Because professions integrate both scientific and value considerations in such a seamless way, a list of basic professional skills can never be a complete account of professional competence. A complete conception of professional competence must include both ethical and technical competence.

These seven factors—autonomy, monopoly, concern for patients, trust, benefits, the nurse-patient relationship, and practical arts—all make it clear that professionals ought to be conscious of ethical considerations. These factors also give professional ethical thinking its special character: self-conscious, institutional, accountable, and formal. The reader should note, however, that the argument is a conditional one: *If* one is professional, *then* one should be competent in professional ethics. I have not argued that everyone should be a professional. The argument also assumes that professionalism is a morally acceptable form of occupational organization despite controversy over the point.

Professional Ethics and Broader Moral Concerns

One's professional *role* is constituted by such things as professional ethics, technical competence, definitions of practice, expectations of others, and actual work activities. This role is limited as a source of principles for making decisions. For instance, it does not tell us what to do when we are not working. It does not tell us whether to accept professional values. Nor does it exclude from consideration at work values and rules extrinsic to professional ethical principles.

---

[11]Jürgen Habermas, *Legitimation Crisis*, trans. Thomas McCarthy (Boston: Beacon Press, 1973), p. 8.

Professional *ethics* is set in the context of broader social and moral principles and the personal convictions of individual practitioners. Professional *work* can be distinguished from personal life outside work. The *institution* of professional practice exists in the context of other institutions. And *practitioners* function in relationship to fellow professionals, members of other professions, clients, and the public. It is thus important to characterize the relationship between professional ethics and ethical issues extrinsic to the professional role. We need to know how much one's professional ethics should affect one's life in general, and how values extrinsic to the profession—those of one's conscience in particular—should be brought to bear on one's work.

In nursing history there has been confusion over the extent to which professional ethics should control personal life and judgment. This confusion has two major sources. First, the borderlines among professional work, personal life, and public duties are unclear. Second, it is not clear how much having "good moral character" should count in our judgments of ethical competence.

Ethics and Extended Roles

It is generally agreed among professionals that their work creates obligations extending beyond the immediate business of providing patients with basic health care. It is easy to move from a simple concern for one's patients' welfare to a general concern with public health and welfare, since these affect one's patients and one's ability to help them. This consciousness is reflected in both the ANA and ICN codes.

> Point 11: The nurse collaborates with members of the health professions and other citizens in promoting community and national efforts to meet the health needs of the public. (ANA, 1976)

> The nurse shares with other citizens the responsibility for initiating and supporting action to meet the health and social needs of the public. (ICN, 1973)

Nurses who have gained fame historically are often best known for their achievements in public health and the development of the profession—Annie Goodrich, Lavinia Dock, Lillian Wald, Mary Nutting, Isabel Robb, Helen Nahm, and so on. At the same time, nurses vary widely in their commitment to public concerns and cannot lose licenses for failing to engage in social or political efforts to improve health.

Private and Professional Life

Conflicting views on the connection between professional ethical competence and one's private moral conduct occur in the development of nursing ethics. A traditional view in nursing's early history held that one's profession should affect both the extent and conduct of one's personal life. As an early nursing text suggests,

A nurse should improve her mind by reading the best books at her command, by going out and visiting friends, and by attending the theater twice a month.[12]

As late as 1953, the ICN code stated:

The nurse in private life adheres to standards of personal ethics which reflect credit upon her profession. . . . In personal conduct nurses should not knowingly disregard the accepted patterns of behavior of the community in which they live and work.[13]

A basic textbook written in 1972 includes in its chapter on "Professional Behavior" a section on "Personal Behavior" giving advice about reputation, social drinking, dating, friendship, manners, and makeup and recommends "that to be morally clean is to bring lasting happiness. . . ."[14]

Another strong tradition holds that one's private life is one's own business and that one's profession should not affect what one does away from work. A profession is unlike a calling in that it permits a separation between professional and private concerns. The move toward separating personal values from patient care is part of our appreciation of privacy for all persons, including nurses. The most recent ICN, ANA, and AMA codes all refrain from making claims on the private lives of their membership.

Separating private and professional roles, however, almost creates two "selves"—a private self and a professional self. These two selves, needless to say, coexist intimately. This creates reciprocal demands, needs, and claims on each self. One's professional self may say to one's private self: "You should work harder; these people need your help; don't worry about such trivia as your weekend, etc." Meanwhile, one's private self complains, "You need rest; the stress is killing you; what about your family; are you still human?" and so on.

Likewise, one's moral conduct in private life and one's ethical competence at work can seem to be related. For example, what if a nurse is arrested for real-estate fraud, murders her husband, beats his wife, engages in prostitution, or sells cocaine? Do these kinds of conduct reflect on one's professional ethical competence?

Licensure boards are sometimes called upon to consider questions like these. "Good moral character" is a condition of licensure in many states, and boards consider felonies substantial evidence of poor moral character. Even though these acts are committed outside work, boards may have good reasons for being concerned with such issues. Their concerns vary:

1. The practitioner may be exploiting her or his position in order to conduct criminal or immoral activities. For example, a nurse may use the respectability of the RN license to endorse a fraudulent product.

[12]Emily A.M. Stoney, *Practical Points in Nursing for Nurses in Private Practice*, rev. by Lucy Cornelia Catlin (Philadelphia: W.B. Saunders Company, 1917), p. 18.

[13]International Council of Nurses, "International Code of Nursing Ethics (1953)" in *Contemporary Issues in Bioethics*, 1st ed., eds. Tom L. Beauchamp and LeRoy Walters (Encino, Calif.: Dickenson Publishing Co., Inc., 1978), p. 139.

[14]Lillian DeYoung, *The Foundations of Nursing as Conceived, Learned, and Practiced in Professional Nursing*, 2nd ed. (St. Louis: The C.V. Mosby Company, 1972), p. 47.

2. Some acts against public welfare may be considered gross violations of the extended role. It is one thing to fail to promote public health, another to hinder it actively. The extended role of nurses may confer upon nurses a special obligation not to harm others.
3. Harming the health of the public can be seen as a form of conflict of interest. It is clearly morally wrong to make people sick in order to drum up business.
4. The confidence of patients is important in nursing practice. If one does things that make patients mistrustful, even if patients mistrust for invalid reasons, one's efficacy as a professional is damaged.
5. The reputation of the profession as a whole is affected by the conduct of its members.
6. Conduct outside of work may affect conduct at work. Alcoholism, for example, may affect one's ability to practice.

It is important for licensure boards to use such considerations with caution, lest they lead to invasions of privacy. Boards should distinguish between the legitimate grounds for concern listed above and the common but mistaken belief that since persons act immorally in one realm of life, they are likely to act immorally in another. In one setting, a person may act generously, considerately, devotedly, and competently. In another, the same person may act cruelly, irresponsibly, or incompetently. Hartshorne and May in extensive studies on lying and cheating found that most people lie in some circumstances and not in others and that these patterns tend to be idiosyncratic.[15] Boards thus should not make general investigations into the moral worthiness of the personal lives of practitioners. A California licensure board, for example, rightly refused to restrict the practice of a nurse who was moonlighting as a topless dancer. Instead, the focus of concern should be on ability to practice according to professional standards or, where needed, defense of the profession.

Conscience in the Workplace

Just as the professional self makes claims on the private self, the latter makes claims on the conduct of the former. I have views about myself as a person that set limits on my conduct in professional life. For me to feel good about myself, I cannot act in my professional capacity in ways that offend my private sense of morality.

One's personal moral judgments enter professional practice in a number of ways, just as personal judgment is important to technical competence: Since professionals practice relatively autonomously, conventional practice requires substantial moral assent and support from practitioners. One must use one's own judgment in applying the basic conventional principles of practice. Practitioners may reasonably differ over applications. And professional ethical principles are necessarily incomplete; they do not address moral issues already clearly addressed by the culture in which the profession functions. Stealing from patients' purses, whispering obscenities to visitors, and shooting the nursing supervisor need not be covered by nursing codes.

Nurses may vary, for example, in their interpretation of confidentiality. Many nurses share medical information about their patients freely with other nurses and

[15]Hugh Hartshorne and Mark A. May, *Studies in Deceit* (New York: Macmillan, Inc., 1928).

physicians; others limit their communications to staff directly involved with the patient. A nurse may feel obligated to communicate some personal information about a patient to the attending physician and to withhold other information. The extent to which a nurse takes professional ethical principles seriously may also reasonably vary.

When things are going well, the personal judgments of practitioners are in substantial harmony with conventional practice. But the present crisis in ethics in health care has been marked by many questions of conscience, such as those about abortion and euthanasia. Nurses have been especially conscious of conflicting feelings over such issues and have found themselves assessing the extent to which they believe they should express and rely on their own moral beliefs at work.

There is no pat answer to whether personal views or professional principles should dominate. Sometimes it is clear that professional principles have more validity than the personal beliefs of some nurses. For example, most nurses would urge that even nurses who honestly believe some creeds are nonsense follow this basic principle:

> Inherent in nursing is respect for life, dignity and rights of man. It is unrestricted by considerations of nationality, race, creed, colour, age, sex, politics or social status. (ICN 1973)

Or, for example, some patients are so obnoxious that nurses rightly judge they deserve punishment. Yet, since it is traditionally held that nursing is a compassionate enterprise, it is wrong and unprofessional to use nursing practice as an instrument of justice. It is unprofessional to respond to such patients by jabbing needles roughly into their flesh and turning them carelessly and painfully in bed.

At other times, it is appropriate that conscience dominate practice. Nurses who believe abortion is morally wrong should not be required to participate in it. Respectable disagreement on the issue is possible and health practice does not require that every nurse perform every conceivable procedure. Much of the work of the field of ethics in the health sciences has attempted to integrate common personal judgments on such issues as abortion and euthanasia with professional practice.

The Hazards of Professionalism

Not everyone has kind words for professionals. Professionals can be seen as self-seeking, hypocritical, divisive, secretive, ambitious, and destructive. Bernard Shaw characterized professions as ". . . conspiracies against the laity."[16] In accepting professionalism, then, we must be cautious with regard to the ways in which it can go wrong.

One of the greatest hazards of professionalism to nurses has been their exploitation. Historically, some nurses have taken their dedication to patients so seriously that they have insisted on referring to nursing as a calling rather than acknowledging the weaker ascription "profession." Florence Nightingale warned nurses against "Making it a profession, and not a calling."[17] Extreme idealism with regard to

[16]George Bernard Shaw, *The Doctor's Dilemma* (1906), Act I.

[17]Nutting and Dock, *A History of Nursing*, p. 277.

patient care can be found in many places in nursing writing. Nightingale, for example, wrote that ". . . a good nurse should be the Sermon on the Mount herself."[18] An early *American Journal of Nursing* article on "Ethics in Private Practice" exhorts nurses:

> Remember the ministering Christ. Was not His whole life one of service? He it was who transformed this lowest form of work into the highest labor.[19]

These sentiments were supported by many physicians, even those so eminent as Sir William Osler.

> There is no higher mission in life than nursing God's poor. In so doing, a woman may not reach the ideal of her soul: she may fall short of the ideals of her head; but she will go far to satisfy those longings of the heart from which no woman can escape.[20]

During the early twentieth century when these claims were made, hospitals were being formed all over the country. Many of them were privately owned by physicians. The hospitals and physicians benefited financially because many student nurses worked long hours in them for free, sometimes over one hundred hours per week,[21] and dedicated nurses were willing to provide patient care for low wages.[22] Even today some nurses fear that to present their needs forcefully for respect, remuneration, and power to make decisions is somehow in conflict with dedication to patient care.

Nurses are right to be concerned about this possibility. The vulnerability of the sick, the structure of hospitals, and the lack of patient participation in health care decision making expose patients to hazards of exploitation by nurses and other health professionals. Misuse of the power of nurses over patients is well illustrated by the character of Big Nurse in *One Flew over the Cuckoo's Nest*.[23] Nurses who exploit patients may not be doing so deliberately or consciously. They need not even do it for their own benefit—they may unknowingly do things to patients that are really for the benefit of others.

Another hazard of professionalism in nursing is disillusionment. Nurses educated for complex professional skills and autonomy sometimes find hospital work boring, repetitive, and far below their ideals. Nurses sometimes have the experience of being "set up" by their professional education for loss, disappointment, and bitterness.

One of the most subtle and pervasive features of professionalism is that of *status* or *prestige*. Many people go into the professions in order to appear worthy in

[18]Ibid., p. 257.

[19]Helen Stuart Thompson, "Ethics in Private Practice," *American Journal of Nursing*, 6, 3 (December 1905), 166.

[20]William Osler, *Aequanimitas: With Other Addresses to Medical Students, Nurses and Practitioners of Medicine*, 3rd ed. (Philadelphia: The Blakiston Company, 1947), "Nurse and Patient," p. 158.

[21]Jo Ann Ashley, *Hospitals, Paternalism, and the Role of the Nurse* (New York: Teachers College Press, 1976), p. 21.

[22]Ibid., p. 6.

[23]Ken Kesey, *One Flew over the Cuckoo's Nest* (New York: The Viking Press, 1972).

the eyes of society and to gain the rewards of respected work, power, and good pay. This motive is so prevalent in the professions that some sociologists refer to status and prestige as essential features of professionalism.[24]

Sometimes people confuse judgments of status or prestige with judgments of moral worth. They associate being better off socially or economically with being a better person and then associate that with being a *morally* better person. Conversely, they may see someone who is worse off as being so because that person is a worse person, specifically, a morally worse person. A nurse with solid old-fashioned virtues of hard work, cleanliness, income, family, frugality, and good health may see herself or himself in contrast to patients who appear dirty, careless, impecunious, selfish, lazy, or the like. Another dimension of prestige-based moral judgments about patients is unwarranted blaming of illnesses on them. This confusion is often termed "blaming the victim." But there is no association between prestige and moral worth. Basic values such as care, honesty, and integrity can be found in all walks of life. Likewise, dishonesty, selfishness, and corruption can also be found among people of any status.

Nightingale recruited her first coterie of nurses from the upper classes in England, apparently partly in order to avoid some common prejudices against the moral character of nurses. It is clear, however, that being a *good* nurse (a concept combining both ethical and technical competence) has no conceptual tie with being a nurse of *high social status*. Neither is improvement in the status of nursing necessarily related to improved patient care. If a professional is of substantially different social status than his or her clients, it may be hard for that clinician to understand their problems and to communicate with them.

As a profession, nursing is of moderate status. It ranks well below physicians, just below clergy and journalists, and above secretaries and flight attendants.[25] I have chosen to exclude the concept of status from that of professionalism so that we do not have to judge nurses as being less professional because of their moderate status. Moreover, in their struggle for greater respect and social appreciation, I would like to see nurses also address the problems of those lower in the hospital hierarchy and not simply join physicians at the top of the status ladder in a marriage of dominance over other hospital staff.

Lastly, professions, like any community, exclude others at the same time that they bring people together within their membership. Professions work closely with "outsiders"—patients, other professions, occupations, and the public. These groups play a role in defining nursing and negotiate relationships with the nursing profession. One problem for nurses is to assert their great strength as a profession with justice and respect and to avoid the hazards of isolation, divisiveness, and secrecy that can come with the exclusiveness of professionalism.

Summary

A profession is a type of occupation represented by organizations which claim that their members have maximal competence in their occupation, practice work of

[24]For example, Eliot Freidson, *Professional Dominance* (New York: Lieber-Atherton Inc., 1970), pp. 155–56.

[25]Margretta M. Styles, "Dialogue across the Decades," *Nursing Outlook,* 26 (1978), 28–32.

significant social value, and possess a high degree of autonomy in their work. Although nursing has lacked autonomy in the past, it now satisfies the criteria of the concept of a profession.

Professional ethics is generally more public, explicit, and subject to scrutiny than personal moral beliefs. Virtually every profession publishes a code of ethics, and professionals are expected to be competent in the ethics of their practice.

The autonomy and monopoly of professionals and the need for their clients to trust them lead professions to make their ethics public and explicit. Moreover, since professions are practical arts and claim to use their techniques (e.g., nursing care) for a social good (e.g., health), they need to be clear about the ethics of their work in order to conduct it well.

Since professional practice only occupies a part of the life of practitioners, professionals are concerned with the relationship of their work to personal views and life outside work. They must consider how their professional ethics should affect their personal lives and extended roles, and how their personal conscience should affect their professional practice.

Professionalism has hazards. Excessively high ideals have been used in the past to exploit nurses. Professionalism can function as a means of mere status seeking and be used to justify domination of clients, and the exclusiveness of professions makes it hard for professionals to cooperate with other workers.

FURTHER READINGS

Professionalism

BAYLES, MICHAEL D., *Professional Ethics*. Belmont, Calif.: Wadsworth Publishing Co., Inc., 1981.

BLEDSTEIN, BURTON J., *The Culture of Professionalism: The Middle Class and the Development of Higher Education in America*. New York: W.W. Norton & Co., Inc., 1977.

FREIDSON, ELIOT, *Professional Dominance: The Social Structure of Medical Care*. New York: Lieber-Atherton Inc., 1970.

————, *The Profession of Medicine*, "The Formal Characteristics of a Profession," pp. 71–84. New York: Dodd, Mead & Company, 1973.

GORDON, LINDA, "The Politics of Birth Control, 1920–1940: The Impact of Professionals," in *The Cultural Crisis of Modern Medicine*, ed. John Ehrenreich, pp. 144–84. New York: Monthly Review Press, 1978.

LINDBLOM, CHARLES E., *Politics and Markets: The World's Political Economic Systems*, pp. 45–50. New York: Basic Books, Inc., Publishers, 1977.

WILENSKY, HAROLD L., "The Professionalization of Everyone?" *American Journal of Sociology*, 70 (1964), 137–58.

Professional Ethics

AMERICAN NURSES' ASSOCIATION, *Perspectives on the Code for Nurses*. Kansas City, Mo.: American Nurses' Association, 1978.

————, "A Suggested Code: A Code of Ethics Presented for the Consideration of the American Nurses' Association," *American Journal of Nursing*, 26 (1926), 599–601.

————, "A Tentative Code for the Nursing Profession," *American Journal of Nursing*, 40 (1940), 977–80.

FLAHERTY, M. JOSEPHINE, "Two Canadian Nursing Codes," *Westminster Institute Review*, 1, 3 (October 1981), 11.

FREEDMAN, BENJAMIN, "What Really Makes Professional Morality Different: Response to Martin," *Ethics*, 91 (1981), 626–30.

GOLDMAN, ALAN H., *The Moral Foundations of Professional Ethics*. Totowa, N.J.: Littlefield, Adams & Co., 1980.

HULL, RICHARD T., "The Function of Professional Codes of Ethics," *Westminster Institute Review*, 1, 3 (October 1981), 12–13.

JARVIS, PETER, "Some Comments on the Rcn Code of Professional Conduct," *Nursing Mirror* (November 24, 1977), 27–28.

JOHNSON, DOROTHY E., "A Philosophy of Nursing," *Nursing Outlook*, 7 (1959), 198–200.

KASERMAN, IMOGENE, "A Nursing Committee and the Code for Nurses," *American Journal of Nursing*, 77 (1977), 875–76.

LIMBERT, PAUL M., "Developing a Code of Ethics for the Nursing Profession," *American Journal of Nursing*, 32 (1932), 1257–63.

MARTIN, MIKE W., "Professional and Ordinary Morality: A Reply to Freedman," *Ethics*, 91 (1981), 631–33.

———, "Rights and the Meta-Ethics of Professional Morality," *Ethics*, 91 (1981), 619–25.

MAY, WILLIAM F., *Notes on the Ethics of Doctors and Lawyers*. Bloomington, Ind.: Poynter Center, Indiana University, 1977.

MOONEY, SISTER MARY MARGARET, "The Ethical Component of Nursing Theory," *Image*, 12, 1 (February 1980), 7–9.

PERRY, CHARLOTTE M., "Nursing Ethics and Etiquette," *American Journal of Nursing*, 6 (1905–1906), 448.

RULE, JUANITA B., "The Professional Ethic in Nursing," *Journal of Advanced Nursing*, 3 (1978), 3–8.

SWARD, KATHLEEN M., "The Code for Nurses: A Guide for Ethical Nursing Practice," *New York State Nursing Association Journal*, 6, 4 (December 1975), 25–32.

Nursing as a Profession

BOSTON NURSES GROUP, *The False Promise: Professionalism in Nursing*. Somerville, Mass.: New England Free Press, 1978.

BROWN, ESTHER LUCILE, *Nursing as a Profession*. New York: Russell Sage Foundation, 1937.

KATZ, FRED E., "Nurses," in *The Semi-Professions and Their Organization: Teachers, Nurses, Social Workers*, ed. Amitai Etzioni, pp. 54–81. New York: The Free Press, 1969.

KRAMER, MARLENE, "Philosophical Foundations of Baccalaureate Nursing Education," *Nursing Outlook* (April 1981), 224–28.

KRUEGER, CYNTHIA, "Do 'Bad Girls' Become Good Nurses?" *Trans-Action* (July/August 1968), pp. 31–36.

MAUKSCH, INGEBORG G., AND MARTHA E. ROGERS, "Nursing Is Coming of Age . . . Through the Practitioner Movement: Pro and Con," *American Journal of Nursing*, 75 (1975), 1834–43.

SCHLOTFELDT, ROZELLA M., "On the Professional Status of Nursing," *Nursing Forum*, 13 (1974), 16–31.

SCHORR, THELMA M., "Yes, Virginia, Nursing *Is* a Profession," *American Journal of Nursing*, 81 (1981), 959.

STYLES, MARGRETTA M., "Dialogue across the Decades," *Nursing Outlook* (January 1978), 28–32.

THORNER, ISIDOR, "Nursing: The Functional Significance of an Institutional Pattern," *American Sociological Review*, 20, 4 (August 1955), 531–38.

WAGNER, DAVID, "The Proletarianization of Nursing in the United States, 1932–1946," *International Journal of Health Services*, 10 (1980), 271–90.

CHAPTER 3

Nursing's Struggle for Autonomy

It is easy to discern in nursing an expression of the first two criteria of professionalism: competence and dedication to an important social good. The third criterion of professionalism, autonomy, has been a center of struggle since the late nineteenth century. This chapter discusses some of the major obstacles to the independent practice and self-government of nurses and suggests that a better understanding of the concept of autonomy could help to overcome these obstacles.

History of the Struggle

Nursing has a strong tradition of ethics teaching. No decade has passed since 1900 without publication of at least one basic text in nursing ethics.[1] The *American*

[1]Textbooks on nursing ethics prior to the "bioethics revolution" include Eva C.E. Lückes, *Hospital Sisters and Their Duties*, 2nd ed. (London: J. & A. Churchill, 1888); Isabel Hampton Robb, *Nursing Ethics: For Hospital and Private Use* (Cleveland: J.B. Savage, 1900); Harriet Camp Lounsberry, *Making Good on Private Duty: Practical Hints to Graduate Nurses* (Philadelphia: J.B. Lippincott Company, 1912); Charlotte A. Aikens, *Studies in Ethics for Nurses* (Philadelphia: W.B. Saunders Company, 1916); Emily A.M. Stoney, *Practical Points in Nursing for Nurses in Private Practice*, rev. by Lucy Cornelia Catlin (Philadelphia: W.B. Saunders Company, 1917); Sara E. Parsons, *Nursing Problems and Obligations* (Boston: Whitcomb and Barrows, 1916); Mary E. Gladwin, *Ethics: A Textbook for Nurses*, 2nd ed. (Philadelphia: W.B. Saunders Company, 1937); Dom Thomas Verner Moore, *Principles of Ethics*, 4th ed. (Philadelphia: J.B. Lippincott Company, 1943, 1st ed. published in 1935); S.A. Rochelle and C.T. Fink, *Handbook of Medical Ethics for Nurses, Physicians and Priests*, 4th ed. (Montreal: The Catholic Truth Society, 1943); Katherine J. Densford and Millard S. Everett, *Ethics for Modern Nurses: Professional Adjustments I* (Philadelphia: W.B. Saunders Company, 1947); Joseph B. McAllister, *Ethics: With Special Application to the Medical and Nursing Professions*, 2nd ed. (Philadelphia: W.B. Saunders Company, 1955). Works early in the rise of bioethics include Francis J. Storlie, *Nursing and the Social Conscience* (New York: Appleton-Century-Crofts, 1970); Loretta Sue Bermosk and Raymond J. Corsini, eds., *Critical Incidents in Nursing* (Philadelphia: W.B. Saunders Company, 1973).

Journal of Nursing published an article on ethics in its first volume (1901), and in the 1920s and 1930s it carried a regular column of nursing ethics cases. Ethics courses were often part of the nursing curriculum until they were pushed aside after World War II by burgeoning courses in sciences and health care technology. By contrast, the tradition of ethics teaching in medicine is weaker. Even the development of bioethics as a teaching subject in medical schools in the late 1970s resulted in large part from outside pressure. Why has there been such a difference?

Three plausible explanations are at hand. First, women have carried the humane tradition in modern Western cultures: they educate children, soften the blows of the world, nurture others, and humanize modern life. Nursing and medicine have reified this stereotype. Nurses stereotyped as "feminine" were expected to be concerned with ethics and humanism while physicians stereotyped as "masculine" toiled with diagnostic tests, science, and instruments. An open concern for ethics was not masculine.

Second, medical ethics has been strongly individualistic. Physicians have not enjoyed being told how to behave; typically, they balked at any suggestion that they did not already know what to do. This attitude is reflected by the introduction to the 1972 American Medical Association Code:

> Ethical principles are basic and fundamental. Men of good conscience inherently know what is right or wrong, and what is to be done or to be avoided. Written documents attempt to express for the guidance of all what each knows to be true.[2]

Third, nursing has carried a tradition of deference. Thus, it has not seemed strange for textbook authors to instruct nurses in their duties. In her 1901 text *Nursing Ethics: For Hospital and Private Use*, Isabel Hampton Robb placed obedience at the center of nursing virtues:

> Above all, let her remember to do what she is told to do, and no more; the sooner she learns this lesson, the easier her work will be for her, and the less likely will she be to fall under severe criticism. Implicit, unquestioning obedience is one of the first lessons a probationer must learn, for this is a quality that will be expected from her in her professional capacity for all future time. Some learn it with more or less difficulty; others never wholly master it; the happy few, who have been fortunate enough to have been trained to it from childhood, accept it naturally and never find it irksome.[3]

Obedience to supervisors and physicians remained a central focus of nursing ethics teaching until the rebirth of feminism in the 1970s. For example, in a 1917 text we find:

> There would be no possible excuse for the nurse to act on her own responsibility in the hospital, as there is always a doctor within calling distance; . . . .[4]

---

[2]Judicial Council, *Opinions and Reports of the Judicial Council* (Chicago: American Medical Association, 1971), p. iii.

[3]Robb, *Nursing Ethics*, pp. 57–58. The example of obedience that Robb offers is the importance of taking a rest when told to do so by the head nurse.

[4]Stoney, *Practical Points in Nursing*, p. 17.

A 1947 text includes, among "some good rules,"

> Carry out the doctor's orders.[5]

In a 1955 text, the author writes:

> Whether the hospital or the patient or the physician employs the nurse, she works *under the instruction of the physician.* . . . In accepting the position, the nurse makes at least an implicit contract to carry out the orders of the physician in charge.[6]

These injunctions, although commonplace, have never been absolute. Nurses have never been called on by these texts to obey physicians making obvious mistakes. Moreover, we can find in nursing history many objections to obedience as a major nursing obligation. As early as 1916 Isabel M. Stewart wrote:

> The traditional virtues of the good nurse are: obedience, the spirit of self-sacrifice, courage, patience, conscientiousness, and discretion. These are good, but under the newer conditions they are not alone sufficient. I think we have not placed enough emphasis on the more positive and vigorous qualities, such as self-reliance, the power of leadership, and initiative.[7]

The struggle against obedience reached an important turning point when the ICN dropped from its 1973 code a point that had lingered in its 1965 version:

> The nurse is under an obligation to carry out the physician's orders intelligently and loyally.[8]

Instead, the ICN confined itself to the more neutral principle:

> The nurse sustains a cooperative relationship with co-workers in nursing and other fields. (ICN, 1973)

The textbook tradition in nursing ethics thus reflects a strong tradition of deference in conflict with the concept of professionalism. In contrast, early nursing leaders were vigorous and outspoken women, improbably cast in a deferential role. This legacy of deference is thus best seen as a price early nursing leaders chose to pay, rightly or wrongly, in order to advance nursing.

At that time, society created many obstacles to leadership by women in health care: Women were supposed to stay in the home; skilled nursing care was confused with unskilled family care; education of women was a new idea for Americans. Other efforts by women to enter health care as professionals were largely defeated. By 1910 only a few women had been able to enter medical practice. Six percent of

---

[5]Densford and Everett, *Ethics for Modern Nurses,* p. 157.

[6]McAllister, *Ethics,* p. 297.

[7]Isabel M. Stewart, "The Aims of the Training School for Nurses," *American Journal of Nursing,* 16 (1915–1916), 319–27.

[8]International Council of Nurses, "International Code of Nursing Ethics," in *Contemporary Issues in Bioethics,* 1st ed., eds. Tom L. Beauchamp and LeRoy Walters (Encino, Calif.: Dickenson Publishing Co., Inc., 1978), p. 139.

physicians were women—a number that declined steadily until the 1950s.[9] Mid-wives, who attempted to practice health care independent of physicians, were driven almost completely out of business by obstetricians and gynecologists. Mid-wives lost this struggle around the turn of the century even though their patients had lower mortality rates than physicians'.[10] Nursing was the only form of health practice which women at that time were able to enter in large numbers. They became the workers that allowed the modern hospital to expand. They did so by avoiding direct conflict with physicians. They stayed within the medical model and used deference to avoid threatening physicians.

Many of the historical influences that once made obedience a prudent choice still operate today, and we should look at them in detail. These include hospitals, physicians, nurses, sexism, and the concept of autonomy.

Opposition from Hospitals

The late nineteenth century was a period of rapid industrialization in the United States. Products previously of handiwork, crafts, small business, and home industry became the products of large organizations. Women who once wove cloth in their homes found themselves weaving and sewing in assembly lines with a consequent degradation in their quality of life and social standing.[11] Early hospitals represented a similar industrialization of the craft industry of health care. At first,

[9]Year   Percentages of women physicians: 1910–1974

1910	6.0
1920	5.0
1930	4.0
1940	4.6
1950	6.1
1960	6.8
1974	8.7

From "Women and Biomedicine: Women as Health Professionals," by Carol C. Nadelson and Malkah T. Notman. (Reprinted with permission of The Free Press, a Division of Macmillan Publishing Company and the Kennedy Institute of Ethics, Georgetown University. From *Encyclopedia of Bioethics,* Warren T. Reich, Editor-in-Chief. Volume IV, page 1716. Copyright © 1978 by Georgetown University, Washington, D.C.) The rates of men in nursing are similarly meager:

Year   Percentages of male RNs: 1949–1972

1949	0.8
1962	0.8
1972	1.4
1980	3.0 (ANA estimate)

Just as more women are entering medicine, more men are entering nursing. The percentage of male LVNs is higher: 3.6 percent in 1970. Aides, orderlies, and attendants have an even higher ratio: 15.2 percent in 1970. Because of the large number of RNs and LPNs, there are more men in nursing than women in medicine, although the *percentage* of women physicians is greater. Nursing figures are from Howard S. Rowland, ed., *The Nurse's Almanac* (Germantown, Md.: Aspen Systems Corporation, 1978).

[10]Neal Devitt, "The Statistical Case for Elimination of the Midwife: Fact Versus Prejudice, 1890–1935," parts I and II, *Women and Health,* 4 (1979), 81–96, 169–86.

[11]Mary P. Ryan, *Womanhood in America: From Colonial Times to the Present,* 2nd ed. (New York: New Viewpoints, 1979), pp. 12–14.

hospitals mainly cared for the poor, but soon people recognized the economic advantages of hospitalization for the well-off sick. As homes became urbanized, the hospital appeared as a convenience for the sick and a "home away from home" in which to be cared for.

Early hospitals followed closely the Victorian concept of the home. The early nurse functioned as "mother."[12] She worked inside the home, in other words, the hospital, and took charge of housekeeping and hospital finances. Cleanliness, orderliness, and frugality were thus major nursing virtues. The nurse as mother also bore direct responsibility for patient care. Like children, patients were the central figures and intended beneficiaries of the hospital family. At the same time, patients were expected to have little say-so in the conduct of hospital affairs. The nurses cared for, cleaned up after, managed, and educated their "children." The physician, to complete this all-too-real image, functioned as "father." Like the typical urban male worker, he spent much of his time absent from home. He only visited briefly to leave instructions with "mother" for care of the "children." In addition, he took major responsibility for the conduct of hospital affairs, was the head of the "household," and often owned the hospital, just as the patriarchal male owned the home. As owner, the physician was the primary financial beneficiary of this arrangement, while nurses made financial sacrifices to support the industrialization of health care.[13]

"Owners" of hospitals have changed since the early foundations, and a large portion of hospital-generated revenue now goes to insurers, investors, builders, suppliers, managers, regulators, and so on. Meanwhile, nurses have taken on many functions initially performed only by physicians: injections, diagnosis, physical exams, medication, drawing blood, record keeping, administration, and so on. Although nurses have acquired these new tasks, control over them has remained mostly with physicians, and the organization of autonomy in the hospital is for the most part unchanged. The main obstacles now facing the autonomy of nurses in hospitals are bureaucratic forms of management and the attending-physician system.

Bureaucracies give authority to their personnel through a top-downward *vertical* mode of authority. Each participant has a limited range of activities and discretion. Each is answerable to someone above, and an administrator or board of directors sits at the top of the pyramid. The legal background of hospital care tends to support this bureaucratic conception of nursing. Under the doctrine of *respondeat superior*, hospitals can be held legally responsible for the actions of nursing staff.[14] Along with an employer's interest in controlling employees' work, this makes hospitals anxious to control the actions of nurses and to discourage autonomy. In contrast, professionals draw their power from a *horizontal* or *collegial* mode of organization. Professionals normally regard each other as having equal authority and do not supervise each other except as teachers. A professional tends to see herself as answerable primarily to the commitments of her profession. Professionals

---

[12]See Anselm Strauss, "The Structure and Ideology of American Nursing: An Interpretation," in *The Nursing Profession: Five Sociological Essays*, ed. Fred Davis (New York: John Wiley & Sons, Inc., 1966), p. 91: "If the doctor was fatherly, the nurse was womanly, and sometimes motherly; . . ."

[13]Jo Ann Ashley, *Hospitals, Paternalism, and the Role of the Nurse* (New York: Teachers College Press, 1976), p. 6.

[14]Helen Creighton, *Law Every Nurse Should Know*, 4th ed. (Philadelphia: W.B. Saunders Company, 1981), pp. 80–83.

claiming increased autonomy can thus be seen by hospital administrators as potential sources of friction and disloyalty.

Professionalism and bureaucracy are different strategies for allocating decision making. The two strategies can be integrated in the hospital by having nursing representatives sit on management and policy committees. The most striking compromise, however, is that between physicians and hospitals. Here, professional autonomy is reconciled with bureaucracy by giving physicians a central place in management and submerging the conflict between professionalism and bureaucracy in medical dominance. In most U.S. hospitals this reconciliation operates through the *attending physician* system. In this system, the physician, not the patient, is the primary client of the hospital. The hospital provides services to physicians who admit patients. Physicians instruct hospitals via orders to provide selected services to these patients. From an institutional point of view, attending physicians do not give orders to individual nurses. They give orders to the hospital, and through its administrative bureaucracy, it directs individual nurses to fill them. Meanwhile, the hospital has its own contract with patients to provide nursing, dietary, and other services independent of but coordinated with services ordered by physicians.

This dual system of authority places conflicting demands on nurses. The hospital may expect one thing of nurses (conserving supplies, ensuring that all patients receive basic services), while physicians expect another (unstinting devotion to their patients). If nurses had a recognized sphere of discretion adequate to reflect their abilities and professional responsibility, then this dual system might not be such an obstacle to autonomy. But the combined tasks of filling physician orders and completing hospital duties exhaust energy that might be used to initiate nursing care plans, bedside care, and patient teaching.

The rewards and sanctions of bureaucracies combine with the dual system of organization to place nurses in a disadvantageous negotiating position with regard to physicians. While physicians are *clients* of hospitals and therefore cannot be fired for their mistakes, nurses are *employees* of hospitals and hold their jobs at the will of the hospital. In negotiations with physicians, nurses are usually more vulnerable than physicians.[15]

The dual system of authority makes it difficult to establish a nurse-patient relationship. In order to define a realm of professional discretion, nurses need a well-defined relationship with their clients, but definition is hard to achieve in the hospital setting. A nurse may work with many patients during a day, and these patients will have different physicians responsible for special medical aspects of their care. Moreover, a nurse may have only certain duties with respect to each patient. It may be the case that no nurse has the overall duty for the nursing care of a patient. Each patient during a shift may receive the care of many nurses, and on each shift, another set of nurses will look after the patient. The patient does not necessarily have one nurse to look to for nursing services. In some hospitals, a mass of nurses thus has a relationship to a mass of patients. The coordination required by this system fragments the provider-client relationship underlying traditional conceptions of professional autonomy. Particularly in large teaching hospitals, intricate divisions of responsibility obscure the physicians' scope of autonomy as well.

These dynamics are not without secondary advantages. The nurse can appeal to hospital duties in reply to physician demands, and to physician duties in reply to hospital demands. The nurse's own decisions can be presented to the patient with

---

[15]In public hospitals with civil service positions, nurses sometimes have stronger negotiating powers.

the weight of hospital policy or physician orders as he or she chooses. Nurses skillful in manipulating such responsibilities may gain power or autonomy by keeping hostile forces in balance in the fashion of a nineteenth-century European diplomat. But this mode of gaining power only offers a cynical and covert autonomy. Full autonomy requires that one's power to make decisions be recognized openly and regarded as legitimate.

These problems with autonomy are not present to the same degree in all nursing settings. In "primary care" systems of nursing, a nurse may have primary responsibility for a certain group of patients, or in intensive care settings, responsibility for just one patient. Nurses on the night shift may act without consultation more than nurses in the day: As one nurse remarked, "To physicians, I am a genius at night, and an idiot by day." Nurse practitioners and private duty nurses may also have a clear nurse-client relationship: one nurse practitioner specializing in cancer chemotherapy exclaimed, "At last, I have a doctor-patient relationship!" Outside the hospital in less bureaucratic settings, nurses may also be able to operate with more autonomy. Public health and registry nurses sometimes have this experience. Acute care hospitals tend to be the settings in which nurses, especially staff nurses, experience the most acute autonomy conflicts.

Opposition from Physicians

Medicine became organized as a profession in the United States in the mid–nineteenth century. In an earlier part of that century it had suffered from a populist movement that supported self-care and damaged the physician monopoly over health care services. With this experience fresh in their history, newly organized physicians were assiduous during the last half of the nineteenth century in protecting their position by limiting entry to their profession and by attacking competing professions.[16] Nursing's growth in the face of this competition has placed the two professions in an intimate relationship of cooperation and conflict. The profession of medicine continues to exercise its decreasing but continuing dominance over the profession of nursing through institutionalized gender discrimination and hospital bureaucracy. To patients and the public, the entire health care organization appears as the doctor writ large.

The use of "medical care" to refer to health care uses the name of a small part to stand for the whole. This language, like the use of "he" to refer to both men and women, tends to conceal less powerful practitioners from view. For example, people use such phrases as "new medical technology" to refer to a variety of machinery and equipment usually operated by nonphysicians.[17] Many procedures and forms of care—using a social worker, getting a hearing aid, administering many medications, creating discharge plans, and others—must be done over a physician's signature even though virtually all of the work, quality control, and decision making

[16]William G. Rothstein, *American Physicians in the Nineteenth Century: From Sects to Science* (Baltimore: Johns Hopkins University Press, 1972), pp. 9–10, 15–18; and Vern L. Bullough, "Licensure and the Medical Monopoly," in *The Law and the Expanding Nursing Role,* 2nd ed., ed. Bonnie Bullough (Englewood Cliffs, N.J.: Prentice-Hall, Inc., 1980), pp. 14–22.

[17]Sandra Harding, "Value-Laden Technologies and the Politics of Nursing," in *Nursing: Images and Ideals: Opening Dialogue with the Humanities,* eds. Stuart F. Spicker and Sally Gadow (New York: Springer Publishing Co., Inc., 1980), p. 52.

is done by nonphysicians.[18] Thus, the successes and failures of health care are often attributed to physicians as though they worked alone when in fact hospital care represents the combined work of a variety of specialists. Some physicians even seem to think of themselves as owning the nurses they work with. Some use such phrases as "I look out for my nurses," or "My nurses are very competent." A physician would never refer to his or her colleagues as "my doctors," nor do nurses often speak of "my doctors."

Medicine has been powerful enough to define its practice on its own terms. This has meant that the standard legal definitions of medicine are so broad that it is very difficult to provide any health care without falling within the meaning of "medicine." Consider, for example, a typical legal definition of medical practice:

> . . . judging the nature, character, and symptoms of disease, in determining the proper remedy for the disease, and in giving or prescribing the application of the remedy to the disease; but the system or method employed, or its efficacy, is immaterial.[19]

Sometimes the definition is not limited to "disease" but includes references to "pain, injury, deformity, or physical condition."[20] In one court decision, the judge said:

> In its broadest sense, the term "physician" includes anyone exerting a remedial or salutary influence.[21]

These broad definitions make it hard to consider any clinical approach to human disorders as outside the province of medical practice. Jack Geiger made humane use of this generality when he prescribed food for hungry patients in Mississippi.[22] But medicine's breadth has been used in attempts to block health insurance programs, flouridating water, midwifery, and holistic health practitioners.

Some of the older statutes give nurses the dubious honor of being the only profession expressly prohibited by law from practicing medicine.

> This chapter confers no authority to practice medicine or surgery or to undertake the prevention, treatment or cure of disease, pain, injury, deformity, or mental or physical condition in violation of any provision of law.[23]

This statute was revised in 1974 with "the legislative intent also to recognize the existence of overlapping functions between physicians and registered nurses and to permit additional sharing of functions. . . ."[24]

[18]Distinguishing the person who actually makes decisions from the one who is responsible for them is a standard managerial device. See Peter F. Drucker, *The Effective Executive* (New York: Harper & Row, Publishers, Inc., 1966), p. 6.

[19]1970 *Corpus Juris Secundum* 834.

[20]New York State Education Department, *Handbook* 13, Art. 131, par. 6501.

[21]U.S. v. 22 Devices, More or Less, Halox Therapeutic Generator, 98 F. Suppl. 914 (D.C., 1951).

[22]H. Jack Geiger, "Hidden Professional Roles: The Physician as Reactionary, Reformer, Revolutionary," *Social Policy*, 1 (March-April 1971), 24–33.

[23]California Business and Professions Code, par. 2726.

[24]Ibid., par. 2725.

By practicing many years alongside medicine so broadly and flexibly defined, nursing has existed largely at the discretion of physicians, and the definition of nursing has proven to be a vexing task.[25] Part of the difficulty in defining nursing comes simply from the size, breadth, and variety of nursing practice. But the broad definition of medicine stands as an obstacle to a similarly broad definition of nursing, since it would inevitably overlap the definition of medicine. As nurses have become more conscious of their own roles, they have been redefining nursing more broadly without such care to avoid areas of medical practice. Yet caution is sounded in such phrases as "nursing diagnosis" and "observing signs and symptoms."

Missing from these efforts is an effort by *nurses* to define *medicine*. Nonphysicians do much of what the definition of medicine says physicians do. Moreover, there are broad areas of health maintenance mostly untouched by medicine, to say nothing of the disease conditions which are engendered by social factors. By observing what physicians actually do, as distinguished from what other health practitioners do, nurses can support definition of their own profession. Not only is this step needed for clarity, but it also meets a principle of fairness. Physicians have been assiduous in defining the role of nurses for years;[26] it would now be suitable for nurses to make public their reflections upon medicine. Until this work has been done, the work of nurses is likely not to be credited to them, and they may continue to be dimly discernible to outsiders, just as contributions of women to the household have often been in the background of the outsider's gaze.

The invisibility of nurses is maintained in part by cooperative interactions between nurses and physicians. One of the classical varieties of such interactions has been analyzed as the *doctor-nurse game*. It is a gender-role game translated into occupational terms. In it, the nurse makes covert suggestions for patient care to the physician. The physician cooperates by giving the order the nurse suggests without seeming to accept her suggestion. Leonard I. Stein, who named the game, renders the following example:

CASE EXAMPLE. The medical resident on hospital call is awakened by telephone at 1:00 A.M., because a patient on a ward, not his own, has not been able to fall asleep. Dr. Jones answers the telephone:

"This is Dr. Jones."

"Dr. Jones, this is Miss Smith on 2W—Mrs. Brown, who learned today of her father's death, is unable to fall asleep."

"What sleeping medication has been helpful to Mrs. Brown in the past?"

"Pentobarbital mg 100 was quite effective night before last."

Dr. Jones replies with a note of authority in his voice: "Pentobarbital mg 100 before bedtime as needed for sleep: got it?"

---

[25]For a brief survey, see the many different models of nursing practice outlined by Catherine P. Murphy, "Making Clinical Judgments: From a Nurse's Point of View," in *Making Clinical Judgments*, ed. Glen W. Davidson (Carbondale, Ill.: Southern Illinois University Press, 1982).

[26]A good example is the American Medical Association Committee on Nursing, "Medicine and Nursing in the 1970s: A Position Statement," *Journal of the American Medical Association*, 213 (1970), 1881–83.

Miss Smith ends the conversation with the tone of a grateful supplicant: "Yes, I have, and thank you very much doctor."[27]

In this dialogue, Dr. Jones asks for and accepts Miss Smith's recommendation. At the same time, the two maintain the verbal forms of the doctor giving orders.

This act of finesse represents a skillful solution to a moral dilemma. The nurse traditionally has both the duty of patient care and the duty of following the physician's orders. How is he or she to meet both duties where physicians are likely to need advice? By these conversational gambits, the nurse can gain influence over the treatment plan by paying the price of deference. When such gambits fail, nurses commonly have the feeling of being "in the middle" since they must either give care they judge inferior or disagree openly with the physician.

Is the nurse who plays the doctor-nurse game any less autonomous than the nurse who makes direct suggestions? It could be argued that the nurse who plays the game is more autonomous than the nurse who does not. The nurse who makes open suggestions runs the risk of a rebuke or loss of influence over some physicians. (Nurses make an effort to know which physicians they can be open with and which not.) So, the more effective control may come from the nurse whose power remains invisible. Invisibility is thus not necessarily identical with powerlessness.[28] It may then seem that the main moral difficulty with the doctor-nurse game is that it uses pretense to solve a moral dilemma. However, a mutual acceptance of pretense in a world imperfect as this one is a peccadillo. In their interaction, Miss Smith and Dr. Jones both recognize in their behavior the importance of Miss Smith's judgment and the need for her recommendation. Why then do they not admit it openly? Because they both believe that it is important to maintain Miss Smith's subordinate position. By using pretense to maintain an appearance of subordination, they give stronger expression to their belief in the system of subordination than they would had Miss Smith's deference been genuine. The game also damages the argument for nursing autonomy. For many years nursing advice about patient care has not been on the record. Thus, the evidence for the consequences of increased nursing discretion has been hidden. The advantage of invisibility is illusory and ephemeral.

A powerful argument for physician dominance is the belief that it is required by the nature of hospital work. Nurses sometimes agree that physicians should be a central source of authority. In discussion, a physician may convincingly claim,

> I am like a captain of a ship or a pilot of an airplane. Someone must have the ultimate authority for decisions here.

There is something right and something wrong about this claim. It is correct that present legal and organizational structure of health care places "ultimate authority" upon physicians for a variety of decisions. A physician facing a malpractice suit would likely not fare well who defended himself or herself by saying, "I know what

---

[27]Leonard I. Stein, "The Doctor-Nurse Game," *Archives of General Psychiatry*, 16 (1967), 699–703. Copyright 1967, American Medical Association.

[28]In Plato's *Republic* Glaucon asks Socrates whether one who had the power of invisibility would both reap the benefits of injustice (such as committing thefts while invisible) and have the appearance of justice (praise, honor). *Selective* invisibility, like selective poverty, is quite different from the enforced invisibility of nurses.

I did was contrary to standard medical practice, but I thought it better to follow the nurse's judgment in this case.'' The physician is expected to make decisions. But this does not mean that we *must* organize our decision-making processes in this way. For example, a small group operating by consensus could equally well take responsibility for decisions. In cases of bad judgments, the law could hold the whole group accountable.

Physicians sometimes argue that since they are *authorities on medicine,* they have a responsibility and a right to direct other health care workers. Again, they are both right and wrong. Physicians are correct when they say that they have special expertise. They are unquestionably authorities on medical diagnosis and therapy. But this kind of authority is simply the authority of expertise; it does not give them the right to order people around. The world is full of experts—engineers, philosophers, seamstresses, roofers, and so on—who do not claim that they therefore have a right or obligation to tell others what to do. Since physicians are the foremost experts on medical diagnosis and therapy, we must take what they have to say on their authority. But this is not the same thing as taking orders.[29] As clients, we can make up our own minds how to use medical information. The physician's expertise is perfectly consistent, theoretically, with the dominance of the nurse over the physician. We only need to see the nurse as deciding upon a treatment plan and coordinating the work of the hospital after taking into account the physician's diagnosis and recommendations for therapy.

Sometimes it is argued that for reasons of efficiency there must be a single decision maker. Where time is critical and many persons must act in close coordination, someone may be needed to orchestrate a performance, as during cardiopulmonary resuscitation or surgery. But these time-pressured activities do not generalize well. Moreover, even though a surgeon has important authority during surgery, this is consistent with the authority of a nurse over proper sterile procedure and with the authority of the patient over whether the operation should be done in the first place.

The traditional nurse-physician relationship is a hindrance to nursing autonomy. But nurses who focus most of their anger, bitterness, and frustration with hospital care on physicians reinforce medical dominance by keeping physicians in the center of the picture. Resentment can also direct attention away from the process of self-examination and analysis of the system that places physicians in power. Moreover, many physicians are aware of these problems and support nursing autonomy. There are many strains among physicians over what medicine should be, and nursing has some influence over the future directions physicians take. Nurses can also work with other health care personnel who have similar autonomy conflicts with physicians.

Opposition from Nurses

The history of deference was made possible partly by the substantial support of nurses. In the past, nurses have not usually sought professional autonomy. Thus, the nurse-physician division of decision making is the combined invention of nurses, physicians, and their milieu. For example, supervisory and administrative

[29]I owe this argument to John Ladd, ''Some Reflections on Authority and the Nurse,'' in Spicker and Gadow, eds., *Nursing: Images and Ideals,* pp. 160–75.

nurses have an interest in maintaining the bureaucratic model of nursing decision making. Although these nurses have power to make decisions themselves, some of them mistrust the increasing autonomy of staff nurses whom they supervise. Staff nurses may also feel ambivalent about autonomy. They are not often anxious to undertake additional responsibilities when physicians and administrators are making decisions of which staff nurses approve. Second-class standing can be seen as safe and undemanding. Nursing ambivalence about autonomy is amply reinforced by patients who look to physicians for decisions.

In recent years, nurses have increasingly worked through *registries*. Registries supply staff to hospitals flexibly through a pool of nurses employed by the registry. Registry nurses usually have more control over their work schedules than those on hospital staff. But this increased *flexibility* should not be confused with increased professional *autonomy*. Because of their peripheral connection with hospitals where they work, registry nurses have less power than staff nurses to control their working conditions and take responsibility for policy formation and patient care. This is one realm in which gains in *personal* autonomy can't be identified with gains in *professional* autonomy. Nurses may express their personal values in their lives through flexibility in managing time, while being less able to express nursing values they identify with in their work.

Nurses are not the only group facing these internal conflicts. Successful corporation engineers, for example, normally become managers in the course of their careers. Yet they continue to belong to professional engineering organizations. As a result, engineering professional associations may represent the bureaucratic viewpoint of corporate engineers. Working people in staff positions of all kinds feel conflict about taking responsibility for difficult decisions and are not sure whether professional autonomy is an attractive concept.[30]

Sexism

Sexism refers to a variety of pervasive practices and beliefs that place women in a secondary standing to men. To see sexism, one can look in the daily paper at the photographs of men in leadership positions in contrast with the illustrations of women predominant in the advertising sections. The obstacles to autonomy described in the last three sections—the birth of the hospital modeled on the Victorian family, the barriers to women in medicine, the exploitation of nurses by hospitals, the identification of nursing as a woman's profession, the doctor-nurse game, and so on—are linked together as elements of sexism. It is hard to identify specific acts which have irrefutable causal antecedents in something as global as sexism; but the division of labor between nurses and physicians as a whole is an important modern expression of sexism.[31] Once the rationality of the present division of labor is questioned, it is transparent that strong and traditional gender expectations have had

[30]We must also make room for the psychological power of obedience. See Stanley Milgram, *Obedience to Authority: An Experimental View* (New York: Harper & Row, Publishers, Inc., 1974).

[31]Virginia S. Cleland, "Sex Discrimination: Nursing's Most Pervasive Problem," *American Journal of Nursing,* 81 (1981), 1542–47; Wilma Scott Heide, "Nursing and Women's Liberation: A Parallel," *American Journal of Nursing,* 73 (1973), 824–27; Martha J. Welch, "Dysfunctional Parenting of a Profession," *Nursing Outlook* (1980), 724–27; and Ashley, *Hospitals,* Chap. 5, "Sexism in the Hospital Family," pp. 75–93.

a profound effect on how the complex tasks of patient care are divided up. Why, for example, is medical diagnosis not simply a branch of nursing practice? Why is there no orderly advancement through experience and education from nursing aide to expert clinician, diagnostician, administrator, pharmacist, or the like?

It is an irony of health care practice that while most health care workers are women, women patients suffer many forms of discrimination. Recognizing sexism in patient care has been an impetus for nurses to examine their own status. Some nurses have sought nurse practitioner degrees in order to express their views on appropriate health care and autonomy in work for women simultaneously. Progress in the autonomy of nurses and of women patients is occurring and should occur together. Each leg of the patient-nurse-physician triangle needs mutual adjustment. Thus, it is important to address briefly how sexism influences the care of patients.

Feminist criticisms of medical care for women have generally fallen into four areas. First, the doctor-patient interaction has been criticized for problems that affect all patients, but particularly women: coldly impersonal or sometimes even crude or degrading behavior, paternalism, authoritarianism, condescension, and the like.[32] A vivid image of such treatment is the gynecologist who discusses his half-draped and uneasy patient with a third person and who never directly addresses the patient. This fault of style becomes a fault of substance when physicians fail to discuss invasive procedures with clients. Complaints are common from women who have had mastectomies, hysterectomies, laparotomies, and other serious procedures without having them adequately explained. Abuses vary and are sometimes subtle, but this story documents a clear case of disrespect for both patient and nursing autonomy:

> CASE EXAMPLE. I observed a Mrs. X was admitted to the obstetric ward with a diagnosis of threatened abortion. She was bleeding, but had not yet miscarried. She was hysterical, and cried, "Save my baby! Save my baby!" The doctor instructed the nurse to prepare the woman for examination, but to tell her nothing about her condition because she was too upset. During the examination, the doctor calmed Mrs. X by telling her that if she stopped being so upset, perhaps she wouldn't lose the baby. Meanwhile he performed an abortion and left . . . the obstetric department justified its policy of not telling a patient she was undergoing abortion "because they get too upset."[33]

Second, medical ideology reflects various cultural prejudices toward women. Psychiatric conceptions of mental health closely parallel conceptions of mental health for *males,* so that females are more often judged deviant.[34] The position that the

---

[32]Karen J. Armitage, Lawrence J. Schneiderman, and Robert A. Bass, "Response of Physicians to Medical Complaints in Men and Women," *Journal of the American Medical Association,* 241 (1979), 2186–87; Gena Corea, *The Hidden Malpractice* (New York: Jove Publications, 1977); and Ellen Frankfurt, *Vaginal Politics* (New York: Bantam Books, Inc., 1972).

[33]Pamela Levin and Eric Berne, "Games Nurses Play," *American Journal of Nursing,* 72 (1972), 486. More telling and subtle examples too lengthy to include here can be found in Nancy Stoller Shaw, *Forced Labor: Maternity Care in the United States* (New York: Pergamon Press, Inc., 1974), pp. 79–80, 91–92.

[34]See Naomi Weisstein, *Psychology Constructs the Female* (Boston: New England Free Press, 1970); and I.K. Broverman et al., "Sex-Role Stereotypes in Clinical Judgment of Mental Health," *Journal of Consulting and Clinical Psychology,* 3 (1970), 1–7.

physician, not the midwife, is the appropriate person to attend at childbirth is sometimes defended by the belief that pregnancy is a disease state. Women are hospitalized, treated, medicated, and incarcerated in mental hospitals significantly more than men.[35]

Third, pain and suffering on the part of women are often inappropriately attributed to psychological and emotional difficulties rather than to "real" physiological causes, particularly with regard to pain in menstruation and childbirth.[36]

Fourth, women are encouraged, pressed, and permitted to accept excessive treatment.[37] For instance, although indications for surgery can be controversial, some argue that many hysterectomies performed in the United States are unnecessary.[38] One indication is that the per capita rate of hysterectomies in England and Wales is less than half the rate in the United States.[39] Another is that hysterectomies are performed for birth control when simpler and less risky procedures such as tubal ligation would suffice.[40] Cost-benefit analyses of hysterectomies as a prophylactic for cancer indicate only marginal benefits.[41] To consider another instance, the rate of cesarean deliveries in the United States tripled in the 1970s, and indications for this procedure are also disputed.[42] Since cesarean sections impose health risks on mothers on behalf of infants,[43] there are indications that the welfare of infants is being given higher priority than the welfare of their mothers without an adequate analysis of the justice issues involved. Cesarean section is a surgical procedure, interferes with mothering, and costs about three times as much as a vaginal delivery.[44] Although it is difficult to pinpoint the causes of the rise in cesareans, some of it may be attributable to increasing use of fetal monitors, which are still not well understood as indicators of fetal distress.[45] Similarly, early developmental research on the birth control pill overlooked indications of health risks to women because researchers believed population control to be the first priority.[46] Other procedures

[35]Phyllis Chesler, *Women and Madness* (New York: Avon Books, 1972), pp. 33, 42–43.

[36]K. Jean Lennane and R. John Lennane, "Alleged Psychogenic Disorders in Women—A Possible Manifestation of Sexual Prejudice," *The New England Journal of Medicine*, 188 (1973), 288–92.

[37]Barbara Ehrenreich and Deidre English, *For Her Own Good: 150 Years of the Experts' Advise to Women* (Garden City, N.Y.: Doubleday & Co., Inc., Anchor Press, 1978).

[38]Carol C. Korenbrot et al., "Elective Hysterectomy: Costs, Risks, and Benefits," in *The Implications of Cost-Effectiveness Analysis of Medical Technology* (Washington, D.C.: Office of Technology Assessment, 1981), p. 3.

[39]John P. Bunker, "Surgical Manpower: A Comparison of Operations and Surgeons in the United States and in England and Wales," *The New England Journal of Medicine*, 282 (1970), 137.

[40]Harold Schulman, "Major Surgery for Abortion and Sterilization," *Obstetrics and Gynecology*, 40 (1972), 738–39.

[41]Korenbrot, "Elective Hysterectomy," p. 24.

[42]Gina Bari Kolata, "NIH Panel Urges Fewer Caesarian Births," *Science*, 210 (1980), 176–77.

[43]Ronald L. Williams and Peter M. Chen, "Identifying the Sources of the Recent Decline in Perinatal Mortality Rates in California," *The New England Journal of Medicine*, 306 (1982), 207–14.

[44]Helen I. Marieskind, "An Evaluation of Caesarean Section in the United States." Final Report submitted to DHEW, Office of the Assistant Secretary for Planning and Evaluation/Health, June 1979, pp. 1–2.

[45]Kolata, "NIH Panel," p. 177.

[46]Carol C. Korenbrot, "Facts and Values in the Testing of Toxic Substances: Experiences with Systemic

that have been questioned include performance of radical mastectomy, prescription of diethylstilbestrol, and use of tranquilizers.[47]

Obstacles to nursing autonomy can be seen as part of a pattern of obstacles to women's autonomy in health care generally. At the same time, the growing understanding of patients' rights gives nurses a more important role in the health care team. As a major source of communication with patients in the hospital, nurses are in a good position to gain power and autonomy through the increasing power and autonomy of patients. And nurses sensitive to the plight of women patients are an increasingly important catalyst for improvements in health care.

The Concept of Autonomy

The deepest obstacle to autonomy is the concept of autonomy itself. It is hard to know what it means. Like the word *taboo,* it is used more often than it is understood. We are told to respect autonomy even though we can't identify it. We often use the concept to contrast with miscellaneous undesirable states, such as dependency, coercion, paternalism, thoughtlessness, and habit. In Chapter 2, I characterized *autonomy* as meaning *self-governed.* More fully stated, *autonomy* can be defined thus:

> My action is autonomous when I choose and carry out my action because of goals or values I perceive as my own.[48]

Although we can speak of the autonomy of groups such as professions, the concept of autonomy is for the most part an expression of *individualism*—of personal liberty and the value of individual persons.

The concept of autonomy was developed partly by Immanuel Kant. Kant saw us as being most ethical when acting purely out of an inward obedience to basic moral principles free of the influences of coercion, desire, impulse, or concern for future consequences. He thus characterized autonomy in terms of an *inner* principle of action. For him, autonomy was a characteristic of the will—our faculty for making choices. A more *outward* conception of autonomy has been developed by John Stuart Mill. In his attack on paternalism, Mill emphasized the value of actions based on personal goals and values in contrast to choices imposed by others. Mill thus emphasized the social conditions of autonomy.

Problems of autonomy arise most often when people with the inner resources for autonomy engage in cooperative actions. If we are all autonomous and respect

Contraceptives,'' *Toxic Substances: Decisions and Values: Conference II, Information Flow* (Washington, D.C.: Technical Information Project, National Science Foundation, 1979).

[47]For brief outlines of treatment of women patients see the article by Mary Rollston Stern and Norma Mera Swenson based on work by Barbara Bridgman Perkins, Lucy Candib, and Nancy Todd, in *Our Bodies, Ourselves: A Book by and for Women,* ed. Boston Women's Health Book Collective (New York: Simon & Schuster, Inc., 1976); Virginia Olesen, ed., *Women and Their Health: Research Implications for a New Era* (Springfield, Va.: National Center for Health Services Research, 1976); and Corea, *The Hidden Malpractice.*

[48]For a similar definition, see Tom L. Beauchamp and James F. Childress, *Principles of Biomedical Ethics* (New York: Oxford University Press, 1979), p. 56.

the autonomy of others, how are we to act when our goals conflict?[49] Voting and consensual group decision-making processes are common modes of resolving conflicts between autonomy and cooperation. In the United States, these modes have not been predominant in work settings. Instead, the traditional solution to the need for cooperation has been respect for authority. When we disagree or don't know what to do, we usually follow the choices made by the person or group in authority.[50] At least three related concepts of authority can be distinguished:

1. *Persuasion:* When the views and reasons of another person are weighty and convincing, these views have authority with me.
2. *Expertise:* Even though I may be unaware of the reasons for another's decision, I may still have confidence in that person's judgment and ability.
3. *Force:* Actions chosen by another may be made reasonable for me by the imposition of sanctions for noncooperation.

Any or all of these forms of authority may be combined in the same person. Even though someone else acts as an authority for me, I may still act as an authority for another. I may be a member of a group with authority over my actions. We may act as authorities for each other. You may be an authority for me on nursing, while I am an authority for you on philosophy. The central question here is: When is authority compatible with autonomy?

In relationship to the authority of *persuasion,* autonomy and authority are compatible. When I am acting on what I regard to be good reasons, even though their source is elsewhere, I am still making choices and performing actions on the basis of goals and values of my own (see the definition of *autonomy* above). For example, if I make choices on the basis of valuing work, I will not be the first person in history to do so. I learned to value work partly through the persuasion of others. The goal or value of work can be mine even though it is also a goal or value of others.

The authority of *force* is incompatible with autonomy. When I perceive someone else as making me do something, this is because I see that person as getting me to do something in conflict with my goals or desires. In the classic paradigm of force—when someone threatens to hurt me badly unless I hand over my purse—we *could* say that I am acting autonomously because I am choosing to give up my purse in order to avoid being hurt. In some sense, I am acting on my own goal of avoiding personal harm. But it is better to describe me as acting on a goal or value *not* my own, since it is *not* my goal to enrich the thief. In this important respect, my act is not autonomous.

The difference between the authority of persuasion and force is not as clear-cut as we might wish. When we adopt goals out of persuasion, we may make them our own because of the overwhelming force of prevailing values or because of irrational motives unknown to ourselves. Acquiring values during maturation is not simply a process of reasoning, and it includes powerful unconscious motifs. Persua-

---

[49]*Goals may be incompatible either by being the same* or by being *different.* We may get incompatibility when the patient seeks comfort and the nurse seeks health for the patient. Or we may get incompatibility when two patients both need a nurse at the same time, and only one is available.

[50]Authority is normally limited in scope. One way to view it is that physicians have authority because they have been given limited *permission* by others to make certain decisions. Exercise of authority beyond a limited scope is sometimes termed *generalization of expertise.*

sion can become less an act of reason and more an act of force. And what counts as force is individual; some people are more easily coerced than others. Fear of open confrontation, for example, may do more to maintain hospital procedures than fear of economic sanctions.

The relationship between autonomy and the authority of *expertise* is less clear. On one hand, an autonomous person will want to rely on the authority of experts when it is wise to do so. On the other, if one treats everyone else as an expert and never oneself, or if one treats a certain class of people as experts automatically and irrationally, then one ceases to be autonomous. If the appearance of expertise is only an illusion created by social dominance, then expertise is reducible to force, not persuasion. The consistency of expert authority with autonomy will thus rest on the presence of an equal and mutual respect among people. Where nurses, patients, and physicians have appropriate trust for the expertise of one another, autonomy is possible. Where the expertise of only one authority is heard, autonomy is reduced.

As nursing increases in autonomy, it is most important that it distinguish *egalitarian* forms of autonomy from *dominant* ones. *Egalitarian* autonomy is consistent with the autonomy of everyone. It emphasizes reason, mutual confidence, identification with others, and avoids coercion of others to obtain one's own goals. *Dominant* autonomy is consistent with subservience of others. This occurs when the dominant person can act on his or her own goals because he or she persuades and forces others to cooperate. It permits one group to develop its goals and values at the expense of groups subservient to it and allows one person to claim autonomy while continuing to impose coercion on others.

Nursing is in a bind with regard to these two forms of autonomy. Nurses tend to look "upward" in the hospital hierarchy for increased autonomy. But at the same time, many early nursing functions such as housekeeping, budget, supplies, and even some bedside care have been taken over to a large degree by other workers and professionals. These are represented by departments like Housekeeping, Laundry, Utilization Review, Dietary, Physical Therapy, Social Service, and others. The head nurse may have considerable responsibility for coordinating the work of these departments on the ward, and within nursing there are various levels of authority. Nurses thus form a highly stratified "middle class" of professionals between the physician and administrative "upper class" and the "working class" of house-keepers, orderlies, and aides. Nurses have the problems of many conscientious workers in hierarchies. Although they suffer from domination by one group of people, they play a part in dominating other groups. This is a very general problem in our work relations. It is not solved simply by placing nurses at the top of the hierarchy with physicians. Yet it would be wrong for nurses to be held back by unrealistic ideals of egalitarian autonomy.

Professionalism is one mode of authority that can be reconciled in principle with egalitarian autonomy. It permits individual professionals to act independently within the sanctions and protection of the profession as a whole. By identifying with and acquiring the goals and values of the profession, the individual professional becomes an autonomous participant in the collective actions of the profession. Professionalism is preferable to bureaucracy as a model for autonomy. Bureaucracies rely on the downward flow of power from central, albeit limited, authority, and operate on the presumption of unequal expertise and power. Bureaucracies support dominant forms of autonomy.

Professionalism is not a conception of unlimited personal autonomy. Self-government for the professional is not the simple power to act upon one's own goals whatever they may be. It is the power to exercise one's professional judgment, that is, use a common understanding of sound practice with which one identifies. This requires good communication, consultation, and consensual decision making among nurses. Although autonomy must also make room for individual conscience, the struggle for autonomy in nursing is primarily for the collective autonomy of the profession.

Professionalism's major defect as a conception of autonomy is the absence of a means to establish egalitarian autonomy between providers and patients. It is one thing to teach professionals the importance of patient autonomy; it is another for patients to have an active part in the formation of professional practice. Moreover, conflicts among different professional groups are not resolved by appeal to the concept of professional autonomy.

The struggle for autonomy in our culture has the flavor of the struggle for wealth and income. We envy those who have more, criticize those we think have too much, and seek ways to obtain more autonomy for ourselves, if only because failure to obtain autonomy for ourselves is likely to result in our being subservient to the dominant autonomy of others. The reconciliation of personal autonomy with respect for the autonomy of others continues as a historical problem. An important intellectual task in ethics for nurses is to work out egalitarian models of autonomy that can be applied broadly in our society.

Is autonomy a "Good Thing?" Do we or should we want to be autonomous? Autonomy is often highly prized by reflective people in our culture. Yet it is not immediately obvious what is good about it. Indeed, there are many autonomous evil actions. The value of autonomy is easiest to see by considering what one risks without it. For instance, it may be hard to pursue one's goals and to exercise personal judgment in treating patients; the world may lose the benefit of one's perception and judgment; one may be exposed to coercion for unacceptable aims; or one may have to cooperate in what one regards as morally wrong acts.

Many nurses desire more autonomous forms of practice and are disappointed by the lack of them in hospital settings. Equality of respect among persons entitles nurses and patients to more autonomy, and the accompanying reduction in sexism would improve health care practice.[51] More adequate autonomy for nurses would involve many things, including power to do the nursing job well and to exercise nursing judgment. Maintaining autonomy also requires a special relationship to ethical principles. Moral codes become oppressive if they contain weighty commands of obedience, or if they are created without conscious participation by nurses. Thus the nursing profession needs to continue to have members who make ethics their focus of attention and to develop programs of education which approach professional principles thoughtfully.

Summary

Autonomy is the third criterion of professionalism. Current obstacles to the professional autonomy of nurses have deep historical roots. During the last century,

---

[51]That nurses are entitled to autonomy and that it would likely have good consequences are very different approaches to the concept. See Chapter 10 (pp. 146–49) for a fuller discussion. For an extended defense

textbooks on nursing ethics have emphasized nursing obedience and deference. Several factors tend to support continuing deference.

First, hospitals were founded primarily on the organizational model of the Victorian family; nurses filled the role of mother, and physicians of father. The subordinate position of nursing in this model is expressed in hospitals today by the attending physician system, hospital bureaucracy, and stratification of staff positions. As employees, many nurses have limited autonomy in relationship to their hospital employers.

Second, physicians have exercised a position of professional dominance in health care. This dominance has operated partly through the legal standing of medical practice, the lack of power of nurses to define and limit medical practice, gender role games such as the "doctor-nurse" game, and the assumption that decision making in health care requires central authority.

Third, many nurses are ambivalent about assuming professional autonomy, and nurses who have been able to obtain power under the present system may be no more willing than physicians to share it with other nurses.

Fourth, the prevailing pattern of gender discrimination in the United States makes the arbitrary division of labor between nursing and medicine seem reasonable and natural. Sexism affects the standing of both nurses and women patients. Sexism is displayed in the lack of nursing autonomy, disrespect for women patients, perception of women patients as deviant, misinterpretations of women's pain and suffering, and excessive and inappropriate treatment.

Fifth, the concept of autonomy is itself complex. It requires both inner maturity to make decisions and outer social conditions supporting these decisions. Autonomy must be limited where many people cooperate in work. These limits are usually set by *authority*. Use of authority by persuasion better respects autonomy than does use of authority by force. Expertise—the common basis for claims of professional authority—sometimes expresses persuasion, sometimes force. Some people become autonomous by dominating others, but if autonomy is to be widespread, it must be shared equally.

Nurses face a challenging intellectual, ethical, and political problem in striving for conceptions of autonomy that can be shared widely in health care among patients and a variety of professions and occupations.

FURTHER READINGS

Historical Aspects

ASHLEY, JO ANN, "Nurses in American History: Nursing and Early Feminism," *American Journal of Nursing,* 75 (1975), 1465–67.
AUSTIN, ANNE L., *History of Nursing Source Book.* New York: G.P. Putnam's Sons, 1957.
CROWDER, ELEANOR, "Manners, Morals, and Nurses: An Historical Overview of Nursing Ethics," *Texas Reports on Biology and Medicine,* 32 (1974), 173–80.
MCISAAC, ISABEL, "Ethics in Nursing," *American Journal of Nursing,* 1 (1900), 483–85.

---

of the claim that patient autonomy would improve the quality of health care, see Wendy S. Schain, "Patients' Rights in Decision Making: The Case for Personalism Versus Paternalism in Health Care," *Cancer,* 46 (1980), 1035–41.

MATEJSKI, MYRTLE P., "Humanities: The Nurse and Historical Research," *Image*, 11, 3 (October 1979), 80–85.
SHOWALTER, ELAINE, "Florence Nightingale's Feminist Complaint: Women, Religion, and *Suggestions for Thought*," *Signs: Journal of Women in Culture and Society*, 6 (Spring 1981), 395–412.
SHRYOCK, RICHARD HARRISON, *The History of Nursing: An Interpretation of the Social and Medical Factors Involved*. Philadelphia: W.B. Saunders Company, 1959.
THOMPSON, HELEN STUART, "Ethics in Private Practice," *American Journal of Nursing*, 6 (1905), 163–66.
WALSH, MARY ROTH, *"Doctors Wanted: No Women Need Apply": Sexual Barriers in the Medical Profession, 1835–1975*. New Haven, Conn.: Yale University Press, 1977.

Sexism in Health Care

ADAMS, MARGARET, "The Compassion Trap," in *Woman in Sexist Society: Studies in Power and Powerlessness*, eds. Vivian Gornick and Barbara K. Moran, pp. 555–75. New York: Basic Books, Inc., Publishers, 1971.
ASHLEY, JO ANN, "Power Structured Misogyny: Implications for the Politics of Care," *Advances in Nursing Science*, 2 (1980), 3–22.
CLELAND, VIRGINIA S., "To End Sex Discrimination," *Nursing Clinics of North America*, 9 (September 1974), 563–71.
FAGIN, C.M., "Professional Nursing—The Problems of Women in Microcosm," *Journal of the New York State Nurses' Association*, 2 (1971), 7.
GREENLEAF, NANCY P., "Sex-Segregated Occupations: Relevance for Nursing," *Advances in Nursing Science*, 2 (1980), 23–37.
GRISSUM, MARLENE, AND CAROL SPENGLER, *Woman Power and Health Care*. Boston: Little, Brown & Company, 1976.
KAISER, BARBARA L., AND IRWIN M. KAISER, "The Challenge of the Women's Movement to American Gynecology," *American Journal of Obstetrics and Gynecology*, 120 (1974), 652–55.
KRITEK, PHYLLIS, AND LAURIE GLASS, "Nursing: A Feminist Perspective," *Nursing Outlook*, 26 (1978), 182–86.
LEWIN, ELLEN, "Feminist Ideology and the Meaning of Work: The Case of Nursing," *Catalyst*, nos. 10–11 (Summer 1977), 78–103.
MUFF, JANET, ED., *Socialization, Sexism, and Stereotyping: Women's Issues in Nursing*. St. Louis: The C.V. Mosby Company, 1982.
NAVARRO, VICENTE, "Women in Health Care," *The New England Journal of Medicine*, 292 (1975), 398–402.
PIRADOVA, M.D., "USSR—Women Health Workers," *Women and Health*, 1, 3 (May/June 1976), 24–29.
REVERBY, SUSAN, "Health: Women's Work," in *Prognosis Negative: Crisis in the Health Care System*, ed. David Kotelchuck, pp. 170–83. New York: Random House, Inc., 1976.
RUZEK, SHERYL BURT, "Medical Response to Women's Health Activities: Conflict, Accommodation and Cooptation," *Research in the Sociology of Health Care*, 1 (1980), 335–54.
SCHULMAN, SAM, "Mother Surrogate—After a Decade," in *Patients, Physicians, and Illness* (3rd ed.), ed. E. Gartly Jaco, pp. 272–80. New York: The Free Press, 1979.
WOMEN'S WORK PROJECT OF THE UNION FOR RADICAL POLITICAL ECONOMICS, "USA— Women Health Workers," *Women and Health*, 1, 3 (May/June 1976), 14–23.
WELCH, MARTHA J., "Dysfunctional Parenting of a Profession," *Nursing Outlook* (December 1980), 724–27.
WILSON, V., "An Analysis of Femininity in Nursing," *American Behavioral Scientist*, 15 (1971), 213–20.

BATES, BARBARA, "Doctor and Nurse: Changing Roles and Relations," *The New England Journal of Medicine*, 283 (1970), 129–34.

BULLOUGH, VERN L., "Licensure and the Medical Monopoly," in *The Law and the Expanding Nursing Role* (2nd ed.), ed. Bonnie Bullough, pp. 14–22. New York: Appleton-Century Crofts, 1980.

CROSS, YVONNE, "Rogue Nurses: The Day of 'Sir' Is Over," *Nursing Mirror*, 134, 12 (March 24, 1972), 16–17.

DOCK, SARAH E., "The Relation of the Nurse to the Doctor and the Doctor to the Nurse," *American Journal of Nursing*, 17 (1916), 394–96.

EDMUNDS, MARILYN W., "Junior Doctoring," *Nurse Practitioner* (September/October 1979), 38.

FORSTER, JEFFREY H., "How Much of Your Turf Do the Non-M.D. Doctors Have?" *Medical Economics* (September 27, 1982), 67–76.

HULL, RICHARD T., "Ethics: Models of Nurse/Patient/Physician Relations," *Kansas Nurse*, 55, 9 (October 1980), 19–24.

KALISCH, BEATRICE J., AND PHILIP A. KALISCH, "An Analysis of the Sources of Physician-Nurse Conflict," *Journal of Nursing Administration*, 7, 1 (January 1977), 51–57.

————, "Slaves, Servants, or Saints? (An Analysis of the System of Nurse Training in the United States, 1873–1948)," *Nursing Forum*, 14, 3 (1975), 22–63.

LEE, ANTHONY A., "Still the Handmaiden," *R.N.* (July 1979), 21–30.

LEWIS, HOWARD L., "Who Makes Decisions about New Technology in Hospitals?" *Hospitals* (March 16, 1979), 114–21.

MAUKSCH, INGEBORG G., AND PAUL R. YOUNG, "Nurse-Physician Interaction in a Family Medical Care Center," *Nursing Outlook*, 22, 2 (February 1974), 113–19.

MEYERHOFF, BARBARA G., AND WILLIAM R. LARSON, "The Doctor as Culture Hero: The Routinization of Charisma," *Human Organization*, 24, 3 (Fall 1965), 188–91.

MITCHELL, CHRISTINE, "Medical Ideology and Nursing Utopia." (Unpublished paper, 1981.)

NUCKOLLS, KATHERINE B., "Who Decides What the Nurse Can Do?" *Nursing Outlook*, 22, 10 (October 1974), 626–31.

OSMOND, HUMPHRY, "God and the Doctor," *The New England Journal of Medicine*, 302 (1980), 555–58.

ROBINSON, A.M., "The Nurse/Doctor Game (New Style): Professional Conflict in the ICU/CCU," *R.N.*, 35, 5 (May 1972), 40–45.

SELMANOFF, EUGENE D., "Strains in the Nurse-Doctor Relationship," *Nursing Clinics of North America*, 3, 1 (March 1968), 117–27.

STEEL, JEAN E., "Putting Joint Practice into Practice," *American Journal of Nursing*, 81 (1981), 964–67.

TAYLOR, CAROL, *In Horizontal Orbit*, "That Fascinating Triangle: Physician, Patient, Nurse," pp. 108–20. New York: Holt, Rinehart and Winston General Book, 1970.

Nursing Autonomy

BANDMAN, BERTRAM, AND ELSIE L. BANDMAN, "Do Nurses Have Rights?" *American Journal of Nursing*, 78 (1978), 84–86.

CHRISTMAN, LUTHER, "Accountability and Autonomy Are More Than Rhetoric," *Nursing Education*, 3 (1978), 4.

HELLEGERS, ANDRÉ E., "Accountability in the Health Care System: To Whom Is the Nurse Responsible?" *Connecticut Medicine* (*Supplement*), 43, 10 (October 1979), 5–6.

KALISCH, BEATRICE J., "Of Half Gods and Mortals: Aesculapian Authority," *Nursing Outlook*, 23 (1975), 22–28.

Krause, Elliott A., *Power and Illness: The Political Sociology of Health and Medical Care,* "Struggle against the Hierarchy: The Case of Nursing," pp. 48–56. New York: Elsevier, North-Holland, Inc., 1977.

Kuperberg, J., "Ethics, Accountability, and Decision-Making," *Journal of Long-Term Care Administration,* 6 (Fall 1978), 25–34.

McClure, Margaret L., "The Long Road to Accountability," *Nursing Outlook,* 26, 1 (January 1978), 47–50.

Mundinger, Mary O'Neil, *Autonomy in Nursing.* Germantown, Md.: Aspen Systems Corporation, 1980.

Murphy, Catherine P., "The Moral Situation in Nursing," in *Bioethics and Human Rights: A Reader for Health Professionals,* eds. Elsie L. Bandman and Bertram Bandman, pp. 313–20. Boston: Little, Brown & Company, 1978.

Newton, Lisa H., "To Whom Is the Nurse Accountable? A Philosophical Perspective," *Connecticut Medicine (Supplement),* 43, no. 10 (October 1979), 7–9.

CHAPTER 4

What Philosophers Do

Like other professionals, philosophers claim to have special skills and to engage in socially important activities. They normally work in academic settings, where they enjoy considerable autonomy with regard to their research and teaching. By 1980, however, philosophers were found increasingly in consulting, teaching, and research roles in nonacademic settings. One of these settings is the hospital, where philosophers are drawn by a wish to be of service, the philosophical interest of ethical problems in the hospital, and the declining availability of attractive academic posts. Philosophers who work in hospital settings are frequently asked what, exactly, they *do*. The question deserves a careful answer. This chapter outlines how philosophers approach ethical problems, philosophers' activities in health care settings, and a decision process for resolving ethical problems in clinical settings.

How Philosophers Approach Ethical Issues

Every normal adult human being is capable of moral thought, and philosophers as a group behave neither better nor worse than most people. It may seem paradoxical that ethicists, who are supposedly experts on ethics, are not therefore especially good people. The paradox is easily resolved when we recognize the independence of the *study of ethics* from leading a *morally good life*. Intellectual appreciation of theory has limited influence on how we live. The immoral ethicist takes an honorable place alongside the sickly physician; the nurse who lives on cookies, coffee, and cigarettes; the judge arrested for growing marijuana; and the debt-ridden economist.

Moreover, the objectives of philosophical ethics usually differ from those of our daily moral inquiries. Most of us use ethics to resolve morally problematic situations and to avoid wrongdoing. Philosophers are usually more interested in discovering, analyzing, challenging, and systematizing the principles, concepts, and reasoning *underlying* our daily choices and conduct. When we study the ethics of philosophers, we study their ideas, not the way they live. In contrast, when we learn the ethics of a profession, we imitate the practice of model clinicians.

What, then, is the philosopher's special relationship to ethical questions? Reflection on ethics requires stepping aside from our commitments and thinking broadly and imaginatively about the basic principles of our cultures. Philosophers have abilities and interests especially suited to such inquiry. They are accustomed to using broad general principles, open to translating questions into radically new terms, willing to treat abstractions formally and systematically, conscious about methodology, and demanding of good reasons for conclusions.

The philosophical study of ethics is not a science. It differs from the work on ethics by sociologists, anthropologists, and psychologists in two important ways. First, there is no consensus among philosophers on methods of experiment or proof in ethics. There is no standard journal format analogous to the "introduction, methods, results, discussion" format of scientific articles. There is only the broadest commitment to speculation in a precise and disciplined manner. Although philosophers therefore do not accumulate a volume of immediate results in ethics, they are more open than scientific fields to radically new discoveries. Important developments in the history of ideas are often identified with the work of philosophers—Socrates, Plato, Aristotle, Confucius, Aquinas, Descartes, Kant, Marx, and others. Second, philosophical inquiry in ethics is basically *normative*. Normative inquiries are directed toward making moral judgments and evaluations, creating policies, and making recommendations. Normative inquiry focuses on what we *should* do. Sociological, psychological, and anthropological work on ethics is more *descriptive*. These fields are more concerned with the moral judgments we *actually* make, and they place moral thinking in the context of sociological, psychological, and anthropological theory.

Philosophical and scientific study of ethics are closely interrelated. Scientists studying moral thinking need to understand important philosophical distinctions and questions about how we *should* think. To consider what we should think in ethics, philosophers need to appreciate our actual daily experience of moral problems and beliefs as well as scientific theories of ethics. Since normative and descriptive inquiries are interdependent, none of these fields can progress without development in both normative and descriptive approaches to ethics.

In the history of philosophy, work on ethics has covered a wide variety of topics, such as happiness, basic values, ideal or virtuous human character, principles governing just societies, our relationship to God, analyses of basic concepts in ethics, and reasoning in ethics.[1] This text takes the philosophical study of ethics to be a broad one that can be roughly divided into three levels of inquiry:

EXPLORING CENTRAL AND BASIC VALUES AND PRINCIPLES THAT WE HOLD, OR FEEL SOME CLAIM ON US TO HOLD, AT THE BEGINNING OF THE INQUIRY. Usually these values and principles will not be merely personal, but will be widely held and referred to often in daily life. They can thus be called *conventional* values and principles. They carry authority through their usefulness to many people in making daily decisions over a long period of time. They refer specifically and concretely to familiar events so that we can feel sure how to use them. They include principles

[1]Maria Ossowska, *Social Determinants of Moral Ideas* (Philadelphia: University of Pennsylvania Press, 1970).

characteristic of professional commitments, such as "The good of patients should be the nurse's primary concern." This and other conventional principles are discussed in detail in Chapters 5 through 9. The most central and most deeply cherished conventional principles of culture are of the most interest to the study of ethics. Their strength comes primarily from the commitment of a culture to them and the ability of its members to interpret them wisely. But since they are often specifically limited in their application and have grown up as historical products of a culture, conventional principles do not meet tests of generality and reason as well as the more reflective principles and concepts of the next two levels.

EXPLORING VALUES AND PRINCIPLES IN A DEEPER AND BROADER WAY.   This involves pressing for greater generality in conventional principles, finding underlying principles and values that embrace more specific ones, testing these for mutual consistency, and connecting them with values and principles expressed throughout history and in various cultures. For instance, this level would include relating "The good of patients should be the nurse's primary concern" to broader principles such as "We should have respect for persons." This level also includes development of concepts like *respect for persons* and others of equal generality like *justice, rights,* and *responsibility.* It includes efforts to tie together such concepts under very general and unified theories of ethics, such as *utilitarianism.* Chapter 10 treats these concepts and others at this level of study.

EXPLORING THE MOST BASIC AND GENERAL DEFINITIONS AND METHODS USED IN THE PREVIOUS TWO LEVELS.   Ethics is a self-reflective discipline. Not only does philosophy study the subject matter of ethics—rules, values, principles, and our modes of reasoning about them—it also studies the study of these things. This is the most general and conceptual realm of philosophical ethics, and it is sometimes called *metaethics.* It includes defining and distinguishing such fundamental terms of ethics as *right* and *good.* It studies the relationship of descriptive theories of ethics to normative theories of ethics. It discusses the nature of reasoning in ethics and attempts to tie it in with philosophical theories about reasoning generally. It connects ethics with general philosophical theories about our relationship to the world in general. Chapter 11 constitutes a largely metaethical discussion of reasoning in ethics. This three-part characterization of the study of *ethics* is itself an instance of metaethics.

These last two levels can be thought of as constituting *reflective* ethics, as distinguished from the *conventional* ethics of the first level.[2] Philosophical reflection on ethics is directed more toward an interest in generality and reason than the conventional level, which meets more strongly the conditions of applicability, consent, and tradition. Just as the study of descriptive and normative theories of ethics are interdependent, the study of conventional ethics and the study of reflective ethics are also interdependent. Consideration of both is needed to understand what constitutes an ethical problem and its solution. Views in ethics and definitions of *ethics* develop partly through changes in conventional ethics and partly through reflective examination and criticism of conventional ethics by philosophers.

Some general features of how philosophers approach ethics are worth describ-

---

[2]For a brief account of differences between convention and reflection, see John Dewey, *Theory of the Moral Life* (New York: Holt, Rinehart and Winston General Book, 1908, 1960), pp. 3–8. For a serious attempt to treat reflective and conventional principles in health care as a single set of principles of the same kind, see Tom L. Beauchamp and James E. Childress, *Principles of Biomedical Ethics* (New York: Oxford University Press, 1979). They discuss beneficence, nonmaleficence, autonomy, and justice.

ing in some detail. Philosophers tend to be especially sensitive to self-examination, methodology, levels of inquiry, unity and generality, and the power of obligation.

Self-Examination

Sometimes students think of ethical inquiry as simply an exercise to clarify what they believe and to distinguish it from what others believe. Once they have found what they believe, they reach a stopping point.[3] They see what they believe as an unchangeable result of their socialization and unique experience of the world. But for philosophers, the inquiry does not stop here. Philosophers presume that what we believe at one time is open to change, that it is possible to learn, grow, and mature in our beliefs. They see this process as influenced not just by what we *do* believe, but also by what we *ought* to believe. It is thus not enough simply to discover what I believe; I must also ask, Should I believe this? Is this a reasonable belief? Is it consistent with other beliefs that I hold? How seriously should I take the objections of those who disagree? Is this what I want to believe? Do people I respect believe this?

Philosophy tests one's personal beliefs. Since one's beliefs about ethics are often very personal and closely associated with one's identity, the experience of examining one's own beliefs can be threatening, anxiety provoking, and painful. But philosophers presuppose that discarded beliefs are replaced by new ones and that a personal identity tested by self-examination naturally reconstructs itself into one stronger and more mature. Ethical inquiry thus includes a personal examination of one's world view.

Methods in Philosophy

When one begins to challenge deeply held personal beliefs, it may seem at first that there are no rules at all and anything can be said. This is not so. It is seldom useful to throw everything into doubt or to make assertions without any basis. Part of the challenge of philosophy lies in artful choice of what to doubt and what to leave untested, what to clarify and what to leave obscure. Since they are not committed to a single method of exploration, philosophers are strongly pressed to keep their inquiry as orderly as possible. In this questioning process, philosophers examine the reasons for conclusions very carefully. It is often not so important to assess the truth of a claim as it is to assess the soundness of reasons explicitly given for it. Philosophers thus attempt two tasks at once: finding answers to questions and examining methods of finding and establishing these answers. Philosophers may even examine manifestly false or unreasonable views in order to clarify the limits of certain methods.

Because of its openness to widely different modes of thought and its self-consciousness about methodology, philosophy is the appropriate mode for responding to issues where no standard method for resolving them is at hand. By being sensitive to methodological alternatives and by avoiding commitment to highly fixed and conventional problem-solving modes, such as the randomized, controlled

---

[3]*Values clarification* exercises appear to be directed primarily to discovering one's own values and observing that some of them differ from others' values.

clinical trial, philosophers play a creative and generative role in the historical development of ideas. Some are committed to the view that reasonable and orderly inquiry into ethics will eventually produce a clear and scientific field of study. How such a field would look is open to debate. In contrast, some philosophers regard the mysteries of how to live as too deep for reason to cope with, and see faith, arbitrary choice, or paradox as more honest approaches. Philosophers thus find themselves in the paradoxical position of discussing reasonably the limits of reason in ethics.

Levels of Inquiry

Philosophers recognize that a general inquiry can be conducted at varying levels of analysis. Care with these levels can reduce the complexity of ethical questions. For example, one could look at judgments in particular cases, such as

In grade school, a girl copied from my paper. Should I have told the teacher?
A child drowned. The lifeguard's defective technique was probably a contributing factor. Should I have told the lifeguard?
Should my mother institutionalize my six-year-old Down's syndrome sister?
My cat is dying of cancer. Should I have it killed?

Or one could see each of these cases as instances of *types* of cases. One could see them as instances of questions of cheating, duty to disclose, care of the mentally retarded, and the treatment of animals. One could then talk in a more general way about these types of cases.

Thinking more generally, one could look at various norms and values of one's culture or seek to identify more general values and norms affecting all people. One might look at concepts like competition, justice, freedom, mercy, and the like. More generally, one could be concerned with highly theoretical and conceptual issues in ethics, such as

What distinguishes ethical values and norms from aesthetic values and norms?
What are the differences between sound and unsound processes of moral reasoning?
Are there any universal moral demands on individuals?
How can we distinguish between true and false moral judgments?
Can a unified theory of ethics be formulated?

These are not the only distinctions of level in inquiry that can be made. One might also distinguish between *clarifying* a norm one accepts and *analyzing* it. For example, it is generally held that stealing the property of others is morally wrong. At one level, one can *clarify* this principle by trying to understand its appropriate applications clearly and to distinguish between cases where the obligation is strong (snatching guide dogs from the blind and statues of St. Francis from the city art museum) from cases where it is weak (taking bread from the rich to feed the poor, taking aspirin from the hospital stock to treat one's headache). At a deeper level, one can analyze the concept of private property by contrasting different forms of control over property, examining the effects of property on the just distribution of goods, clarifying the meaning to our lives of exchanges and contracts, and so on.

Unity and Generality

Philosophers strive for unity and generality in their accounts of ethics, if only because generality is a methodological presupposition of reasoning. They admit that each case encountered is unique, and yet insist that among cases there are important similarities. It is thus necessary to use generalizations, typical cases, and analogies. For instance, if a patient persistently refuses lifesaving treatment, it is relevant to consider what the patient's reasons are and whether or not the patient is mentally competent. Competence should be considered even though a unique constellation of factors is present in every case and myriad states of consciousness are possible. In a particular case it may be justifiable to override a competent refusal or to accept an incompetent one, but it would be irresponsible simply to disregard the factor of competence. Even in complex "gray" areas of ethical decision making, professional responsibility and personal integrity require an effort to follow general principles unifying a series of decisions; otherwise, one is open to charges of arbitrariness and irrationality. Similarly, moral principles involved in health care are connected with considerations applicable to other settings. Exploitation in health care should be treated with attention to our views on exploitation in other realms of life. Telling a lie to a patient should be treated in the context of our understanding of lying generally—in business and personal relations.

Unity and generality can also be seen in philosophers' efforts to relate their conceptions in ethics to their theories about logic, language, reasoning, and the nature of the world and human beings. Philosophical approaches to ethics are often tied to general perspectives on the world as a whole. This *synthetic* motive can be seen most strongly in attempts by philosophers to create unified theories of ethics.

The Power of Obligation

Philosophers tend to view thinking as more than an individual process. Where I disagree with others, their reasonable views have to be considered, and others must consider my reasonable views. Philosophy, no less than science, is a collective inquiry. One person may seem to be first and alone with a good idea, but a good idea is rarely completely unprecedented. If an idea is sound, some support can be found for it in the reasonable principles to which others assent if not in the direct assent of others.

Likewise, philosophers assume that ethical conduct, although to some degree personal, is not *merely* personal. Philosophers presume that moral claims can place obligations on other people. What I think is right for me is not necessarily right. It is not necessarily even right for me. We could show that Dr. Norse should not practice surgery because she is all thumbs, even though she disagrees. I can validly claim a right not to be degraded, abused, or manhandled even though someone claims a right to do these things to me. In such areas of conduct, it is generally agreed that claims on the conduct of others are so strong that it is morally appropriate to use force to bring their conduct within acceptable limits. The legal system is the best instance of the defense of some moral principles by force, and it is thus open to analysis from a moral point of view.

Since philosophy is highly self-reflective, all of these characterizations of ethics are open to debate among philosophers. However, these presumptions are a good starting point for the study of ethics from a philosophical standpoint. Nurses are likely to hear these concerns reflected in the work of philosophers who consult in hospitals.

Philosophers in Health Care Settings

Within a hospital, a philosopher may work in many different settings and perform a variety of functions. These include

Daily bedside rounds: Philosophers accompany physicians or nurses on rounds and teach ethics or raise ethical questions during discussion.

Case consultations: Philosophers are sometimes asked to assist in making decisions about the management of a case presenting difficult ethical issues.

Periodic conferences devoted to ethics: Health professionals gather regularly to discuss pertinent ethical issues.

Grand rounds and in-service training: Hospitals carry on a variety of educational services for their staff. Discussion of ethical issues important to staff can be part of such training programs.

Ethics committees: A hospital may set up a committee to consult on ethical issues. Such committees are usually available on request to attending physicians and other staff.

Public forums on health issues: When hospitals hold public meetings on medical issues, it is appropriate for philosophers to present ethical aspects of these issues.

Philosophers also work in nonhospital health care settings. They teach in professional schools. They assist professional associations in preparing codes of ethics and fair standards for assessing practitioners. In general, philosophers play the role of outsiders with a humanistic perspective. They are not usually needed to identify moral problems because professionals are usually aware of the moral problems in a situation. However, on those occasions when a problem is not perceived, the philosopher can be helpful in pointing it out. Also, after some diagnostic analysis by a philosopher, the presenting ethical problem may be displaced by a less apparent but more significant one.

One of the most important things that philosophers have to offer is the occasion for health professionals to take time for ethics discussions. This by itself allows them to work through moral problems and come to satisfactory solutions. Here, philosophers do not so much lecture on ethics as facilitate discussion among staff.

Philosophers add significant information to a decision-making process either by asking questions to elicit knowledge health professionals already possess but have not considered relevant or by contributing new data. For this function, hospital philosophers have to be generalists familiar with economics, sociology, psychology, and law. They also need the special skills of philosophy—making distinctions, bringing in new ideas, clarifying concepts and issues, focusing on what is problematic, and being familiar with arguments in ethics.

Hospital philosophers are divided on whether they should give recommendations when consulted. Those against it appeal to philosophers' lack of knowledge about nursing and medicine. They also note the hazard that philosophers may invite or have thrust upon them the cloak of *moral expert* and acquire authority inappropriate to their role and expertise. As counselors and facilitators, it may be wise for them to keep their views in the background. Proponents of making recommendations point out that the customary role of the consultant in health care is to give recommendations. A person engaged in the decision process should be willing to share responsibility for the outcome by making judgments. Those who favor making recommendations also see health professionals as far less likely than some ethicists imagine to give philosophers' views undue weight. Group decision processes tend to resolve this conflict. When clinicians and consultants work together for a consensus, it is important for everyone to express a judgment. Comparison of judgments is needed for a reasonable group process, but no single judgment should be given undue weight.

It is difficult to say when a philosopher should be consulted. "Whenever anyone wants to," is one answer, while "Whenever an ethical issue comes up," is another. Ethics rests on the assumption that people can choose courses of action themselves, so one tends to think of talking with philosophers only when one perceives a problem about moral values and principles. A nurse may want to consult a philosopher when he or she has

1. Conflicting ideas about what to do because of tension between different values or principles (a nurse may not be sure, for example, whether to support the patient's freedom of choice or the patient's health)
2. No ideas about what to do (one may ask, for example, "What am I doing here?"); or clear ideas of what to do, but no ideas of *why*
3. Ideas about what to do which conflict with those of others (the nurse may say, "I think the baby should be allowed to die," while the medical resident says, "I think we should make every effort to keep this baby alive")

These types of questions—which I have labeled earlier as dilemmas, uncertainty, and distress—are appropriate for consultation with a philosopher. But these are not the only occasions appropriate for philosophical discussion of ethics. One may simply want corroboration of one's thinking or an opportunity to reflect on ethics away from the bedside. A philosophical perspective on the ethics of practice should be an integral part of education in professional ethics, and thus an integral part of professional education as a whole. Although philosophers need not be ubiquitous, they should be encountered at important points during the development of one's professional career.

Philosophers are by no means the only "ethicists" or "ethics consultants" practicing in health care. Ministers, priests, rabbis, and theological scholars give close attention to ethics in health care and sometimes combine ethics teaching for clinicians with pastoral care for patients. Anthropologists and sociologists provide important details of patients' cultural values and sensitize practitioners to cultural and social elements in patient decision making. Lawyers combine ethical analysis with legal advice. Most importantly, nurses and other health professionals with an interest or education in ethics enlighten decision making by combining clinical experience with ethical theory. Conversely, philosophers teaching in health care settings are not confined to ethics. They also teach philosophy of science, theory of knowledge, clinical reasoning, philosophy of nursing, and social philosophy in health care.

Of course, philosophers also have limitations. Like health professionals, hospital ethics consultants face ethical conflicts. Though they have no obligation to be paragons of virtue, they face moral dilemmas when unethical practices come to their attention. If philosophers are to have free and open discussions of ethical issues with staff, they cannot also act as "police" or be eager to blow the whistle. Most ethics consultants think of their consultations as confidential. Yet, in 1980 there was no official "Association of Consulting Ethicists (ACE)" to lend the weight of convention to that opinion. There may be confusion about who the ethicist's client is, or who should pay for the consultation and how much. Indeed, the hospital ethicist may be a transitional figure marking the moral crisis in health care and may pass away as new modes of health care practice develop.

Philosophers may also have difficulty appreciating the need for rapid decisions, since they normally work with issues that take centuries to resolve. They may be ignorant of important health considerations or miss the point of a discussion. Most hazardously, like specialists who see a need for their work everywhere, they may label issues as ethical when the real issue is a careless or incomplete diagnosis or treatment plan. The question Should we terminate life support for this dying patient? may arise before a more careful look shows that the patient is not in fact dying. As with any consultant, knowing the limitations of philosophers is useful in getting the best from them.

Ethics case conferences can have a variety of goals and outcomes. They can be oriented to making a decision. They may analyze a prior decision to improve future ones. The outcome may be a checklist of things to remember. Since moral dilemmas create distress, it can be a relief for staff members to discuss an issue even if no decision is made. Indeed, some philosophers think of their discipline as therapeutic rather than problem solving. The outcome may be a feeling of enlightenment or a feeling of more focused frustration. Staff may find words with enough magic to transform the institution in which they work, recognize the futility of blaming themselves, gain a sense of art in their work, or strengthen their ideals. Used rightly, philosophers can assist health professionals in maintaining and developing a sense of moral competence in their work.

A Method for Resolving Nursing Ethics Problems

In most clinical situations, nurses have a clear idea of how to proceed in solving problems. But ethics problems appear to intrude opaque and complex issues into an otherwise orderly setting. Nurses therefore often hope to learn from philosophers how to make decisions in cases presenting ethical issues. Is there some orderly method by which clinicians can find the "right" answers to ethics questions?

There are many such decision methods, and I will outline one next.[4] But nurses should be aware of their limitations. Clinical situations raising ethical questions often involve suffering or deep personal conflicts. Anxiety, guilt, and doubt are almost inevitable reactions. It is illusory to hope that being right or having a

[4]For additional decision procedures, see Ruth B. Purtilo and Christine K. Cassel, *Ethical Dimensions in the Health Professions* (Philadelphia: W.B. Saunders Company, 1981); Howard Brody, *Ethical Decisions in Medicine*, 2nd ed. (Boston: Little, Brown & Company, 1981); Mila A. Aroskar, "Anatomy of an Ethical Dilemma: the Theory, the Practice," *American Journal of Nursing*, 80 (1980), 658–63; Mary Catherine S. Halloran, "Rational Ethical Judgments Utilizing a Decision-Making Tool," *Heart & Lung*, 6 (1982), 566–70; and Bernard Lo and Albert R. Jonsen, "Clinical Decisions to Limit Treatment," *Annals of Internal Medicine*, 93 (1980), 764–68.

method will relieve all difficult feelings in these cases. Even if one chooses the right pole of a dilemma, one still must forgo the lesser value. Good decisions remain open to new doubts and reexamination.

A careful approach to ethical problems in the clinic will usually involve the following steps:

IDENTIFY THE PROBLEM. State the problem as clearly as you can. (1) Is there an ethics issue you are *unclear* about? Do two or more important values or principles appear to be in *conflict?* Is something going on that you have moral *objections* to? (2) What is your relationship to the decision? Are you responsible for it? Has it been delegated to you? Are you a consultant, advisor, intermediary, voter, participant, authority, supervisor, or the like? (3) What are your time parameters? Do you see a problem coming up ahead that can be *avoided?* How much time do you have to consider this problem? Will you have to make a decision while you are still *uncertain* about important features of the case?

GATHER DATA. Describe the situation that gives rise to the problem. What is its history? What additional facts do you need? What facts are irrelevant and unimportant to consider? (1) Who are the main people involved? What are their views and interests? What is the patient's overall nursing, medical, and social situation? What does the patient want? Are there any relevant legal, administrative, and staff considerations? How is this case like and unlike similar cases? (2) The result of this step will be a *story* or *case study* that identifies main characters and events.

IDENTIFY OPTIONS. (1) What courses of action are open to you? Can you imagine any new or surprising courses of action? What is the probable impact of each possible course of action on those most involved? (2) Each course of action may involve several possible *outcomes,* depending on circumstances beyond your control. Who will be helped and who will be hurt by each possible outcome? How likely is each of these outcomes? (3) What is the probable impact on those peripherally involved or the probable long-term impact on institutions and society? (4) What future decisions are likely to come up, given a course of action? For example, if you perform CPR on a patient, are you likely to have to do so repeatedly while the patient becomes increasingly moribund? Or if you put a patient on a respirator, will you be able to wean the patient later?

THINK THE ETHICAL PROBLEM THROUGH. This is the "black box" of the method. What one considers at this step will vary widely depending on the case problem. One good way to proceed here is first to consider basic *conventional principles* of professional ethics and see whether they address the issue and resolve the problem. For example, does the primacy of the patient, a professional ideal, the futility of further treatment, cooperation on the health care team, maintaining competence, respecting the wishes of the patient, or some similar consideration appear to be of overriding importance in the case? Appropriate conventional principles will be discussed in Chapters 5 through 9.

If these fail, see if any reflective ethical considerations clarify and resolve the problem. Do broad considerations of respect for persons, equality, justice, responsibility, rights of individuals, or basic values such as health, personal liberty, and simplicity of life appear to be of overriding importance in the case? Useful reflective concepts and principles will be discussed in Chapter 10.

Rely on those principles you judge most important and of which you feel most sure. It is important to remember that in ethics case problems one normally faces two different kinds of problems: making a decision in the particular case and resolving the broader conflict or unclarity in principle that gives rise to the decision problem. A reflective person will strive to make a decision on a specific case by resolving the broader issue of principle.

MAKE A DECISION. Choose a course of action that best reflects your judgment informed by the considered judgments of others, after carefully considering controversial issues. At some point, one must cease pondering and make a choice. One rarely has time to consider an ethics problem fully, and one has to use judgment in finding closure to uncertain issues. It is appropriate to discuss ethical issues with other health care staff. It is sometimes helpful to appeal to models and ask questions like What would my grandmother have done? Where appeals to ethics still leave the decision open, it is acceptable to take into account one's more personal moral beliefs or one's professional and personal hopes, aspirations, and wishes.

ACT AND ASSESS. Carrying out the chosen action may be full of surprises. Compare the actual outcome with what you considered and hoped for in advance. How can you improve the decision process next time? It is important to assess and remember outcomes so that subsequent cases can be approached with more efficiency, sensitivity, and sophistication. The reflection on broader issues in thinking the problem through can also be resumed, and one can use what one has learned in making decisions in specific cases to make progress with unresolved questions of principle. As one encounters a series of situations where similar ethical issues arise, one soon acquires a ''checklist'' of important case considerations and issues needing further study. Such case considerations will be discussed in Chapters 12 through 18.

Philosophers in hospitals participate in all aspects of the decision process. They aid in making particular case decisions, maintain attention to unresolved issues of principle, keep track of prior related decisions, and remind staff of relevant case considerations. These are extremely important contributions, but their value can be appreciated only when one recognizes that decision methods in ethics do not yield definite answers and that the study of ethics is an inexact enterprise. One can sometimes only discover vague or conflicting indications of the right direction or action, and even the clearest articulation of a moral point of view may leave a range of choices that can be seen as right. This inexactness in ethical inquiry was noted long ago by Aristotle:

> Our discussion will be adequate if it achieves clarity within the limits of the subject matter. . . . For a well-schooled man is one who searches for that degree of precision in each kind of study which the nature of the subject at hand admits. . . .[5]

Those who turn to ethics in the hope of finding a secure and definite action are bound to be disappointed. There is no way to escape the final responsibility of saying, ''This is my choice.''

Summary

This chapter discusses how philosophers approach the study of ethics and the roles they play in health care settings. The study of ethics can be divided roughly

[5]Aristotle, *Nicomachean Ethics,* trans. Martin Ostwald (Indianapolis: The Bobbs-Merrill Co., Inc., 1962), p. 5 (para. 1094b).

into three parts: (1) the study and application of conventional principles and values associated widely with practice, such as professional codes of ethics; (2) the study of fundamental concepts and principles important in the history of philosophical ethics, such as respect for persons, justice, values, rights, and responsibilities, and the development of theories of right and wrong; and (3) reflections on the study of ethics, such as examining reasoning methods in ethics and defining basic concepts such as *ethics, morals, right,* and *good.* The first of these three interrelated levels can be called *conventional* ethics, and the second two can be called *reflective.* The second level is called *normative* ethics and the last level *metaethics.*

Much philosophical work begins with *self-examination* and doubting one's own beliefs, since discovering one's mistaken assumptions and the reasons for one's own assurance are both important to philosophical inquiry. Philosophers are not committed to a single *method* of discovering knowledge. They try out different methods depending on the question they have formulated, and discovering the important questions is a common philosophical aim. Philosophers have to be careful about *levels of inquiry* in order to keep complex abstract issues from becoming too obscure. Philosophers try to address problems *generally* and in a *unified* way. Philosophers take *obligations* of morality seriously and do not regard them as mere expressions of personal opinions. Philosophers assume that ethics is an area of study worthy of serious and reasoned examination.

Increasing numbers of philosophers work in health care settings, partly because health professionals increasingly recognize that ethical competence is an important part of overall professional competence, and partly because they face difficult ethical issues. Philosophers are active in teaching, consultation, bedside rounds, hospital committees, and so on. Philosophers act as humanists and generalists in these settings and take an active role in resolving ethical questions faced by staff. Whether consulting philosophers should give their judgments on issues is a matter of debate.

When facing ethical problems in a clinical case, a nurse can follow one of several orderly processes for making decisions on the ethical issues. One such process outlined in this chapter has six steps: identify the problem, gather data, identify options, think the ethical problem through, make a decision, and act and assess.

FURTHER READINGS

About Bioethics

BERGMAN, REBECCA, "Ethics—Concepts and Practice," *International Nursing Review,* 20, 5 (1973), 140.

CAPLAN, ARTHUR L., "Ethical Engineers Need Not Apply: The State of Applied Ethics Today," *Science, Technology, and Human Values,* 6, 33 (Fall 1980), 24–32.

CHURCHILL, LARRY R., "The Professionalization of Ethics: Some Implications for Accountability in Medicine," *Soundings,* 60, 3 (Spring 1977), 40–53.

CLOUSER, K. DANNER, "Medical Ethics: Some Uses, Abuses and Limitations," *The New England Journal of Medicine,* 293 (1975), 384–87.

———, "What Is Medical Ethics?" *Annals of Internal Medicine,* 80 (1974), 657–60.

DAVIS, LENNARD J., "The Ethics of Medical Ethics: A Radical Perspective," *Radical Teacher,* 19 (1981), 9–11.

ENCYCLOPEDIA OF BIOETHICS, 1978 ed., s.v. "Bioethics," by K. Danner Clouser.

ENCYCLOPEDIA OF BIOETHICS,   1978 ed., s.v. "History of Medical Ethics: North America in the Twentieth Century," by Albert R. Jonsen, Andrew L. Jameton, and Abbyann Lynch.

GOROVITZ, SAMUEL,   "Bioethics and Social Responsibility," *Monist,* 60, 1 (January 1977), 3–15.

HULL, RICHARD T.,   "Defining Nursing Ethics Apart from Medical Ethics," *Kansas Nurse,* 55, 8 (September 1980), 5.

LADD, JOHN,   "Legalism and Medical Ethics," in *Contemporary Issues in Biomedical Ethics,* eds. John W. Davis, Barry Hoffmaster, and Sarah Shorten, pp. 1–35. Clifton, N.J.: Humana Press, 1979.

Bioethicists

CLARK, MATT, WITH SUSAN AGREST,   "Moral Specialist," *Newsweek* (January 8, 1979), 67.

JAGGAR, ALISON,   "Philosophy as a Profession," *Metaphilosophy,* 6, 1 (1975), 100–16.

JONSEN, ALBERT R.,   "Can an Ethicist Be a Consultant?" in *Frontiers in Medical Ethics,* ed. Virginia Abernathy, pp. 157–71. Cambridge, Mass.: Ballinger Publishing Co., 1980.

LEVINE, MELVIN D., LEE SCOTT, AND WILLIAM J. CURRAN,   "Ethics Rounds in Children's Medical Center: Evaluation of a Hospital-Based Program for Continuing Education in Medical Ethics," *Pediatrics,* 60 (1977), 202–8.

RUDDICK, WILLIAM, ED.,   *Philosophers in Medical Centers.* New York: Society for Philosophy and Public Affairs, 1980.

SINGER, PETER,   "Can Ethics Be Taught in a Hospital?" *Pediatrics,* 60 (1977), 253–55.

VEATCH, ROBERT M.,   "Hospital Ethics Committees: Is There a Role?" *Hastings Center Report* (June 1977), 22–31.

Teaching Ethics

AROSKAR, MILA ANN,   "Ethics in the Nursing Curriculum," *Nursing Outlook,* 25, 4 (April 1977), 260–64.

————, AND ROBERT M. VEATCH,   "Ethics Teaching in Nursing Schools," *Hastings Center Report* (August 1977), 23–26.

BAKER, ERIC,   "On Teaching Ethics to Nurses," *Nursing Times* (May 24, 1973), 683–84.

BRIDSTON, E.,   "An Educational Strategy for Enhancement of Moral-Ethical Decision Making," *Topics in Clinical Nursing* (April 1982), 57–65.

DICKOFF, JAMES, AND PATRICIA JAMES,   "Beliefs and Values: Bases for Curriculum Design," *Nursing Research,* 19 (1970), 415–26.

LANGHAM, PAUL,   "Open Forum: On Teaching Ethics to Nurses," *Nursing Forum,* 16, 3-4 (1977), 221–27.

STENBERG, MARJORIE JONES,   "Ethics As a Component of Nursing Education," *Advances in Nursing Science,* 1, 3 (April 1979), 53–61.

WIEDENBACH, ERNESTINE,   "Comment on 'Beliefs and Values: Bases for Curriculum Design,'" *Nursing Research,* 19 (1970), 427.

WILSON, HOLLY SKODOL,   "A Case for Humanities in Professional Nursing Education," *Nursing Forum,* 13 (1974), 406–17.

ZUZICH, ANN,   "Some Frameworks for Ethical Development," in *Teaching and Evaluating the Affective Domain in Nursing Programs,* ed. Dorothy E. Reilly, pp. 1–8. Thorofare, N.J.: Charles B. Slack, Inc., 1978.

CHAPTER 5

Conventional Principles and Values

When we enter new situations we often make decisions guided by values or principles. Consider a distressed family gathered in the waiting room for news of a daughter unconscious in the intensive care unit. The task of discussing her condition with the family has fallen to the nurse, who wonders how best to report the emotionally intense mixture of good and bad news. The nurse may use some general principles for guidance as the conversation develops. These may include such advice as, "At least, don't tell any lies;" "Don't worry too much about saying anything wrong; they will hear selectively anyway;" "Be responsible for the consequences of your actions;" or "Let your feelings show, but not too much." In such principles one can find intermingled ethical and practical considerations.

Many people in our culture think such principles vary a lot from individual to individual.[1] We say things like: "These are my personal principles of action, but I would not impose them on others," and "No two people have the same values." Indeed, a thorough inventory of the beliefs, decisions, and doubts of any two persons would probably reveal at least one interesting disagreement. Equally significantly, however, many moral principles are widely held. The situation is analogous to variation in clothing. Hardly any two people in the noninstitutionalized population wear exactly the same clothing. Yet each item is mass-produced. We don't invent new principles any more often than we make our own clothing. We learn, accept, endorse, embrace (and reject, interpret, counter, and overlook) principles widely held in our culture.

Rules for action—and related principles, ideals, standards, and values—that are widely held, commonly used as standards of praise and criticism, and followed in practice may be thought of as *conventional* principles. To term them *conventional* is not to belittle them. Even if they are arbitrarily chosen, like driving on the right side of the road rather than the left, they are important.

---

[1] In this chapter, I use the term *principles* as a surrogate for *rules, standards, ideals, values, and principles*.

Adopting the principles of a group is part of the process of *identifying* with it. Some groups have self-conscious and explicit codes of ethics or statements of belief, such as professional codes of ethics or religious confessions and commandments. Other groups are more diffuse and have less well formulated sets of principles. A street fighter may take pride in never hitting women; stool pigeons may be frowned upon by thieves. We can use the word *ethos,* a cognate of the word *ethics,* to identify principles characteristic of a group.[2]

In making health care decisions, one needs principles useful in action and on which health professionals agree. For example, nurses agree on the importance of competence and the need to regard the good of the patient highly even though nurses may have very different philosophical perspectives on the fundamental sources of moral obligation. Conventional ethical principles meet this need because they carry with them a history of interpretations and cases which guide their application. Since they have the assent of health professionals, they are backed up by the active participation of many people. This creates practical support for adherence: incompetent nursing practice, for example, is *imprudent* as well as unethical.

Not all conventional principles are morally right, nor are all conventional principles even moral principles. Some conventional principles and practices, such as racism, are clearly immoral. Some simply result from habit and superstition, serve special interests, or represent partial or hypocritical commitments.

In spite of these problems, conventional principles are an excellent starting point for studying ethics. Not only are they necessary for efficient and cooperative decision making; they satisfy an important condition of moral obligations: Moral principles should be part of the ethos one identifies with; they should not seem external and unresponsive to one's particular concerns. As one embarks on a reflective philosophical investigation of ethics, it is important to take initial stock of one's consciously accepted principles and values.[3]

Conventional principles are not simply applications of philosophical reflective principles to daily life. Consider for example the obligation of *confidentiality* so common in the health professions. It is stated as Point 2 of the ANA "Code for Nurses:"

> The nurse safeguards the client's right to privacy by judiciously protecting information of a confidential nature. (ANA 1976)

This principle is often justified by saying that it is important to maintain trust between provider and client, and patients might not work with providers if confidentiality were not promised. Thus, confidentiality has positive consequences. Confidentiality is treated here as an application of the reflective principle that we should do acts that maximize positive consequences.

Overlooked in this account is the way in which confidentiality serves the emotionally powerful nurse-patient relationship. What is it like to hear the secrets of patients? Such intimate knowledge of others poses two problems. First, in the absence of a conscious and explicit vow to keep such matters silent, the nurse will feel an obligation to expose information that may help others. Without Point 2,

[2]Fittingly, more formal groups often symbolize their ethos by a uniform manner of dress.

[3]Values clarification exercises facilitate this stock-taking. Useful exercises can be found in Shirley M. Steele and Vera M. Harmon, *Values Clarification in Nursing* (New York: Appleton-Century-Crofts, 1979).

nurses would be unable to work long without encountering conflicts between feelings of loyalty to patients and to others. This desire to avoid conflict can be seen in common regulations on child abuse: Laws do not *permit* violations of confidentiality in order to report child abuse; they *require* it. By creating conventions, nurses minimize the frequency of painful moral conflicts. Second, if Point 2 were not in the code, patients would be *indebted* to nurses who kept their secrets. The code protects nurses from acquiring a list of patients with intangible secret debts of gratitude. Thus Point 2 does not so much *reflect* an obligation engendered by general moral principles as *create* one in order to foster the nurse-patient relationship.

In the next four chapters, we will draw attention to and discuss four basic and conventional ethical principles of the nursing profession:

1. Nurses have an obligation to be competent. (Chapter 6)
2. The good of patients should be the nurse's primary concern. (Chapter 7)
3. Nurses should not use their positions to exploit patients. (Chapter 8)
4. Nurses should be loyal to each other. (Chapter 9)

These principles summarize a variety of fundamental and common principles of nursing practice and are consistent with more general philosophical ethical concepts. They are characteristic of the nursing profession in that many nurses appeal to these and similar principles to justify their actions. Moreover, sanctions may be imposed on those who deviate greatly from their requirements, and feelings of self-esteem and meaningfulness of practice often rest on meeting them. They are also stated in a form characteristic of professions generally. We could formulate principles of other professions by substituting words like *social workers* and *clients* or *engineers* and *clients* for the words *nurses* and *patients* in the principles above.

Roots of Conventional Principles and Values

These four principles are not the only ones that the nursing profession follows. Since nurses are also members of nations, cultures, and religions, they bring external principles to bear on practice. For example, popular values of individual responsibility, hard work, courage, and honesty shape nursing practice. Moreover, as popular moral views change on contraception and abortion, nursing practice changes. Nor can nursing prevent regrettable principles from affecting practice. When racism flourished in this country, nurses worked in hospitals and doctors' offices which maintained separate wards and waiting rooms for blacks and whites.[4]

General cultural convictions about ethics also shape scientific theories of health care practice, and such theories support and modify current cultural practices. There are many examples of this. In the nineteenth century, the health problems of blacks were often explained by practitioners as the result of vices thought to be common among that race.[5] Victorian physicians found medical justifications both for the idleness of wealthy women and the long hours of women factory workers.[6]

[4]*Encyclopedia of Bioethics*, 1978 ed., s.v. "Racism and Medicine," by James H. Jones.

[5]Ibid.

[6]Barbara Ehrenreich and Deirdre English, *Complaints and Disorders: The Sexual Politics of Sickness* (Old Westbury, N.Y.: The Feminist Press, 1973).

Principles appear sometimes as moral principles, sometimes as medical, sometimes as both. *Cleanliness* is perhaps the paradigm case of a value associated sometimes with morality, sometimes with health. Masturbation, regarded as morally wrong in the nineteenth century, was also considered to be a disease.[7] Madness, once regarded as a spiritual disorder rooted in evil, is now seen largely as a medical or psychiatric problem.[8] Falling in love and being in love have begun to receive psychological and physiological analysis.[9] Placebos received more respect from physicians when they were found to have physiological mediators.[10] The success of the germ theory of disease did much to undercut blaming-the-victim theories of poor health among blacks,[11] but recent medical work on life-styles as a source of poor health has supported a renaissance of blaming the victims of disease.[12]

Moral conceptions may enter the health professions by means of individuals who choose and are chosen to enter them. People with certain ideals about their lives and work may choose to become nurses more often than others. There have been many studies on why nurses choose their profession and on what sorts of people choose to become nurses. One study, for example, asked women just admitted to a two-year diploma program to rank their reasons for choosing nursing school from a list of possible motives. Leading items chosen were helping people, interest in science and medicine, excitement, challenge, and improvement of health care.[13] Olesen and Whittaker identified students' nursing ideals such as "demonstrating care and concern for others in an immediate and tangible way," "high technical skill," "emotional control and restraint," and "job security."[14] Recent studies of people entering nursing later in life find a frequent interest in "frontiering," that is, moving into new areas of practice and extending and changing health care practice.

In addition to these sources of the health care ethos, the health professions maintain principles closely associated with their histories. There is a "subculture" of health care which fosters certain principles, values, and virtues; teaches them in professional schools; and uses them in assessments of work. These are articulated in written oaths and codes and communicated verbally and by example. The day-to-day conditions of work serve to give meaning to these principles and to show how they may be applied in practice. If one does not already possess these values on

[7]H. Tristram Englehardt, Jr., "The Disease of Masturbation: Values and the Concept of Disease," in *Contemporary Issues in Bioethics,* eds. Tom L. Beauchamp and LeRoy Walters (Encino, Calif.: Dickenson Publishing Co., Inc., 1978), pp. 109–13.

[8]Thomas Szasz discusses this issue in a number of works such as *The Myth of Mental Illness,* rev. ed. (New York: Harper & Row, Publishers, Inc., 1974).

[9]*Time,* January 21, 1980, p. 52, and *Newsweek,* February 25, 1980, p. 90. See also Theodore D. Kemper and Roslyn Wallach Bologh, "What Do You Get When You Fall in Love? Some Health Status Effects," *Sociology of Health and Illness,* 3 (1981), 72–88.

[10]Jon D. Levin, Newton C. Gordon, and Howard L. Fields, "The Mechanism of Placebo Analgesia," *Lancet* (September 23, 1978), 654–57.

[11]Jones, "Racism and Medicine."

[12]Johanna Shapiro and Deane H. Shapiro, "The Physiology of Responsibility: Some Second Thoughts on Holistic Medicine," *The New England Journal of Medicine,* 301 (1979), 211–12.

[13]Peter B. Morris and Norma Grassi-Russo, "Motives of Beginning Students for Choosing Nursing School," *Journal of Nursing Education,* 18, 5 (May 1979), 34–40.

[14]Virginia L. Olesen and Elvi W. Whittaker, *The Silent Dialogue: A Study of the Social Psychology of Professional Socialization* (San Francisco: Jossey-Bass, Inc., Publishers, 1968).

entering health care, one will tend to acquire them as one matures in the field. The four principles listed earlier, as important summary ethical principles of health care traditions, are linked to the history of nursing more than they are linked to the values of a national culture or to the personal biographies of nurses.[15]

Regulation and Adherence to Principle

The four principles mentioned may indeed be principles that nurses *ought* to follow, but are they in *fact* part of the conventional system of principles and actions of nursing? We actually have three questions here: Do nurses *express* these principles in thought and language? Are there *sanctions* and rewards affecting actions that accord with or deviate from these principles? And, do nurses generally *act in accordance* with these principles?

Expression

Of these three questions, the first is the easiest to answer. We can read codes, laws, regulations, publications, and so on. We can interview people or listen to their conversations. In the chapters on specific principles, I will include relevant statements supporting and elucidating them. Sanctions and actions are harder to assess.

Sanctions and Rewards

These consist of rewards we receive for doing the conventionally right thing and punishments for doing wrong. Sanctions may be formal or informal, conscious or unconscious, vague or precise, severe or mild, written or unwritten, and so on. Among the most informal yet powerful sanctions are the feelings and comments of other professionals. Being told, "You are doing a great job!" can be very encouraging. Being told, "You are clumsy and have bad breath!" can disrupt the rest of a procedure. The law provides the most formal sanctions. Dressed up in documents and rituals, it imposes defined punishments such as fines and sentences. There are many sanctions intermediate in formality: hospital procedures, conditions of employment, state administrative regulations, licensure proceedings, examinations, assessments by teachers, supervisors, and peers, economic rewards and costs, publicity, and so on. Some of these are closely associated with more or less formal rules and principles and are imposed with a consciousness of rule following. Others simply affect actions, and it may be hard to say whether a rule or principle is involved.[16]

[15]The International Council of Nurses' "Code for Nurses" (see Appendix) is a good example of a professional code of ethics that transcends national boundaries.

[16]Observing that an action accords with a rule and that people give the rule as a reason for acting is not sufficient to establish that the rule is being *followed*. It is also a condition of the concept of rule-following that the rule be a significant cause of the action. Both expressing the rule and performing the action may have a third cause in common, such as institutional constraints, or expressing the rule may be dependent on performing the action, as in a rationalization.

Particular sanctions do not affect everyone equally. Some who would gladly be eaten by ants for a good cause cannot bear to be scolded. Others thrive on confrontation, scurry for every personal advance, or shriek over the slightest disadvantage. It is thus hard to tell how sanctions will affect practice, and they are no substitute for widespread personal support of principles.

The Law

Of these sources of sanctions, the law is usually the most significant for ethical thinking. The impact of the law on our conduct goes well beyond formal procedures. Few people encounter the law directly by actually being sued or going to jail. People seldom even consult lawyers or read lawbooks in order to answer their legal questions, and most health professionals seem to get their legal information from other health professionals. There are doubtless many reasons why lawyers are not often consulted by nurses: Lawyers cost more than ethicists; the most available lawyer may work for the wrong party, that is, the hospital; and many lawyers dwell on all the things one could be sued for, just as gloomy physicians dwell on all the diseases one could have. Meanwhile, lawyers look to health care practice for guidance on making laws and decisions on health care.

One consequence of this is that rumors and mythologies about the law abound in hospitals. In 1978 for example, most staff at one hospital believed that "do not resuscitate" orders *must* legally be written in the chart. At another hospital, the popular view was that in order to avoid legal risks, these orders must *not* be written down. One hospital ward preferred to have written in charts, "Call resident in case of respiratory arrest" as a code for "do not resuscitate." The picture of the law expressed by hospital staff may thus reveal more about the needs of the staff than about the law. These legal myths may make it possible for staff to create conventional practices without taking responsibility for them. Instead of admitting, "Our procedure is as follows," the staff collectively shifts responsibility: "The law makes us do it this way."

Even when we know the law, it is often not a helpful guide to moral conduct. It may say nothing about, or give conflicting interpretations of, important issues. Since each event is particular, it may be hard to identify appropriate legal precedents for a question. The legal principle a judge uses to express a sense of justice in one case may be hard to generalize to other cases. Even when the law takes a definite position, what the ethical professional should do is still not established. The law compromises among many interests: Like the law on packaging for food and drugs, some protections are for the consumer, some for the provider. Conventional ethical principles of health care or one's private conscience may conflict with the law.

Some nurses pay close attention to the law in order to avoid malpractice suits, since nurses are increasingly named in them. Excessive suit-consciousness becomes "defensive nursing," drawing attention from good nursing practice and making one defensive toward patients. However, even books on malpractice remind practitioners that a good relationship with patients is the most important factor in avoiding suits. Instead of thinking about avoiding suits, it is better to practice in terms of sincere concern for patient good, consulting in doubtful cases, acting openly and on the record, and having good reasons for one's decisions. In the unlikely event of a legal dispute, consultation, openness, and carefully considered reasons are good defenses against charges of acting negligently. Although legal cases contain much ethical thinking, and we may learn much about ethics by studying and criticizing the law, the law provides only a background for thinking about ethics.

Adherence

It is hard to say whether conventional principles are being adhered to. In the first place, conventional moral principles in health care are not unconditional orders to be obeyed like the Ten Commandments or many rules we obeyed as children. Neither do they carry with them clear, step-by-step instructions which tell us whether or not we are following them. They function as general guides for deciding what to do. They require interpretation, consideration of their relevance to particular situations, and individual judgment. Interpreting conventional rules is an important part of ethical competence.

And it is not clear how high a standard conventional principles set. If the requirement of competency were fulfilled only if one never made a mistake, everyone would fall below the standard. In contrast, if competence were simply doing something right now and then, all of us would be competent. Conventional principles both set minimum standards and express ideals. When we see them as minimum standards, we would say they are being followed when these minimum standards are met. When we see them as ideals, we can follow them the way that travelers used to follow stars: We are "following" them even though we never reach them. Whatever the actual conduct of health professionals has been historically, they have a strong tradition of idealism. Self-sacrifice, relief of suffering, concern for human welfare, and compassion are part of the rationale of the everyday practice of nursing.

Part of what it means to say that health care is in crisis is to say that the principles governing its delivery are under severe strain. This strain takes a variety of forms. First, because of new technological advances and institutional changes, it is hard to interpret the rules. Familiar examples of their applications become obsolete. For example, the old nursing virtue of frugality does not readily apply to cost-containment. The good of the patient is often a puzzle given the current pharmacopoeia and array of tools. Second, changing external moral values affect how we perceive health care conventions. The requirement of informed consent conflicts with traditional paternalist interpretations of patient good. Confidence in technology has had to confront the problems of short resources, harmful consequences, and high costs. Ideals of equality, strengthened by the civil rights and women's movements, conflict with strongly hierarchical loyalties in the health professions. Third, it is hard to fulfill all of these principles at once in the present institutional context. Competency sometimes conflicts with patient welfare. Loyalty and patient good sometimes conflict. These new conflicts press us to reflect on these traditional principles. We can reinterpret them for a new setting; we can replace them with others; or we can change the work setting to make it easier to follow these rules. The next four chapters will treat each of the four principles mentioned in this chapter, in order to indicate how they are used in reasoning about health care and how they work out in practice.

Summary

In order to make decisions efficiently and with the cooperation of others, we need conventional and customary principles which we all can understand and apply. Four summary conventional principles of nursing ethics are the following:

1. Nurses have an obligation to be competent.
2. The good of patients should be the nurse's primary concern.
3. Nurses should not use their positions to exploit patients.
4. Nurses should be loyal to each other.

The conventional ethics of nursing practice is shaped partly by principles like these arising from the experience of nurses. Practice is also influenced by the moral views of the culture in which nursing is practiced and by the moral views of individuals choosing to go into nursing.

We can identify the ethical principles of nursing practice as the ones nurses follow, express in their discussions, and back up with sanctions, whether they be legal sanctions such as loss of licenses, or informal ones such as praise and criticism.

Using conventional professional principles requires good personal judgment since they can never cover all cases explicitly. Conventional principles function to indicate both professional ideals and minimally acceptable standards of practice. Being able to use and interpret the conventional principles of nursing is essential to professional ethical competence. Increasing inapplicability of and conflict among conventional ethical principles is one dimension of the current crisis in health care.

FURTHER READINGS

Legal Aspects

BULLOUGH, BONNIE, ED., *The Law and the Expanding Nursing Role.* New York: Prentice-Hall, Inc., 1980.
CREIGHTON, HELEN, *Law Every Nurse Should Know* (4th ed.). Philadelphia: W.B. Saunders Company, 1981.
FENNER, KATHLEEN M., *Ethics and Law in Nursing: Professional Perspectives.* New York: D. Van Nostrand Co., 1980.
HEALTH LAW CENTER AND CHARLES J. STREIFF, EDS., *Nursing and the Law* (2nd ed.). Rockville, Md.: Aspen Systems Corporation, 1975.
MURCHISON, IRENE A., AND THOMAS S. NICHOLS, *Legal Foundations of Nursing Practice.* New York: Macmillan, Inc., 1970.
SHORT, EMILE F., "Revocation of Nurse's License to Practice Profession," *American Law Review,* 3rd Series, vol. 55, 1141–50.
WARREN, DAVID G., *Problems in Hospital Law,* chap. 5, "Nurses," pp. 71–80. Germantown, Md.: Aspen Systems Corporation, 1978.

Values and Occupations

BERGER, PETER L., BRIGITTE BERGER, AND HANSFRIED KELLNER, *The Homeless Mind: Modernization and Consciousness,* chap. 3, "Pluralization of Social Life-Worlds," pp. 63–82. New York: Random House, Inc., 1973.
HUGHES, EVERETT CHERRINGTON, "Dilemmas and Contradictions of Status," *American Journal of Sociology,* 50 (1944–1945), 353–59.

Rosenberg, Morris, *Occupations and Values*. New York: The Free Press, 1957.
Zimmerman, Donald, "The Practicalities of Rule Use," in *Understanding Everyday Life,* ed., Jack Douglas, pp. 221–38. Chicago: Aldine Publishing Co., 1970.

CHAPTER 6

Competence:

Nurses
Have an Obligation
to Be Competent

Competence lies at the heart of the concept of professionalism. The other parts of the concept, social good and autonomy, would be empty without some special skill giving specific form to professionals' aspirations. Skill and craft are part of the classical image of professionals, and pride in one's work is an important source of professionals' satisfaction. Nursing takes the competence of its members seriously. Five of the eleven points of the American Nurses' Association code are closely related to issues of competence, the simplest being

Point 5: The nurse maintains competence in nursing. (ANA, 1976)

This emphasis on competence can be seen in nursing education. A certain level of special training is required as a condition for entry into the profession, in contrast with occupations that require no special education or admit practitioners upon passing a test or paying a fee. Since long periods of education require considerable commitment from novices, confidence in the value of education is necessary for nurses to maintain their motivation. During the educational process, much emphasis is placed on the acquisition of skills. Instructors impress upon students that mistakes can kill patients. Sociologists observing a nursing class reported:

> The instructor said again, rather sharply . . . that no one in the class was going to give medications for quite a while because of the extremely poor performance the class had given on the arithmetic test. She put it very forcefully, "We cannot trust you in giving medication and we feel that we simply cannot take these risks." This news about the medications was greeted by the girls with what I can only describe as shocked silence.[1]

Students may suffer considerable anxiety as they encounter new procedures. Many

[1]Virginia L. Olesen and Elvi W. Whittaker, *The Silent Dialogue: A Study in the Social Psychology of Professional Socialization* (San Francisco: Jossey-Bass Inc., Publishers, 1968), pp. 140–41.

nurses recall helpful and sympathetic patients who stoically endured their first attempts at procedures.

The focus on competency in nursing and medicine grows partly from the need to assess the quality of patient care. Concern for the patient's good is hard to assess directly, since it is often difficult to obtain information on the outcomes of patient care. Even such straightforward measures of outcome as recovery, mortality, and sick days are hard to obtain and take a long time to collect. Hospital staff frequently never see their patients after they leave the hospital and so have little feedback on whether their work helped or harmed patients in the long run. To assess their work, practitioners have to look at more immediate elements such as skill in performing procedures and ability to exercise judgment according to the standards of the profession. One assesses the work itself, not its outcome.

Like most conventional obligations, practices surrounding professional competency are imbued with formal and informal sanctions, strong feelings, and elements of self-interest. Thus, competency is not only an ethical concern but also a practical one. Susan R. Gortner places "Become competent in what you do" first on her list of "Strategies for Survival in the Practice World."[2] Incompetent acts make one vulnerable to formal and informal repercussions. Obvious competence is an element in success and promotion. Incompetence creates work for others and imposes risks on them, thereby inspiring their criticism.

To the cynical eye, only the *appearance* of competence is needed to survive within the system of sanctions. Yet most of us have a strong need to feel genuinely competent. Mistakes cause acute feelings of shame and guilt. Nurses struggle to assess whether their level of commitment and effort is adequate to patients' needs. Intensive care unit nurses smolder with anger at surgeons who don't wash their hands before examining a patient. When a patient is dying as the result of a hospital error, staff may make heroic attempts to save the patient partly because of excruciating guilt feelings. Strong feelings like these show a genuine concern for real competence, not merely for looking good.

It is difficult to ascertain from the exercise of sanctions how seriously competence is taken by a profession. Medicine displays strong internal controls over competence, as for instance in the practice of holding Morbidity and Mortality Conferences, where physicians critique their work. The Board of Medical Quality Assurance, which has the main responsibility for California state review of medical licensure, uses a range of disciplinary procedures from reprimands, through probation and suspension, to revocation. The major infraction in 1982 was indiscriminate prescribing of medications without prior examination. Prescribing medications for oneself and alcohol abuse were being handled by a program treating impaired physicians rather than by disciplinary action. Other actions were based on criminal convictions, especially fraudulent claims against state reimbursement programs. Gross negligence is also a disciplinary category, such as overlooking an obvious cancer or performing plastic surgery without having done a residency in it. The Board of Registered Nursing has the main responsibility for licensing nurses in California. Between January 1981 and March 1982, sixty-two licenses were revoked and seventy-three nurses placed on probation. Forty-seven of these revocations and sixty-four of the probations were for medication infractions, such as diverting demerol or morphine for personal use, and for mischarting medications on

---

[2]Susan R. Gortner, "Strategies for Survival in the Practice World," *American Journal of Nursing*, 77 (1977), 618.

patient records. Other infractions were for incompetence or negligence, such as nonnarcotic medication errors and inadequate patient care.[3]

People are often reluctant to punish people for isolated mistakes. The harm has already been done, and we all make mistakes sometimes. Our cultural concept of responsibility focuses more on the goodness of our intentions than on our ability to carry them out perfectly. It is thus common to forgive mistakes unless they are seen as resulting from overall incompetence or character defects such as inattentiveness to patient welfare, lack of dedication, or disrespect for others.[4]

Competence and Context

Most judgments of competence focus on the individual, and we each must supply something of our individual resources to be competent. However, individual competency depends on outside factors beyond our individual control and is to some degree contextually determined. This is a vulnerability we all share with patients. A patient may manage well at home but be psychotic in the hospital. In a setting with good support, nurses may be very competent. In a context short of staff and with conflicting concepts of nursing tasks, nurses can function poorly even though individual nurses in the second setting are just as skilled as those in the first.

In order to function competently, one needs the definition of one's *role* or *scope of practice* to be congruent with one's skills. This is expressed in the ANA code:

> Point 6: The nurse exercises informed judgment and uses individual competence and qualifications as criteria in seeking consultation, accepting responsibilities, and delegating nursing activities to others. (ANA, 1976)

There are two ways to increase competency: one can improve one's skills or one can adjust one's role to fit one's skills.

The work setting affects competency through the cooperation of others. The competence of surgeons depends on the competence of nurses working with them, suppliers of equipment, nurses who prepare the surgical stage beforehand, nurses who care for the patient afterwards, and patients who care for themselves. For example, a study by Katherine Jones on renal transplant patients showed that patients whose care was planned and managed by one nurse throughout their hospitalization recovered more quickly from surgery and had fewer complications than patients who received less personalized nursing care.[5]

Failure to maintain adequate staff and supplies reduces the competency of staff and causes nurses ethical distress. At a large underfunded county hospital, staff nurses spend much of their time looking for gurneys, sheets, hypodermics, and other necessities in short supply, with the result that it is hard to move beyond the most basic nursing services. The following case illustrates vividly how disaster can

[3]Figures are from verbal communication with state officials.

[4]For a detailed account of how surgeons handle errors, see Charles L. Bosk, *Forgive and Remember: Managing Medical Failure* (Chicago: University of Chicago Press, 1979).

[5]Katherine Jones, "Study Documents Effect of Primary Nursing on Renal Transplant Results," *Hospitals*, 49, 24 (December 16, 1975), 85–89.

arise from short staffing combined with imprudent timing of a coffee break. A forty-year-old postsurgical patient suffered irreversible brain damage from a respiratory arrest in the recovery room. Detection of the arrest was delayed due to inadequate observation in the following circumstances:

> CASE EXAMPLE. The recovery room, in this case, was usually staffed by three nurses but, on the day in question, only two nurses were on duty. When one nurse went for coffee, the other was alone in the recovery room with two patients. Shortly thereafter a third patient arrived. The nurse's care of that patient was interrupted by the arrival of the plaintiff. Before the nurse could complete the assessment of the plaintiff's immediate condition, yet another patient arrived accompanied by his anesthetist who ordered the nurse to give this patient a STAT injection of Demerol. The nurse, still alone with all five post-op patients, went to carry out the order. After doing so, she also took a telephone call before returning to the plaintiff. . . . On her return, the nurse observed that [the plaintiff] was not breathing and put through a call for assistance to another anesthetist. At about the same time another patient was brought to the recovery room and another physician was summoned. The absent nurse returned about this time.[6]

Who Judges Competence

In keeping with the concept of professionalism, peer and supervising nurses are the primary judges of nursing competence. Other health professionals, patients, educators, and administrators also have input. Because of their dominant position in health care, physicians also have had an important role in judging nursing competence.

Our ability to handle suffering and to affect the course of disease is limited. Nursing and medicine are vast fields which no single person can master, so health care professionals maintain their sense of competence against a background of uncertainty. Yet in a bureaucracy, the work of many people needs to be coordinated with definiteness. In hospitals, physicians traditionally play an important role in coordinating work. Physicians are trained to make diagnoses and decisions in spite of uncertainty.[7] They create certainty with the magic of medical language. Their decisions make it possible for large numbers of people to work with some feeling of controlling death, disease, and pain. Purveying certainty is an important source of medicine's power and an important source of its vulnerability.

This power to define clinical situations, together with the tradition of physician dominance, has given physicians considerable influence in judging nursing competency. This has had unfortunate consequences for the nursing profession. It has hindered professional autonomy of nurses, and nurses are too often seen as less knowledgeable than doctors. Physicians tend to focus on the dependent functions of

---

[6]Corinne L. Sklar, "You and the Law: The Coffee Break: Potential Pitfall for Nurses," *The Canadian Nurse*, 75, 5 (May 1979), 15. The case cited is Laidlaw v. Lions Gate Hospital et al., 8 D.L.R. 3d 730 (B.C.S.C., 1969).

[7]Renée C. Fox, "Training for Uncertainty," in *Dominant Issues in Medical Sociology*, eds. Howard D. Schwartz and Cary S. Kart (Reading, Mass.: Addison-Wesley Publishing Co., Inc., 1978), pp. 189–202.

Table 6.1. Importance of Nursing Tasks: Ratings by Nurses and Physicians

Nurses' Ranking	*Physicians' Ranking*
1. Notice changes in patient's condition and report them. (2)	1. Carry out the doctor's orders. (5)
2. Observe the effects of treatments ordered by the physician. (5)	2. Notice changes in patient's condition and report them. (1)
3. Take time to listen to patient. (7)	3. Give prescribed medication on time.*
4. Explain about diagnostic tests ahead of time so patient will know what to expect.*	4. Notice when patient has pain and give him medication if ordered.*
5. Carry out the doctor's orders. (1)	5. Observe the effects of treatments ordered by the physician. (2)

NOTE: Numbers in parentheses indicate rank in the other list.
*Item is not in first eight of other list.
SOURCE: Reprinted with permission of American Hospital Publishing, Inc., and the author, from David M. Ambrose, "Physicians and Nurses Rank Importance of Nursing Activities," *Hospitals, J.A.H.A.,* published by the American Hospital Association, November 1, 1977, Vol. 51, No. 21.

nursing and to have different ideas of what nursing should be. For example, David M. Ambrose asked both nurses and physicians to list nursing functions in order of importance and averaged their responses to get two rank lists for comparison. It is clear from the lists that physicians and nurses conceive the role differently (see Table 6.1). Since physicians and nurses conceive of nursing roles differently, we can expect them to disagree in general on what counts as competent nursing. Some nurses regard a physician's judgment that, "She is a good nurse" with suspicion. The judgment may mean merely that the nurse is good at following doctors' instructions.

Physicians have a history of opposing increasing nursing competence and supporting tight medical control over nurse training and assessment. This view is very much alive among physicians according to Jo Ann Ashley:

> Today physicians still assume that nurses will remain in their "logical place at the physician's side" functioning "under the supervision of physicians" for the purpose of "extend(ing) the hands of the physician," (according to) statements of the American Medical Association's Committee on Nursing approved by the association in 1970.[8]

Not only do physicians misidentify nursing competencies, but they also sometimes fail to notice nursing competence at all and so are in a tenuous position to assess it. For example, it was found in one study that when psychiatric patients were asked to list what helped them most during hospitalization, 31 percent identified nursing as the most helpful, and another 59 percent mentioned it as helpful. In contrast, only 1 percent of physicians mentioned nursing as most helpful, and 2 percent listed nurses as helpful.[9] These problems remain a source of conflict in nurse-physician relations.

[8]Jo Ann Ashley, *Hospitals, Paternalism, and the Role of the Nurse* (New York: Teachers College Press, 1976), p. 129.

[9]Marshall O. Zaslove, J. Thomas Ungerleider, and Marielle Fuller, "The Importance of the Psychiatric Nurse: Views of Physicians, Patients and Nurses," *American Journal of Psychiatry,* 125 (1968), 482–86.

Valued Competencies

We observed in Chapter 2 that some competencies are more valued than others. The *cure* function stereotypically associated with medicine is generally more valued than the *care* function similarly pegged to nursing. However, these values hardly correspond to the competencies most strongly affecting patient good.

If health professionals were mainly concerned with public health and overall welfare, then they would develop and honor the skills most useful in maintaining these. Public health measures, screening campaigns, epidemiology, political skills, and ability to encourage patients to manage their lives better would probably be most honored.

If health professionals were mainly concerned with doing the most obvious and immediate good for patients, they would emphasize skills in caring for and comforting the sick, that is, palliation of symptoms and relief of pain, since most diseases are still either incurable or self-limiting. If bedside care were in fact the most honored specialty, the prestige of the health professions would likely be the reverse of its present standing: LVNs, LPNs, aides, orderlies, and attendants would rank highest in prestige. Next in line would be RNs, interns, and residents. Last would be attending physicians.[10] Among physicians, specialties emphasizing patient contact, such as family practice and geriatrics, would be more respected than specialties like cardiology and immunology, noted for their scientific interest and achievements. Among nurses, ward staff would enjoy the same prestige as critical-care nurses.

The most valued forms of competence currently tend to reflect scientific and technological interests—what people consider intellectually difficult, exciting, and challenging—rather than what is most directly related to patient good or to public health. This has the effect of making patients whose problems are not readily accessible to current technologies and conceptions of competence seem uninteresting to clinicians. In this way, values with regard to professional competence affect who gets the most attention and the best care.[11]

The moral value of a skill ultimately rests on patient good, while the ability of professionals to pursue a particular skill may depend on its challenge and interest. In order to encourage forms of competence that serve patient good, it may be necessary to create new intellectual challenges in more appropriate areas of skill, so that clinicians pursuing excellence can achieve in these areas. This is difficult to do in such areas as chronic disease, dementia, degenerative diseases, and complex social and psychiatric problems. Nurses generally seem to be less vulnerable than physicians to the seduction of technology, and so have an important role in directing new forms of health care competence toward patient good.

Task Orientation

The high regard for the professions in our culture indicates a high regard for competence. Our cultural conceptions of competence tend to be oriented to visible

---

[10]See Chapter 1, n. 10.

[11]Joseph E. Hardison, "The Importance of Being Interesting," *American Journal of Medicine*, 68 (1980), 9–10.

activities with tangible products. Health professionals are often seen as good examples of this *task orientation*. Contemplation, meditation, study, and the arts may have their place in the life of the health professional, but only in the context of a life devoted to "accomplishing something."

Doing nothing about a health problem is probably one of the most difficult things for a health practitioner to do. It is a rare patient who is told by a physician that nothing can be done and is sent home without a prescription. The common treatment of minor viral infections with antibiotics—which do not affect the virus but may help prevent complications—can be seen as having its origins in both patients' and physicians' convictions that something must be done. Patients are often anxious about their health, and offering them nothing for it, even where nothing would be effective, may seem like a rejection. But even when the patient is not personally involved, health professionals have a reluctance to remain passive.

> CASE EXAMPLE. Mr. S., unconscious for several weeks in the ICU had suffered lengthy and heroic efforts to rescue him from a variety of system failures. He had been saying while conscious that he wanted to die. It is now clear to everyone that he is going to die, that he is dying, and that any attempts at recovery are futile. It has been decided not to try to resuscitate him if his heart should stop beating. His heart stops beating. The intern announces, "Mr. S. is flatlining." (Actually, the record of electrical activity in Mr. S.'s heart is showing a flat line; Mr. S. is not "flatlining.") The entire energy of the staff on the ward becomes involved in doing nothing. They stay away from the patient for a while. They pretend to discuss other matters; but their entire attention is focused in their minds on the patient. They move slowly; the atmosphere is like molasses.

When patients are given a choice of treatment, doing nothing at all is seldom mentioned or encouraged as a treatment. A policy of doing *something* accomplishes two things: First, if I do something and the patient does not recover, at least I tried. It is part of a task-oriented set of values to see doing nothing as not trying. Second, I can maintain an illusion of control by being involved in the process. As long as I am involved in doing something with regard to the disease, I have some responsibility in connection with it. To do nothing is to admit my inability to control it and to see responsibility in forces outside my control.

Task orientation can thus be seen as reflecting a broad social value in our culture in favor of control. Part of the respect that professionals and experts receive rests in the hope that they can control such phenomena as economic cycles, production, and education of children. In our strongly individualistic culture, most of us experience anxiety in reaction to our isolation and the prospect of death. The use of technology, task orientation, and technical approaches to problem solving gives us a means of creating the illusion that we might escape isolation and death. We create machines and techniques which we can predict and control, and about which we can develop a science, while our ability to influence societies, organisms, biological systems, and the massive elements of the physical world remain limited. As long as we are surrounded by machines and techniques, we can maintain confidence in control over our lives. Thus, nurses who try to slow down the intense pace of medical intervention find themselves in fruitless conflict with this strong and marginally rational impulse.

Task orientation also reflects the value of productivity. Doing productive work is one of the important sources of individual legitimacy in our culture. Even people who do not work because of a handicap, a chronic illness, or the like suffer discrimination, stigma, and loss of support. Health professionals are in the paradoxical position of being supremely competent and productive individuals committed to people who are sick and sometimes therefore unproductive. Nursing is less vulnerable than medicine to these excesses of task orientation, but it is strong in both professions.

How Competent Nurses Are

Because of multiple factors in competence, and because the obligation of competence calls for both minimal levels of competence and striving for higher levels, assessing adherence to the principle of competence can barely be attempted meaningfully. Nevertheless, nurses generally have feelings about how competent they, their colleagues, and their institutions are. Judgments on hospitals, for example, are not completely positive. When asked if they would choose to be patients in the institution where they were employed if seriously ill, 68 percent of those in large hospitals (more than two-hundred beds) and 59 percent in smaller hospitals answered affirmatively. Nurses who worked in nursing homes and extended care facilities were more negative: Only 45 percent said they would choose to be patients in their own institutions.[12]

But when nurses were asked to judge their own abilities, 96 percent responded that they felt moderately or very competent. Four percent said "Somewhat" and none said "Not very" or "Not at all." Nurses were more critical in judging each other. For example, in the same study, nurses judged that 23 percent of nurses gave fair or poor patient care and that 64 percent of nurses gave fair or poor patient psychological support. They judged that 19 percent of physicians gave fair or poor patient care and 77 percent of physicians gave fair or poor psychological support.[13]

In brief, competence is preeminently valued in health care practice, but in ways uncertainly related to the good of the patient. Linking nursing skills more clearly to patient good is part of the problem of maintaining the conventional principles of nursing ethics.

Summary

The obligation to be competent is central to nursing practice and to the concept of professionalism. Nursing education is largely directed to acquiring the skills necessary to meet this obligation.

The ability of individuals to be competent and to display competence depends on the context in which they work. For example, to be competent a nurse must work in a hospital that is adequately staffed. Disagreements about which skills are most

[12]G. Ray Funkhauser and *Nursing 76*, "Quality of Care," Part I, *Nursing 76*, 6, 12 (December 1976), 26.

[13]Ibid., pp. 24–25.

important to nursing work lead staff to conflicting judgments of competence. One important conflict is between the value of highly technological skills versus interpersonal and emotional skills.

In health care, the task orientation of professionals requires them to express their competence through action and intervention. Since the outcomes of care are distant in time, this active conception of competence can be harmful to patient welfare in the long run.

Very few nurses think they are not very competent, and most nurses think highly of those they work with. But patient psychological support by nurses and physicians is often criticized, and many hospital and nursing home nurses would prefer not to be cared for in institutions where they work.

FURTHER READINGS

BENNE, K.D., AND W. BENNIS, "Role Confusion and Conflict in Nursing: The Role of the Professional Nurse," *American Journal of Nursing*, 59 (1959), 196–98.

CHRISTMAN, L., "The Influence of Specialization on the Nursing Profession," *Nursing Science*, 3 (December 1965), 446–53.

COLAVECCHIO, RUTH, BARBARA TESCHER, AND CYNTHIA SCALZI, "A Clinical Ladder for Nursing Practice," *Journal of Nursing Administration* (September/October 1974), 54–58.

CORWIN, RONALD G., "The Professional Employee: A Study of Conflict in Nursing Roles," *American Journal of Sociology*, 66 (1961), 604–15. Reprinted in *Sociological Perspectives on Occupations*, ed. Ronald M. Pavalko, pp. 261–75. Itasca, Ill.: F.E. Peacock Publishers, Inc., 1972.

CUSHING, MAUREEN, "The Legal Side: A Matter of Judgment," *American Journal of Nursing*, 82 (June 1982), 990, 992.

DAVIS, FRED, *Illness, Interaction, and the Self*, pp. 92–103. Belmont, Calif.: Wadsworth Publishing Co., Inc., 1972.

CHAPTER 7

Patient Good:

The Good of Patients Should Be the Nurse's Primary Concern

Nurses usually justify their clinical activities by referring to the needs and welfare of patients; nursing competence finds its basic rationale in its effect on patients. While at work, nurses normally set aside other concerns and devote their attention, time, and energy to work intended to help patients. In this chapter, I examine what thinking about the good of patients usually involves. I address such questions as Who decides what is good for the patient? How should we balance harm and benefit? How should we allocate care among patients with conflicting needs? The next chapter will focus on *other interests* that may conflict with patient good such as the nurse's concern for his or her own welfare or conflicts between teaching and patient care.

The American Nurses' Association code only passingly addresses the issue of patient good. Point 1 ("The nurse provides services with respect for human dignity . . .") addresses nondiscrimination. Point 3 enjoins the nurse to ". . . safeguard the client and the public . . ." Points 10 and 11 refer to the health of the public and do not focus on individual patients. Codes sometimes refer to patient good in the "statement of purpose." The ICN and ANA codes do this:

> The fundamental responsibility of the nurse is fourfold: to promote health, to prevent illness, to restore health and to alleviate suffering. (ICN, 1973)

> Nursing encompasses the promotion and restoration of health, the prevention of illness, and the alleviation of suffering. (ANA, 1976)

These statements also specify with what aspects of patient good nurses should be concerned.

Concern for the good of patients creates a paradox for nurses. *Good* is a broad concept. Nurses cannot claim to have maximal competence in everything that leads to patient good. On one hand, a nurse who emphasizes a specific competence must show how that competence is related to the overall good of the patient. However, such evidence may not be available. For instance, skill in managing patients on respirators may or may not lead to the overall good of these patients. On the other hand, if the nurse claims to be able to provide the patient with a variety of goods which support *overall* patient welfare, the nurse risks being unable to claim maximal competence in a specific arena. In each area of activity, it will be possible to find a specialist more competent at that task.

Indeed, conventional forms of health care competence can conflict painfully with a nurse's judgments about patient welfare. For example, a nurse commented on her stressful experience in a newborn intensive care unit:

> CASE EXAMPLE. A child was kept alive mechanically for weeks because the parents could not accept his dying. I started avoiding him and then felt guilty for it. I started questioning much of our unit's work: "Is this what we are really here for? Doesn't quality of life mean something?" I had to resuscitate him once, which was particularly stressful—I didn't want to succeed but I had to look like I was trying hard enough.[1]

When conflicts arise over what is good for patients, nurses often ask: Who should say what is best for the patient? Whose conception of patient good should I follow? My own? The patients'? The physicians'? Blue Cross's? The court's? A philosopher's?

Paternalism

Nurses generally work in settings where the question of Who is to decide? is frequently answered by "the doctor." For some clients, the views of physicians carry great authority, and this authority may extend beyond medical matters to counseling on personal and moral issues. Many people believe, however, that this question should be answered more often by "the patient."

When the nurse, physician, or anyone other than the patient decides for the patient what to do, we encounter an area of great controversy in ethics—*paternalism*.[2] The meaning of *paternalism* is "making people do what is good for them" (and conversely, "preventing people from doing what is bad for them"). Some people think that it is sometimes morally right to make people be good to themselves; others think that it is never, or almost never, right to do so.

[1]Sharol P. Jacobson, "Stressful Situations for Neonatal Intensive Care Nurses," *MCN: The American Journal of Maternal Child Nursing*, 3 (1978), 144–52.

[2]Paternalism should be distinguished from the authority physicians have traditionally had over nurses. The latter form of authority can be distinguished from paternalism because it is not intended to benefit nurses. Since the nurse-physician division of labor has historical roots in sexist cultural practices, the authority of physicians over nurses can be described by the related concept of *patriarchy*.
Some prefer to use the term *parentalism*, rather than *paternalism*, in order to neutralize implications of gender. I have no objections to this practice. Women act paternalistically or parentalistically as well as men. But I prefer the more historically common usage, since I believe the forms of dominance common in medicine are linked to sexism and sex role traditions. For an early discussion of paternal versus parental terminology, see John Locke, *The Second Treatise of Government* (Indianapolis: The Bobbs-Merrill Co., Inc., 1952), "Chapter VI: Of Paternal Power," pp. 30–31.

Nurses often treat postsurgical patients paternalistically. Although they are mentally sound and alert, such patients may be reluctant to face the pain and discomfort of breathing deeply, coughing, getting up, or walking. Nurses know that coughing and moving around are essential to recovery. Thus, nurses encourage, cajole, push, prod, tease, press, and threaten patients until they cough or get up. Such acts by nurses are analogous to legislative acts imposing penalties on those who fail to take care of themselves. Examples of laws that are at least partly paternalistic include those requiring motorcycle drivers to wear helmets and laws restricting the sale of prescription drugs.

People who believe that it is morally acceptable to force *competent* people to act for their own good are sometimes labeled *strong* paternalists. They differ from *weak* paternalists, who believe that it is only morally permissible to force people with diminished mental capacity to take care of themselves. Some common reasons people are held to be *incompetent* to decide for themselves include immaturity, insanity, mental retardation, stress, and confusion. Sometimes people are so incapable that making decisions for them is unavoidable. For instance, people in comas must be acted upon. Children can be so uncomprehending and psychotics so incapable of decision that manipulation is necessary. Since many health professionals are weak paternalists, determining patient competency is an important problem for them.

Paternalism is not limited to deliberate or conscious coercion by clinicians. Many factors present in settings for care of the sick may create an atmosphere of paternalism. Hospital structure and procedures, respect for medical authority, dependent feelings of the sick, fantasies of reprisal, fear of illness and death, mystification, and the commitment of nurses and others to professional standards and values all combine to create coercive effects on competent and incompetent patients. Figure 7.1 illustrates graphically the imbalance of power between patients and hospital structure which inevitably introduces coercive elements into patient care.

Nurses have generally shown less paternalism in their professional practice than physicians; indeed, many nurses express strong advocacy of patients' rights and models of self-care.[3] This is partly because paternalism and patriarchal authority have been associated historically, and nurses have had little access to the latter. Feminists have identified many social arrangements that purportedly exist for the good of women but which are really for the benefit of men. Such critiques have given substance to arguments against paternalism. Since nurses have not been the main decision makers in health care, they have had less opportunity to impose their own views on patients; instead, they have acted as accomplices to physicians when they have unduly pressed patients to accept medical advice.

The traditional patriarchal doctor-nurse relationship creates obstacles to the autonomy of both nurses and patients. Consequently, nursing has not had the opportunity to explore fully its conceptions of patient advocacy and autonomy. At the same time, nursing has not stated its view of the limits on patient autonomy, nor have nurses said when they think the Who is to Decide? question should be answered by "the nurse." (For a more philosophical assessment of paternalism, see pp. 126–29.)

---

[3]See, for example, Dorothea Orem, *Nursing: Concepts of Practice,* 2nd ed. (New York: McGraw-Hill Book Company, 1980).

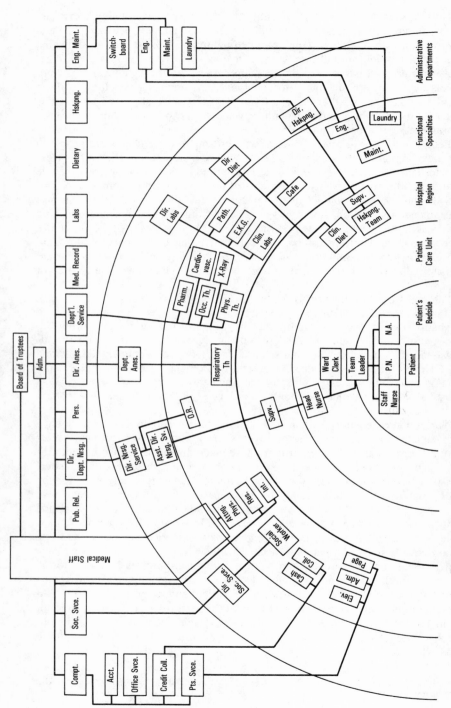

Figure 7.1. The Functional and Territorial Organization of a Hospital

SOURCE: Reprinted with permission of the publisher from p. 119 of Hans O. Mauksch, "The Organizational Context of Nursing Practice," in *The Nursing Profession: Five Sociological Essays*, ed. Fred Davis. © 1966 by John Wiley and Sons, Inc.

Assessing Pros and Cons of Procedures

The question of *who* decides what is good for patients is compounded by the problem that many good acts also have risks of bad consequences. Few medical procedures are so simple as to be free from harmful side effects. A few interventions—such as a back rub, a bed bath, a cup of tea, quiet company—can be administered respectfully, caringly, and professionally without hesitating over the goals of treatment. Most courses, however, are riskier.

Some antibiotics, although they treat infections, can also cause fatal disorders such as kidney failure or aplastic anemia. Other drugs, such as cancer chemotherapy, will certainly damage patients, via nausea, hair loss, and loss of appetite, even if they save their lives. Cardiopulmonary resuscitation or major surgery may be the only lifesaving options in some circumstances, but these procedures carry substantial health risks.[4] Sometimes clinicians are completely uncertain whether a therapy will be beneficial. For instance, in a debilitated intensive care unit patient, a respirator may assist in a dramatic recovery or it may lengthen a period of declining quality of life and increasing suffering. How should patients and health personnel weigh these pros and cons?

One traditional answer found in both nursing and medicine is *do no harm,* or in its Latin phrasing, *primum non nocere.* It is often attributed to the Hippocratic Oath, but its origins lie in another Hippocratic work, *The Epidemics.*[5] Though most often cited in medical ethics, it appears in the nursing ethics literature. Florence Nightingale wrote: "It may seem a strange principle to enunciate as the very first requirement in a Hospital that it should do the sick no harm."[6] Taken literally, this principle would be impossible to follow in practice, since only the simplest forms of treatment do no harm. This principle should be read as: *It is more important to avoid doing harm than it is to do good.* The do-no-harm principle warns against excessive risk taking with patients—a hazard of task-oriented competence. For example, in the late 1970s a surgeon was doing prophylactic breast surgery in women without breast lumps but with several risk factors for breast cancer. The physician *may* have saved the lives of these patients, but all we are *sure* that he did was to surgically maim his patients. The do-no-harm principle warns against procedures like this that do harm for the sake of speculative benefits. The do-no-harm principle is also expressed by conceptions of nursing competence that emphasize patient safety and care in checking doses of medications.

Another common principle for handling risks and benefits is *treat the whole person.* To treat the whole person is to attend to all the consequences of treatment to the patient and to see the patient as a whole individual who cannot be divided into independent sets of concerns or independent specialties. If approaches to care are too specialized, the wound specialist may treat the surgical incision and neglect harm to digestion, or the specialist in diabetes may be less interested in whether the patient dies than in what the blood sugar level was at death. This dehumanization is displayed by such language as, "I'm taking care of bed eight tonight."

[4]For a study of the risks of surgery, see John P. Bunker, Benjamin A. Barnes, and Frederick Mosteller, eds. *Costs, Risks, and Benefits of Surgery* (New York: Oxford University Press, 1977).

[5]*The Genuine Works of Hippocrates,* trans. Francis Adams (Melbourne, Fla.: R.E. Krieger Publishing Co., Inc., 1972), p. 104.

[6]Florence Nightingale, *Notes on Hospitals,* 3rd ed. (London: Longman, Green, Longman, Roberts, and Green, 1863), p. iii.

By calling attention to the whole picture in an integrated fashion, the treat-the-whole-person concept forces us to attend to the wide range of harms and benefits possible from health care. These considerations may be very diverse. Treatment of lower back pain may be hindered by psychological factors arising from the patient's unconscious fears that recovery will require resuming burdensome tasks. Financial cost may be an important concern to some patients. An overweight man may have to adjust his whole life-style in order to obey the doctor's order to "lay off the beer." A Jehovah's Witness mother may bleed to death in childbirth, happy to die in the cause of her faith. The treat-the-whole-person principle does not tell us how to balance these considerations of risk and benefits, but it reminds us to pay attention to them.

Our most common means of *calculating* the balance of pros and cons is *risk-benefit* analysis. This mode of calculation takes two factors into account. It considers the *value or disvalue of an outcome* measured in dollars, cases found, lives saved, lives lost, an estimate of utility, or any relevant measure of value that can be quantified. And it considers the *probability of the outcome*. It combines these two factors arithmetically (value times probability) in order to give an overall *expected value* of an outcome. To make choices by this method, one compares the expected values of different choices and selects that course of action yielding the highest expected value or the lowest expected disvalue.

For example, consider deciding to have a baby when there is some risk of birth defects. First, we assign a measure to the value of our overall life experience. For example, we could rate the best sort of experience as a +10, and the worst sort of experience as a −10. One possible calculation for the question Shall I have a baby? might look like this:

Choice		Value ×	Probability =	Expected Value
Having a baby	if it is normal	+10	.75	7.5 } Sum = 6.2
	if it is abnormal	−5	.25	−1.2
Not having a baby		+5	1.00	5.0

The Expected Value of Having a Baby Is Higher by 1.2

In this case, the outcome of the calculation was to give a risk-benefit argument for choosing to have a baby. If the risks of a birth defect were higher, the value of having a baby lower, or the disvalue of a defective baby greater, then the calculation would quickly balance toward not having a baby.

Home versus hospital births are a common controversy and could conceivably be subjected to risk-benefit analysis using primitive "value-of-life-experience" estimates. The question is, Should I have my baby at home or at the hospital? The calculation might look like this:

Choice		Value ×	Probability =	Expected Value
In hospital	good outcome	6	.95	5.7 } Sum = 5.6
	bad outcome	−2	.05	−0.1
At home	good outcome	10	.90	9.0 } Sum = 8.5
	bad outcome	−5	.10	−0.5

The Expected Value of a Home Birth Is Higher by 2.9

Since in this case the expected value of the home birth outweighs the expected value of the hospital birth, it would be the choice favored by risk-benefit analysis. If the risks of home birth were higher, or if it made little difference whether one experienced birth at home or in the hospital, then the balance might shift in favor of hospital births. I have made up figures to illustrate the method, but the reader can make similar calculations using figures based on appropriate probabilities and personal value judgments. The methods presented here are very simple, but complex realities can be better analyzed by a variety of more sensitive mathematical tools.[7]

These analytic methods have the advantages of forcing us to display our choices, possible outcomes, and values clearly. Yet they also have limitations. For instance, it is not clear that linearly calculated ratios represent truly rational judgments. If one takes the do-no-harm principle seriously, one would want most of all to avoid harm. One would then not be concerned with maximizing the benefit-to-risk ratio. Instead, one would give extra weight to ratios that involve lower risk figures irrespective of the benefits. This method does not distinguish people who like to take risks from those who prefer a surer course of action. For example, decisions on cancer therapy are sometimes made by calculating risks and benefits. A study on choosing between surgery and radiation treatment for thoracic cancer showed that the usual calculation of survival in terms of five-year survival may not represent the whole story. Although surgery has a better five-year survival rate than radiation, patients may prefer radiation to surgery. This is because hardly anyone dies immediately of radiation treatment, but there is about a 15-percent immediate postsurgical mortality rate for this condition. Once they survive, surgical patients are likely to live longer than irradiated patients. But very few patients are gamblers with their longevity: They would rather have the guaranteed life now than more probable life later. (Quality of life is about the same in both treatments.) More conservative patients would therefore prefer radiation to surgery despite worse five-year survival rates.[8]

Moreover, it is difficult to put a numerical value on many important considerations; indeed, numerical representations often do not even make sense. What is the value of having a baby? How much is a year of life worth compared to a week of intense pain? How much money is it worth to save a human life?[9] How should the pleasures of smoking be balanced against the health risks? The disparities of human values defy numerical analysis. Finally, these forms of analysis often do not make clear who receives benefits and who bears risks. One should distinguish in the home-birth dispute between risks to the mother and risks to the infant. Cost-benefit analyses often neglect to compare *who* pays the costs under different options.[10]

[7]A basic outline of methods of calculating costs, risks, and benefits is Richard Zeckhauser and Edith Stokey, *A Primer for Policy Analysis* (New York: W.W. Norton & Co., Inc., 1978).

[8]Barbara J. McNeil, Ralph Weichselbaum, and Stephen G. Pauker, "Fallacy of the Five-Year Survival in Lung Cancer," *The New England Journal of Medicine*, 299 (1978), 1397–1401.

[9]According to the "Ethical Aptitude Test," *Harper's* (October 1976), pp. 20–21, $28,000 is the value of a human life. Other estimates vary from this figure, mostly upward.

[10]For a discussion of ethical issues in the use of cost-benefit analysis, see The Hastings Center, "Values, Ethics, and CBA in Health Care," in *The Implications of Cost-Effectiveness Analysis of Medical Technology* (Washington, D.C.: Office of Technology Assessment, 1980), pp. 168–82.

Allocating Care among Patients

Hospital nurses are usually responsible for the care of several patients at one time. The nursing staff in a unit or on a ward may be collectively responsible for many patients. Nurses have considerable discretion in timing medications, administering tests, teaching, counseling, and consulting, and in managing indirect forms of patient support such as keeping records and ordering supplies. Nurses may have considerable control over patient access to physicians, and, where there are no telephones in patient rooms, to outside support. Nurses may decide how many patients they can adequately care for, and the head nurse of an intensive care unit may play an important role in deciding whether a patient can be admitted to the unit.

Thus nurses in the hospital must take a broad view and consider the needs of many patients. While traditional medical ethics creates the illusion that physicians can devote their entire attention to one patient, nurses are generally aware that they must allocate care among them. Finding the fairest way to allocate care is one of the first ethical problems that a nurse faces in the hospital. Respecting the good of patients thus becomes a complex exercise in balancing the good of many and requires of nurses a good sense of justice.

Patients do not normally participate in these decisions. There is no political process in hospitals by which patients can decide among themselves who needs the most care. Instead, nurses have the main responsibility for assessing patients' needs. Even where physicians speak for patients through their orders, nurses still must decide which orders are to be given priority. Because nurses are responsible for these decisions, they can be unforgiving of patients who are demanding, who claim to have needs they do not have, or who expect special favors. Uncomplaining patients may be seen as "good" patients because they facilitate work on the ward, just as a physician may perceive a nurse as "good" because he or she is obedient.

Nursing responsibility for allocating resources is most explicit in the role of the triage nurse in the emergency room.[11] The concept of *triage* originated in French military field hospitals, where a "triage officer" sorted wounded soldiers according to the amount of care they needed and the ease with which they could be returned to battle. The triage nurse determines the order in which patients will be treated, to maximize the good done by the emergency room. An emergency room sorting in one hospital is as follows:

Category 1: Care is urgently needed. The patient is to be seen right now.

Category 2: The patient presents serious problems that can nevertheless wait a little. The patient is to be seen within half an hour.

Category 3: The patient presents complex and nonurgent problems. The patient is referred to a special section for training interns and residents.

Category 4: The patient's problem is not serious. The patient is seen on a first-come-first-served basis when staff are free from treating patients in other categories. Much of the notorious emergency room waiting time falls, appropriately, on this group of patients.

An intuitively harsh but justifiable triage decision is sometimes made to let the most seriously hurt patients die. When staff is very short during a disaster, full-time devotion to those most likely to die keeps staff from attending to other patients who

---

[11]For a good study of triage, see Gerald R. Winslow, *Triage and Justice* (Berkeley, Calif.: University of California Press, 1982).

could survive with less care. A subtler form of this practice is that of a head nurse who practices triage by assigning the least competent nurse to the least salvageable patients.

Budgetary pressures tend to make staff shortages a common nursing problem. This policy is apt to create moral dilemmas for nurses by increasing the pressure on allocation decisions. These can sometimes be difficult.

> CASE EXAMPLE. The nurse is alone on a twenty-bed postcardiac surgery ward because the aide is out to dinner. Mrs. S. has been discussing her experience with the nurse. She is in crisis, about to "let go." At just that moment the food cart arrives on the ward. It is the nurse's job to serve it. The patients need their food while it is warm, and the food cart will be needed soon on other wards. The nurse is sure that if she leaves Mrs. S. for just a minute, the opportunity to help her will be lost.[12]

In this case, the nurse must balance justly the needs of one patient for communication in a crisis against the needs of twenty patients for dinner. There may be no good answer to this moral dilemma except to prevent its occurring.

Actual Practice

Is the good of the patient the highest concern of nurses? As with competence, this is difficult to answer. We have here at least two questions. One is a question about motivation. The other is about the actual impact of nursing work. The motivational question is concerned with what nurses desire, intend, or wish for in their interactions with patients. There is every reason to think that nurses are initially and consciously very concerned about the welfare of their patients, as indicated in a number of studies. For example, Olesen and Whittaker found that "demonstrating care and concern for others in an immediate and tangible way" was an important motive nursing students attributed to themselves in more than three-quarters of their sample.[13]

As was pointed out in the discussion of competence, it is hard to say whether this motive is realized in fact. Outcome studies assessing the actual impact of nurses on patient health are hard to find. In fact, some major demographic studies show a tenuous relationship between health care and health.[14] Yet health is not the only good nurses provide. Care and comfort, help for pain, protection during illness, encouragement and support, hope and humane concern are all immediate values arising from the nurse-patient relationship. These are good in themselves even if nurses do not affect patient health very much. Nor should we think that if nurses do not affect health much, they cannot. Historically, nurses have played an important

---

[12]Adapted from Marlene Kramer, *Reality Shock: Why Nurses Leave Nursing* (St. Louis: The C.V. Mosby Company, 1974), p. 1. About 70 percent of nurses regard serving meal trays as a nonnursing function, according to Karen Davis, "Non-Nursing Functions: Our Readers Respond," *American Journal of Nursing*, 82 (1982), 1858.

[13]Virginia L. Olesen and Elvi W. Whittaker, *The Silent Dialogue: A Study in the Social Psychology of Professional Socialization* (San Francisco: Jossey-Bass, Inc., Publishers, 1968), pp. 126–28.

[14]Thomas McKeown, *The Role of Medicine: Dream, Mirage, or Nemesis* (Oxford: Basil Blackwell, Ltd., 1979).

role in public health movements such as the Settlement House movement.[15] By pressing for improvements in the institutions delivering care, nurses can do much to make patient care more available and more effective.

Summary

Health is a basic value important to the overall welfare of patients. The value of nursing competence ultimately rests on the good it does for patients. By supporting clients' health, nurses work on behalf of the good of patients; supporting the good of patients is a major principle of nursing practice. This principle is expressed in such phrases as *do no harm* and *treat the whole patient*.

A major problem in serving the good of patients is that of *paternalism*. Paternalism is coercing others to do what is good for them. Most people support *weak* paternalism, that is, pressuring or manipulating *incompetent* people into doing what is good for them. *Strong* paternalism, directed to *competent* people and practiced widely in health care, is more controversial.

It is generally held that it is more important to avoid harming patients than it is to do them positive good. Since many procedures do both beneficial and harmful things to clients, methods have been developed for balancing harm against benefits. *Risk-benefit* analysis, for example, balances the *expected value* of benefits against the expected disvalue of harm.

Since resources are limited, benefits must be distributed among many patients. Patients should receive appropriate care, and no one should be unduly deprived. *Triage* is a policy of selecting patients for therapy in order to deliver the greatest overall good to patients when resources are scarce.

FURTHER READINGS

Patient Care

CALLAND, CHAD H., "Iatrogenic Problems in End-Stage Renal Failure," *The New England Journal of Medicine,* 287 (1972), 334–36.

CARPER, BARBARA A., "The Ethics of Caring," *Advances in Nursing Science,* 1, 3 (April 1979), 11–19.

COUSINS, NORMAN, "Anatomy of an Illness (As Perceived by the Patient)," *The New England Journal of Medicine,* 295, 26 (1976), 1458–63.

FIORE, NEIL, "Fighting Cancer—One Patient's Perspective," *The New England Journal of Medicine,* 300 (1979), 284–89.

LEONARD, CALISTA V., "Patient Attitudes toward Nursing Interventions," *Nursing Research,* 24, 5 (1975), 335–39.

ROTH, JULIUS A., "The Necessity and Control of Hospitalization," *Social Science and Medicine,* 6 (1972), 425–46.

UJHELY, GERTRUD B., *Determinants of the Nurse-Patient Relationship.* New York: Springer Publishing Co., Inc., 1968.

YEAWORTH, ROSALEE C., "The Agonizing Decisions in Mental Retardation," *American Journal of Nursing,* 77 (1977), 864–67.

[15]Lillian D. Wald, *Windows on Henry Street* (Boston: Little, Brown, & Company, 1934).

Nurses as Advocates

ABRAMS, NATALIE, "A Contrary View of the Nurse as Patient Advocate," *Nursing Forum*, 17 (1978), 258–67.

BANDMAN, ELSIE L., "The Rights of Nurses and Patients: A Case for Advocacy," in *Bioethics and Human Rights: A Reader for Health Professionals*, eds. Elsie L. Bandman and Bertram Bandman, pp. 332–38. Boston: Little, Brown & Company, 1978.

BANDMAN, ELSIE L., AND BERTRAM BANDMAN, "The Nurse's Role in Protecting the Patient's Right to Live or Die," *Advances in Nursing Science*, 1, 3 (April 1979), 21–35.

BANDMAN, ELSIE, AND BERTRAM BANDMAN, "There Is Nothing Automatic about Rights," *American Journal of Nursing*, 77 (May 1977), 867–72.

BELL, NORA K., "Whose Autonomy Is at Stake?" *American Journal of Nursing*, 81 (1981), 1170–72.

CLEMENCE, SISTER MADELEINE, "Existentialism: A Philosophy of Commitment," *American Journal of Nursing*, 66 (1966), 500–505.

CURTIN, LEAH L., "The Nurse as Advocate: A Philosophical Foundation for Nursing," *Advances in Nursing Science*, 1, 3 (April 1979), 1–10.

GADOW, SALLY, "Existential Advocacy: Philosophical Foundation of Nursing," in *Nursing: Images and Ideals: Opening Dialogue with the Humanities*, eds. Stuart F. Spicker and Sally Gadow, pp. 79–101. New York: Springer Publishing Co., Inc., 1980.

SKLAR, CORINNE, "Patient's Advocate—A New Role for the Nurse?" *Canadian Nurse* (June 1979), 39–41.

SMITH, CHRISTINE SPAHN, "Outrageous or Outraged: A Nurse Advocate Story," *Nursing Outlook* (October 1980), 624–25.

ZUSMAN, JACK, "Think Twice about Being a Patient Advocate," *Nursing Life* (November/December 1982), 46–50.

CHAPTER 8

Nonexploitation:

Nurses Should Not
Use Their Positions
to Exploit Patients

The last chapter examined thinking about the patient's good when it is the center of attention. This chapter focuses on how the interests and goals of nurses and other health care providers create hazards to patients. The therapeutic interaction takes place in a social context that introduces factors not directly related to patient care: Nurses earn salaries, teach students, conduct research, gain emotional satisfactions, address personal needs, and so on. When these concerns override patient good or when nurses or others take advantage of their special relationship to patients, we become concerned with the potential for exploitation. *Exploitation* occurs when exchanges between patients and health care providers become unfair or too costly to patients, especially when patients are in a relatively poor position to make choices. The ANA code refers in passing to the potential for exploitation, but mainly in relationship to the use of the RN title outside of regular professional practice:

> The title and other symbols of the profession should not be used, however, for personal benefit by the nurse or by those who may seek to exploit them for other purposes. (Point 10.2, ANA, 1976)

No ethical inconsistency or inevitable conflict stands between compensating nurses for patient care and providing good care to patients. A nurse might seek to be famous as the world's best nurse by providing exquisite patient care. But the interests of health care professionals and institutions can become too powerful and threaten the quality of patient care or take too much from patients. The resolution of problems of exploitation does not lie in determining whether the self-interest of professionals or altruistic devotion to patients should prevail. Instead, such conflicts require creating real situations in which the potential for conflicts of interest between patient and professional are reduced and where fair and voluntary exchanges—nonexploitative exchanges—are fostered.

The present setting of health care delivery, however, provides many occasions for exploitation. These do not normally arise from conscious intentions of health professionals. They are instead natural products of the character and power imbalance of the professional-patient relationship as determined by current forms of health care delivery. Scrupulousness is needed in order to avoid exploitation of patients, and a good sense of irony is needed to cope with situations where it is unavoidable.

The following sections outline issues in some common areas of potential exploitation of patients. They treat gifts and tips; fees, salaries, and profits; theft; experimentation; education and training; emotional exploitation; and hospital routine.

Gifts and Tips

Gifts play an important role in personal reactions to death and disease. Volunteers are common in health care; large charitable funds support research on the diseases of children; blood donorship[1] and organ donorship[2] are widespread practices. Grateful clients sometimes show appreciation through tangible gifts. But should nurses accept gifts or tips? Is doing so fair to patients?

We should first distinguish gifts from tips. Both gifts and tips may be either in money or in kind. Although tips are partly intended as expressions of gratitude for service, they are different from gifts in that they are expected and part of the basic compensation for work. Tips are like fees—they are charges for services rendered— but they are different from fees in that they are not fixed in advance. Gifts are given over and above basic compensation for work performed. Gifts should not be expected, and work should not be done in order to obtain them.

Should nurses accept tips? In most hospitals, nurses cannot accept tips as I have defined them. In most hospitals, nurses receive their full financial compensation in salaries and benefits, so that small presents of money are gifts, not tips. Would it be professional or ethical for a nurse to practice by relying on tips? Such a relationship would place considerable economic power in patients' hands and would probably not harm them. On the other hand, accepting tips is usually a symbol placing the recipient lower in status than the tipper. Those who associate professionalism with prestige would regard accepting tips as unprofessional. And if relying on tips led to low levels of compensation for nurses, this would be unfair to them and threaten their welfare.

Should nurses accept gifts? Of course, but accepting them takes some consideration. Six areas of concern are:

1. One should first ask whether the offering is really a gift and not a bribe or purchase.
2. One should then consider the principle of *reciprocity*.[3] Gift giving is an ancient and deeply rooted human custom. In the complete transaction, gifts are *ex-*

[1]For an excellent discussion of blood donorship, see Richard Titmuss, *The Gift Relationship: From Human Blood to Social Policy* (New York: Random House, Inc., 1972).

[2]H. Harrison Sadler et al., "The Living, Genetically Unrelated Kidney Donor," in *Psychiatric Aspects of Organ Transplantation: 3. Seminars in Psychiatry,* ed. Pietro Castelnuevo-Tedesco (New York: Grune & Stratton, Inc., 1971).

[3]Marcel Mauss, *The Gift* (New York: W.W. Norton & Co., Inc., 1967).

changed. If one receives a gift, one must *reciprocate* in order to bring the relationship back into balance. A gift from a patient to a nurse should normally be the second half of a reciprocal transaction: The patient gives a gift *in return* for one given the patient by the nurse. It is important to ask what the nurse gave in the first place. If the nurse gave little or has already been compensated, then the gift would be inappropriate.

3. One should next appreciate the distinction between tangible and intangible exchanges. A tangible gift is often a symbol of an intangible gift of care and compassion. But as gifts become larger, their tangible features become more important. One needs to ask, What does this gift mean to the donor? What does it mean to the recipient? Families who give the nurse a $100 bill in advance for special care of a patient are offering bribes, not gifts. A hospital that places pressure on nurses to provide special care to wealthy patients turns potential gifts to the hospital from these patients into tips or purchases.

4. The gift, in some cases, may be a sacrifice to the gods in gratitude for safe passage. In such a case, it is most appropriate for the nurse to pass the gift on as a donation to a good cause.

5. One should also notice whether one has in some way solicited or invited the gift. One can grow to expect gifts from clients. An obstetrician who had delivered the baby of an opera singer wistfully complained, "And she didn't even give me any tickets to a performance."

6. One should consider what refusing the gift would mean to the patient. Caring for patients can result in a deep human relationship that transcends professional roles. To refuse a gift may be to deny that relationship. Refusals may say, "I gave you nothing" or "I am in power here, not you."

Many nurses accept gifts. Units are mined with boxes of candy. Nurses find $5 bills stuffed in their pockets. Items made by patients, such as ceramic candlesticks, works of needlepoint, and small paintings, are common gifts.[4] *Nursing '74* posed the following question in a survey of its readers:

> Nurse Sharon receives a letter with $100 from a former patient who was very pleased with Sharon's care and concern. If you were in Sharon's place, what would you do?[5]

Overall, the survey found the respondents divided on whether they would accept the money. Thirty percent said they would have kept the money. Fifty-one percent thought they would return it. Fourteen percent would give it to charity and 5 percent would have shared it with other nurses.

The higher nurses ranked in administration and the longer they had been in nursing, the more likely they were to say that they would accept the $100 in Sharon's case. Twenty-three percent of nurses under twenty-two years old would keep the money, while 46 percent fifty years or older would do so. Twenty-eight percent of staff nurses said that they would keep the money, while 38 percent of nursing administrators said that they would. It would be interesting to study these differences. Do they represent growing disillusionment, shifting conceptions of the

[4]Helen E. Gordy, "Gift Giving in the Nurse-Patient Relationship," *American Journal of Nursing,* 78 (1978), 1027–28.

[5]Reprinted with permission from "Nursing Ethics: The Admirable Professional Standards of Nurses, A Survey Report, Part II," p. 65, from the October issue of *Nursing '74.* Copyright © 1983 Springhouse Corporation. All rights reserved.

nurse as a professional, increasing sensitivity to clients' needs, or better self-knowledge?

Fees, Salaries, and Profits

Nurses do not pay patients for the opportunity to work with them. Neither do they work as unpaid volunteers. Instead, they receive and are entitled to payment for their services. What patients pay for these services, whether out-of-pocket or by insurance and taxes, should be neither excessive nor beyond public control. The professional ideal of providing socially worthwhile services should be balanced against the public costs of maintaining the health professions. Many have argued that health care is too costly, too profitable, and insufficiently controlled by consumers (see pp. 267–70). They charge, in short, that health care exploits patients economically. This charge is highly controversial, and discussion covers a wide range of economic features of health care.

CONTROL. Some economists claim that health care prices and services are effectively determined by providers, not clients.[6] For instance, government and insurance programs may reimburse hospitals on a cost-plus basis; physicians may agree among themselves on fees; and insurance companies may set rates of reimbursement without consulting patients. Since decisions about diagnostic tests and therapies are made largely by physicians, some economists claim that increasing the supply of physicians tends to increase the costs of care rather than increase competition and reduce prices.[7] Increasingly, health care services are provided by large national organizations, such as hospital and nursing home franchises and health maintenance organizations.[8]

COSTS. A significant and increasing proportion of the Gross National Product is devoted to health care. This proportion was 9.8 percent in 1981, and annual health expenditures in the U.S. were about $1,225 per capita, 42.7 percent of which was paid by public funds.[9] In 1981, the daily charges for a semiprivate hospital room in San Francisco ranged from $197 to $302, and intensive care unit charges were from $406 to $995 per day.[10] Although figures vary widely, a representative study found that mean hospital charges for the last two weeks of patients' lives ranged from $3,333 to $11,645 and averaged $6,180. The last two weeks of dying at home ran from $137 to $1,162 with a mean of $586.[11]

PROFITS AND INCOME. Whether some health care providers make too much money is a common subject of dispute. Physicians, whose average annual net

[6]Victor R. Fuchs, *Who Shall Live? Health, Economics, and Social Choice* (New York: Basic Books, Inc., Publishers, 1974), p. 11.

[7]Charles T. Stewart and C.M. Siddayao, *Increasing the Supply of Medical Personnel: Needs and Alternatives* (Washington, D.C.: American Enterprise Institute for Public Policy Research, 1973), p. 10.

[8]Arnold S. Relman, "The New Medical-Industrial Complex, *The New England Journal of Medicine*, 303 (1980), 963–70.

[9]Robert M. Gibson and Daniel R. Waldo, "National Health Expenditures, 1981," *Health Care Financing Review*, 4 (1982), 1.

[10]"Your Bill of Health," *San Francisco Examiner*, November 30 and December 3, 1981.

[11]Bernard S. Bloom and Priscilla D. Kissick, "Home and Hospital Cost of Terminal Illness," *Medical Care*, 18 (1980), 561.

income was $86,000 in 1982,[12] are often mentioned, but attention is seldom drawn to other highly salaried beneficiaries of health care, such as executives of hospitals and of pharmaceutical, equipment, and insurance companies. In 1981, top executives of large national companies of these types received annual salaries in a range of about $200,000 to $600,000, and benefits and stock options brought figures for some of these officers to more than $1,000,000 per year.[13]

Providing health care can also be profitable for investors. As one study charges,

> Analyzed in terms of all of its functions, the medical industry emerges as a coherent, highly organized system. One particular function—patient care—may be getting slighted, . . . The most obvious function of the American medical system, other than patient care, is profit-making. When it comes to making money, the health industry is an extraordinarily well-organized and efficient machine.[14]

Eighteen pharmaceutical companies were on the "Fortune 500" list in 1982 and rated high among industry medians in returns on sales and stockholders' equity. Measuring, scientific, and photographic equipment companies, many of which manufacture medical equipment, also rank favorably according to these indications.[15] A private company which in 1980 treated 17 percent of the nation's approximately 48,000 dialysis patients had profits in 1979 of $19 million on revenues of $190 million.[16]

NEW TECHNOLOGY. Highly technological forms of patient care, such as intensive and coronary care units, tend to develop and become widely used without having been shown to be beneficial to clients overall.[17] How and why they develop is a controversial issue, but it is clear that economic factors play an important role.[18]

CORRUPT PRACTICES. The debate over the legitimacy of normal and standard fiscal exchanges in health care is barely distinguishable from the debate over what constitutes corrupt health care practices, that is, practices most of us could agree exploit patients. Because there is so much latitude in expert judgments of appropriate health care, charges of corrupt practices are difficult to substantiate. A clear example might be a hospital that regularly reuses supplies intended for one use

[12]Arthur Owens, "Where Do You Fit In?" *Medical Economics* (September 13, 1982), 247.

[13]"How Much Does the Boss Make?" *Forbes,* 127 (June 8, 1981), 114–46; and "Annual Survey of Executive Compensation," *Business Week* (May 11, 1981), 58–59+.

[14]From p. 21 of Barbara Ehrenreich and John Ehrenreich, *The American Health Empire: Power, Profits, and Politics,* copyright © 1970 by Random House, Inc., New York.

[15]"Fortune 500," *Fortune Magazine* (May 3, 1982), 258–86.

[16]Gina Bari Kolata, "NMC Thrives Selling Dialysis," *Science,* 208 (1980), 379–82.

[17]Arnold S. Relman and Drummond Rennie, "Treatment of End-Stage Renal Disease: Free but Not Equal," *The New England Journal of Medicine,* 303 (1980), 996–98; Howard Waitzkin, "How Capitalism Cares for Our Coronaries: A Preliminary Exercise in Political Economy," in *The Doctor-Patient Relationship in the Changing Health Scene,* ed. Eugene B. Gallagher (Washington, D.C.: John E. Fogarty International Center for Advanced Study in the Health Sciences, 1978), pp. 317–32; Louise B. Russell, *Technology in Hospitals: Medical Advances and Their Diffusion* (Washington, D.C.: The Brookings Institution, 1979); Richard E. Brown, *Rockefeller Medicine Men: Medicine and Capitalism in America* (Berkeley, Calif.: University of California Press, 1979), pp. 228–35.

[18]Howard Waitzkin, "A Marxist View of Medical Care," *Annals of Internal Medicine,* 89 (1978), 264–78.

only or that purchases defective equipment in order to obtain discounts. There is wide agreement that overuse of diagnostic tests is widespread and that many therapies are prescribed excessively, but there are many disputes over specific instances.[19] One drug company executive testified that he estimated about half of all prescriptions were not medically indicated.[20] A 1972 study found that anti-microbiological medication was prescribed irrationally in over 65 percent of cases according to a review team.[21] A consumer group charged that one out of five pacemakers is installed unnecessarily.[22] Wheelchair manufacturers have been said to manufacture substandard equipment at inflated prices.[23] Government officials have estimated that fraud and abuse account for about 10 to 25 percent of Medicare costs.[24] Some alcohol treatment centers have been charged with shipping clients from one state to another and duplicating diagnostic tests in the process to evade government reimbursement limits.[25] Some have charged nursing homes with colluding with physicians and pharmacy companies to take advantage of government-funded cost-plus contracts.

> Medicaid alone pays out an estimated $200 million a year for drugs for its nursing home patients. From the evidence already accumulated about this business, it is a fair estimate that at least half of that bill is padding: that is, if only the needed drugs were ordered, and if the price was right, the government would be paying out less than half what it pays now—and patients who are now overdrugged would be healthier.[26]

BUSINESS ETHICS.   Not only is it difficult to determine what constitutes a legitimate health care service, but it is also difficult to determine whether business transactions in health care should be assessed by the standards of business ethics or health care ethics. Practices commonly accepted in business may appear ethically tainted in health care.[27] For instance, a manufacturer may donate a large piece of

[19]Stephen J. McPhee, Lois P. Myers, and Steven A. Schroeder, "The Costs and Risks of Medical Care: An Annotated Bibliography for Clinicians and Educators," *Western Journal of Medicine*, 137 (1982), 145–61. Section II "The Problem of Overutilization," pp. 148–50, contains good references to instances of overutilized tests and therapies. See also Brendan Phibbs, "The Abuse of Coronary Arteriography," *The New England Journal of Medicine*, 301 (1979), 1394–96.

[20]*Encyclopedia of Bioethics*, 1978 ed., s.v. "Drug Industry and Medicine," by Harris L. Coulter.

[21]Andrew W. Roberts and James A. Visconti, "The Rational and Irrational Use of Systemic Antimicrobial Drugs," *American Journal of Hospital Pharmacy*, 29 (1972), 1054.

[22]Mary Knudson, "Pacemakers Held Unneeded in 1 Case in 5," *Baltimore Sun*, July 8, 1982; Kevin P. Helliker, "Pacemaker Firm Has a Few Palpitations As Its Profits Shrink," *Wall Street Journal*, December 30, 1982, pp. 1, 12.

[23]Betty Medsger, "Most Captive Consumers," *Progressive*, 43 (March 1979), 34–39.

[24]"Those High Hospital Bills Aren't Always Right," *U.S. News and World Report* (May 17, 1982).

[25]Paul Jacobs, "Raleigh Hills Patients Shifted to Escape Medicare Limits," *Los Angeles Times*, April 15, 1982.

[26]From p. 177 of Mary Adelaide Mendelson, *Tender Loving Greed*, copyright © 1975 by Random House, Inc., New York.

[27]Robert M. Cunningham, Jr., "Changing Philosophies in Medical Care and the Rise of the Investor-Owned Hospital," *The New England Journal of Medicine*, 307 (1982), 817–19; Richard Quinney, "Occupational Structure and Criminal Behavior: Prescription Violation by Retail Pharmacists," *Social Problems*, 11 (1963), 179–85; and Roxane Spitzer, "The Nurse in the Corporate World," *Supervisor Nurse* (April 1981), 21–24.

equipment to a hospital for research and patient care in the hope that this will result in future purchases. From the perspective of business ethics, this is a perfectly acceptable practice, but the clinicians who accept the equipment could be accused of allowing a financial rather than a health concern to determine the course of care.

Advertising is widely accepted as a legitimate business practice, but its effect on sound health care is questionable. In the mid-1970s, pharmaceutical companies spent about $5,000 annually per physician on advertising. They devoted about 25 percent of their gross income to advertising and only 9 percent to research. About 80 percent of the 9 percent spent on research was for packaging, flavoring, and designing pills and liquids. Four of the five trade journals with the largest advertising income in the United States were medical journals. Occasionally, drug companies have distorted research results indicating medication hazards.[28] In countries less restrictive than the U.S. about publishing indications and contraindications of medications, drug companies publish more indications and fewer contraindications in physicians' reference manuals.[29] As one critic observed,

> When the so-called morals of the marketplace are applied to drugs that can be invaluable when used properly, the result is not only the prostitution of science. It also means that physicians and pharmacists are uninformed or misinformed. Moreover, it means that patients are needlessly harmed.[30]

However, it is clear that hope of profit and economic development play an important role.

Nurses work amid these broad economic influences. As the "middle class" among hospital workers, they cooperate in acts producing economic abuses. At the same time, nurses have historically been more exploited than exploiting, and they have been paid poorly in comparison with others with similar educational backgrounds and tasks. In recent years, increased activism by unions and professional organizations has begun to increase salaries rapidly. A survey by *R.N.* indicated that in 1979 staff nurses were paid an average annual salary of about $13,000, while nursing administrators received about $20,000 and head nurses and supervisors about $17,700.[31] In 1982, the Veterans Administration, which tends to pay nurses slightly above average salaries, used a salary schedule ranging from $14,328 to $36,723, with a mean in the $22,000 to $23,000 range.[32] In a period of concern over health care costs, how should nurses press for economic equity without joining overpaid providers in exploiting clients? As workers in a financially inequitable system of rewards, can nurses keep their hands clean of exploitation?

These are difficult and important questions. The problems of economic exploitation in health care are linked with similar problems throughout society. As long as we accept gross economic inequality as a social norm, it will be difficult to

[28]Summarized from Coulter, "Drug Industry and Medicine," and Milton Silverman and Philip R. Lee, *Pills, Profits, and Politics* (Berkeley, Calif.: University of California Press, 1974).

[29]Milton Silverman, *The Drugging of the Americas* (Berkeley, Calif.: University of California Press, 1976).

[30]Ibid., p. xi.

[31]Andrea L. Lucas, "What's Nursing Worth?" *R.N.*, 43, 1 (January 1980), 31–39, 83.

[32]"VA Raises Show Where Nursing Pay Is Up (and Where It Isn't)," *American Journal of Nursing*, 82 (1982), 1188, 1197.

distinguish exploitative from nonexploitative financial exchanges. Economic exploitation is an ethical problem that is insoluble within the limits of the four basic conventions of health care ethics. Exploitation arises from factors that go well beyond the borders of health care.

Theft

Since nurses customarily administer medications, they have opportunities to take them for their own use. Half of a dose of morphine may go to the patient and the other half to the nurse, while the placebo effect takes up the slack. Nurses have also been known to take money and other property from patients. These acts of theft illustrate well the distinction between the *nonexploitation* and the *patient-good* principles. Taking patients' medications is not nursing practice that fails to respect the good of the patient; it is not nursing practice at all—one takes personal advantage of one's relationship with patients at their expense.

Stealing from patients is not usually addressed in codes of ethics, since its prohibition is well established as a conventional principle of the culture in which nurses practice. Abuse of medications is a common reason that nurses lose their licenses (see pp. 81–82); not because it is a common practice, but because it is a clear violation of professional responsibility.

Taking medications, equipment, and supplies from hospital stock, however, is a more common practice. Although it involves taking unauthorized advantage of one's position, it does not involve exploiting patients directly. The *Nursing '74* survey found that 1 percent of women nurses and 3 percent of men said that they had taken prescription drugs from their work place. Eighty percent think that, in general, "nurses take *medication* (other than aspirin and antacids) from hospitals for their own use."[33] Taking aspirin for a headache while on duty is too common to survey and a conventionally acceptable practice.[34]

Experimentation

Clinical experimentation introduces a second motive to patient care, that of finding out something. Where research dominates patient good, patients may be exploited. As clinical investigators and as participants in selecting and caring for subjects during research done by others, nurses should be aware of the ethical hazards of this enterprise.

Ethical problems in research have an ancient history. In this history, extremes of ethics can be found. On one hand, experimenters have occasionally sacrificed their own lives heroically for the sake of knowledge.[35] On the other, they have

---

[33]"Nursing Ethics: A Survey Report," p. 56.

[34]The issue of theft arose early in the nursing profession. On the theft of alcohol from hospital stock, see Irene Sabelberg Palmer, "Florence Nightingale and the Salisbury Incident," *Nursing Research*, 25 (1976), 370–77.

[35]Lawrence K. Altman, "Auto-Experimentation: An Unappreciated Tradition in Medical Science," *The New England Journal of Medicine*, 286 (1972), 346–52.

occasionally sacrificed unconsenting subjects painfully to satisfy their curiosity. For instance, prisoners have been the subjects of vivisection by physicians.[36] It was commonly believed in the 1950s and 1960s that medical experiments in the United States were immune to abuse due to the high ethical standards of the profession. However, in 1966 Harvard medical professor Henry Beecher was able to document a number of questionably ethical studies,[37] and further abuses came to public attention. Among the most well known instances were:

JEWISH CHRONIC DISEASE HOSPITAL.   Physicians injected live cancer cells into hospitalized elderly patients without telling them about it. They wanted to study the immune response and were sure that the patients would not get cancer. They were also sure that patients, were they informed, would not consent to the study.[38]

WILLOWBROOK.   Mentally retarded children were inoculated with hepatitis in order to study the disease. Parents or guardians consented, often because participants in the study could gain earlier admission to the hospital. Conditions in the institution were such that the children would have contracted hepatitis anyway.[39]

TUSKEGEE.   Rural black men were chosen as subjects in a longitudinal study of syphilis. The study began in the 1930s. Although a cure for syphilis was later found, it was decided not to treat them in order to complete the study.[40]

EXPERIMENTAL PREGNANCY.   Mexican-American women were given placebo birth control pills to study psychological side effects of oral contraceptives. They were not told of the placebos and many became pregnant.[41]

When these scandals came to light, medical research was being increasingly funded by the federal government. This created an opportunity for regulation. The Department of Health, Education, and Welfare (now the Department of Health and Human Services) established guidelines for the ethical conduct of experimentation and established a system of institutional review boards to oversee their application.[42] All experimentation in institutions receiving DHHS funds must be reviewed

[36]*Encyclopedia of Bioethics*, 1978 ed., s.v. "Human Experimentation: History," by Gert H. Brieger.

[37]Henry K. Beecher, "Ethics and Clinical Research," *The New England Journal of Medicine*, 274 (1966), 1354–60.

[38]Elinor Langer, "Human Experimentation: New York Verdict Affirms Patient's Rights," *Science*, 151 (1966), 663–66.

[39]Samuel Gorovitz et al., eds., *Moral Problems in Medicine* (Englewood Cliffs, N.J.: Prentice-Hall, Inc., 1976), pp. 123–42.

[40]United States Public Health Service, "Final Report of the Tuskegee Syphilis Study Ad Hoc Advisory Panel (1973)," in *Ethics in Medicine: Historical Perspectives and Contemporary Concerns*, eds. Stanley Joel Reiser, Arthur J. Dyck, and William J. Curran (Cambridge, Mass.: The MIT Press, 1977), pp. 316–21.

[41]Robert M. Veatch, "Experimental Pregnancy," *Hastings Center Report*, 1 (June 1971), 2–3.

[42]The National Commission for the Protection of Human Subjects of Biomedical and Behavioral Research, *Report and Recommendations: Institutional Review Boards* (Bethesda, Md.: Department of Health, Education, and Welfare, 1978).

by these boards. The review boards are dominated by physicians and scientists, although some nurses, other health care practitioners, lawyers, philosophers, and "outsiders" are normally included.[43]

Scientific progress is an important element in medical ideology. It is easy for experimenters to look beyond the patient's good to the good of future patients. For example, older consent forms given to subjects sometimes used such phrasing as, "in order to better understand your disease." Was the patient to read this as a reference to his or her *own* case, or as a reference to *others* who had the same disease? Medical and nursing school faculty depend on research for support and advancement, and the schools are dependent on research to maintain their budgets. These factors create incentives for practitioners to impose risks upon patients for motives extrinsic to patient good.

Because practitioners have become aware of this potential, the literature on the ethics of experimentation is extensive, and sensitive analyses of its problems are not hard to find. The ANA code lists general guidelines outlining obligations of nurses participating in research.

1. To ascertain that the study design has been approved by an appropriate body.
2. To obtain information about the intent and nature of the research.
3. To determine whether the research is consistent with professional goals (Point 7.2, ANA, 1976).

Nurses interested in conducting research or cooperating in research should keep a number of precautions in mind.

1. Ascertain how realistic intentions to benefit the patient are blended with the interest in research. When research is clearly nontherapeutic in intent, this can be made clear to subjects and researchers alike. But when therapy is conducted partly in the hope of benefiting clients as well as gaining knowledge, as is often the case in cancer chemotherapy research, it is important for nurses to delineate clearly how experimental procedures modify patient care.[44]
2. Participation in research should never be a condition of receipt of care. This needs to be made clear to patients.[45]
3. The knowledge sought should be worthwhile; the experiment, well designed; and the experimenter, competent to perform the study.[46]
4. The experimental design should impose the least risk possible to subjects. Sometimes risks are so great that they should not be undertaken, even if the knowledge gained is important and even if subjects consent.[47]
5. Potential subjects with special vulnerabilities warrant special protection. For example, young children, mentally ill persons, retarded persons, prisoners,

---

[43]Bradford H. Gray, "An Assessment of Institutional Review Committees in Human Experimentation," *Medical Care,* 13 (1975), 318–28.

[44]For a brief discussion, see Joseph V. Brady and Albert R. Jonsen, "The Evolution of Regulatory Influences on Research with Human Subjects," in *Human Subjects Research: A Handbook for Institutional Review Boards,* eds. Robert A. Greenwald, Mary Kay Ryan, and James E. Mulvihill (New York: Plenum Publishing Corporation, 1982).

[45]Robert J. Levine, *Ethics and Regulation of Clinical Research* (Baltimore: Urban & Schwarzenberg, Inc., 1981), pp. 84–88.

[46]LeRoy Walters, "Some Ethical Issues in Research Involving Human Subjects," *Perspectives in Biology and Medicine,* 20 (1977), 193–211.

[47]Ibid.

institutionalized elderly persons, dying persons, and desperate persons require special protection.[48] Some argue that they should never be subjected to experimentation.[49]

6. Patients should be fairly selected for treatment.[50] One's most vulnerable patients should not be chosen for one's riskiest study.[51]
7. Patients should neither be undercompensated nor overcompensated for participation in a study. Compensation should be available for those injured in a study.[52]
8. Termination and follow-up should be considered. If the proposed new treatment does not work and the study comes to an end, what will you do for your clients afterward?
9. Risks to others besides the patient should be considered. For example, who will use the information? Will it be used for the benefit of people?[53]
10. Subjects must give their informed consent to participation.[54] Signing a form is not enough. Most consent forms make difficult reading,[55] and a complex experiment may require time-consuming and careful explanation.[56]
11. Subjects should be free to drop out of a study at any time.

Nurses are frequently aware of the moral ambiguities in research and have cooperated reluctantly in procedures they felt would not help their patients. Sometimes nurses are dubious about the benefits of "high-tech" medicine, and this increases their reluctance to assist in or undertake studies. Since patients are not morally obligated to participate in experiments, nurses sensitive to these issues may

[48]For thorough reports on some vulnerable populations see the *Reports and Recommendations,* with *Appendices,* of the National Commission for the Protection of Human Subjects of Biomedical and Behavioral Research on *Research Involving Children* (Bethesda, Md.: Department of Health, Education, and Welfare, 1977), *Research Involving Prisoners* (1976), *Research Involving Those Institutionalized as Mentally Infirm* (1978), and *Research on the Fetus* (1976).

[49]Paul Ramsey, *The Patient As Person: Explorations in Medical Ethics* (New Haven, Conn.: Yale University Press, 1970).

[50]Levine, *Ethics,* pp. 49–68; and Walters, "Some Ethical Issues."

[51]Ward patients end up in risky studies more often than private patients. See Bernard Barber, "The Ethics of Experimentation with Human Subjects," *Scientific American,* 234 (February 1976), 25–31.

[52]President's Commission for the Study of Ethical Problems in Medicine and Biomedical and Behavioral Research, *Compensating for Research Injuries: A Report on the Ethical and Legal Implications of Programs to Redress Injuries Caused by Biomedical and Behavioral Research, Volume One: Report* (Washington, D.C.: U.S. Government Printing Office, 1982).

[53]Margaret Mead, "Research with Human Beings: A Model Derived from Anthropological Field Practice," in *Experimentation with Human Subjects,* ed. Paul A. Freund (New York: George Braziller, Inc., 1969); and Edward Diener and Rick Crandall, *Ethics in Social and Behavioral Research* (Chicago: University of Chicago Press, 1978), pp. 195–212.

[54]John Fletcher, "Human Experimentation: Ethics in the Consent Situation," *Law and Contemporary Problems,* 32 (1967), 620–49; Jay Katz, with the assistance of Alexander Morgan Capron and Eleanor Swift Glass, *Experimentation with Human Beings* (New York: Russell Sage Foundation, 1972), pp. 521–608; and Levine, *Ethics,* pp. 69–116.

[55]Gary R. Morrow, "How Readable Are Subject Consent Forms?" *Journal of the American Medical Association,* 244 (1980), 56–58.

[56]Bradford H. Gray, *Human Subjects in Medical Experimentation* (New York: John Wiley & Sons, Inc., 1975) is an excellent study of the failure of explanation.

be able to protect patients from studies that impose on them.[57] Nurses who initiate studies in the psychosocial aspects of nursing practice need to consider issues particularly associated with social science research, such as avoiding deception and psychological consequences of inquiry.[58]

Education and Training

Every skilled occupation needs opportunities to educate its future practitioners. In nursing, many skills can only be learned by working with patients. This poses an ethical problem, because work done by student nurses is presumably less skilled than work done by experienced clinicians. What if teaching motives dominate patient-care motives, and patients receive worse care so that nurses can be trained? What if risks sometimes have to be taken for teaching purposes? Would we say this is clinically acceptable because without students there are no future practitioners? Fortunately, there need be little conflict in actual practice. Students can be well supervised and gradually introduced to increasingly difficult problems. Where a health care team functions well as a whole, students improve overall patient care. Students keep practitioners honest by asking questions and having time for tasks, such as talking with patients, that busier practitioners neglect.

Yet abuses occur. Interviews, tests, and procedures are sometimes performed largely for teaching purposes. Nurses working in hospitals with medical teaching programs are frequently able to report anecdotes of such procedures.

CASE EXAMPLE.　The team was performing CPR on a patient. In senior resident Dr. McCally's judgment, the rescue was hopeless and the patient definitely dead. The junior resident, Dr. Lake, wanted, however, to try an injection of epinephrine into the heart. Dr. McCally allowed Dr. Lake to go ahead, because in her judgment Dr. Lake needed experience in intracardiac injection and the patient was beyond being harmed.

Nurses feel that patients are treated cruelly when a student attempts a painful procedure, such as inserting a catheter into a vein, ten or twelve times before succeeding. These nurses judge that two or three times should be the student's limit before being relieved by more skilled practitioners. In teaching hospitals, patients' rooms may be crowded during rounds and patients may lack privacy. The case of a patient is sometimes discussed *by name* and without consent at grand rounds before several hundred people, although no effort is made to ascertain who is present at these occasions. A teaching hospital may be unwilling to undertake a service to patients, such as adding a hospice unit, unless it can be made part of a teaching program.

Patients may be disvalued and exposed to emotional hazards as a result of teaching. When death and dying were first introduced as important teaching sub-

---

[57]For additional outlines of principles see Robert J. Levine and Karen Lebacqz, "Ethical Considerations in Clinical Trials," *Clinical Pharmacology and Therapeutics,* 25 (1979), 728–41; and American Nurses' Association, *Human Rights Guidelines for Nurses in Clinical and Other Research* (Kansas City, Kans.: American Nurses' Association, 1975).

[58]A review of the issues special to social science research is Diener and Crandall, *Ethics in Social and Behavioral Research.*

jects, some dying patients found themselves undergoing endless discussions of death with students. Or a patient may be made to feel "special" as a teaching subject in order to obtain the patient's consent to be examined in front of students.[59] Vulnerable patients may become the object of risky teaching. For example, a prominent pediatric surgeon and director of a reputable university hospital department reported that he had never performed surgery on a Down's syndrome infant; this work was always reserved for residents. Patients are not the only parties at risk in teaching situations. Students may be exploited as cheap labor or thrust into situations for which they are unprepared at understaffed institutions. They may even be deliberately overprepared in order to set them in conflict with regressive institutions.

The practice of health care institutions has tended to leave this ethical problem unresolved. The "Statement on a Patient's Bill of Rights," for example, makes no explicit reference to teaching but instead says:

> The patient has the right to every consideration of his privacy concerning his own medical care program. Case discussion, consultation, examination, and treatment are confidential and should be conducted discreetly. Those not directly involved in his care must have the permission of the patient to be present. (AHA, 1973)

Are students directly involved in care? Does this mean that a patient may *not* refuse someone directly involved in his or her care? Lest patients be confused on this subject, a prominent west coast teaching hospital includes the following statement in the "Conditions of Admissions" that the patient signs:

> The University of . . . is a teaching institution. Consequently, attending physicians may be assisted by medical students, interns, residents and postgraduate fellows during the care of each patient. The patient agrees to treatment by these persons while under the direction of the attending physician.[60]

It is not difficult to identify principles for limiting use of patients for teaching purposes. It is clear that *patient good* must dominate teaching needs. As we have already mentioned, supervision and gradual acquisition of skills can help. Sometimes simulated patients can also be helpful in avoiding problem situations. Simulations include "Resusci-Annies" and other mechanical imitations of patients.[61] Venipuncture can be introduced by simulation. At one university teaching hospital, the nursing students have their first venipuncture experiences with mechanical simulations, while medical students do their first venipunctures on patients. Actors and "expert" patients may be hired to act out mock interviews.[62]

[59]For a vivid description of this, see I.S. Cooper, *It's Hard to Leave While the Music's Playing.* (New York: W.W. Norton & Co., Inc., 1977), pp. 100–11.

[60]This university includes a nursing school. Nursing students are trained on the wards. Why are nursing students not mentioned? Why is a *teaching hospital* always a *medical* teaching hospital? There are many nursing teaching hospitals without medical education programs.

[61]Are cadavers simulated patients?

[62]Howard S. Barrows and Robyn M. Tamblyn, *Problem Based Learning: An Approach to Medical Education* (New York: Springer Publishing Co., Inc., 1980); and Howard S. Barrows *Simulated Patients (Programmed Patients): The Development and Use of a New Technique in Medical Education* (Springfield, Ill.: Charles C. Thomas, Publisher, 1971).

Since the health professions strongly emphasize competence, and its institutions are sometimes economically dependent on teaching programs, it is difficult to keep teaching risks to patients within the bounds of patient good.

Emotional Exploitation

Illness, death, and hospital settings often give rise to strong feelings. Important emotional interchanges can arise in the nurse-patient relationship. Part of nursing education teaches nurses how to use these feelings for the good of patients. For example, one writer advises with regard to compassion:

I believe that the natural spark of compassion should be professionally utilized for the benefit of the patient. It is reasonable to assume that in most cases showing compassion for the patient will probably make him feel better, although it is not necessary to feel the compassion too emotionally.[63]

Sociologists have observed how feelings and their expression receive attention in professional training:

Ellen did not know how to manage her face when giving a shot . . . she winced and let the patient see this wince.[64]

And, teachers take the ability of students to handle emotional situations into account:

The psychiatric nursing instructors were talking about Harriet Yates and her schizophrenic patient and whether Harriet could go upstairs with this seductive man, after hours, so that he could practice the piano. Miss MacDuff refused to sanction this, saying she didn't like the idea of Harriet alone with this patient in the secluded semidarkness of the music room.[65]

Patients' feelings about disease, death, nurses, or physicians can be sources of power or pleasure which practitioners may consciously or inadvertently misuse. For example, health practitioners reluctant to share bad news with patients sometimes give patients excessive hope. Misplaced hope sometimes leads patients into intensive treatments and experimental therapies, when learning to live with chronic disease or accepting death might have been the soundest choices. The first recipient of a successful heart transplant, Dr. Philip Blaiberg, described his impressions of the surgeon, Dr. Christiaan Barnard.

He was tall, young, good-looking with features that reminded me a lot of General Jan Christian Smuts in his later years. His hands were beautiful; the hands of the born surgeon. . . . He inspired me with the greatest confidence, . . . [Later, after the death

[63]R.D. Ryder, "Feelings in Physical Illness," *Nursing Mirror* (August 18, 1972), 20.

[64]Virginia L. Olesen and Elvi W. Whittaker, *The Silent Dialogue: A Study of the Social Psychology of Professional Socialization* (San Francisco: Jossey-Bass, Inc., Publishers, 1968), p. 145.

[65]Ibid., p. 139.

of an earlier transplant patient] he no longer resembled the handsome Smuts, . . . but more a martyred Christ. I felt a twinge of pity for him when I noticed the pain in his face and eyes. [Asked if he still wanted to go through with the transplant, Dr. Blaiberg said,] "I want to go through with it now more than ever—not only for my sake but for you and your team who put so much into your effort to save Louis Washkansky."[66]

It is clear from this description that Dr. Blaiberg is undertaking this risk not only for his own sake but also for the sake of Dr. Barnard.

Or emotional exploitation may appear in the form of emotional domination and manipulation of patients. Emotional exploitation may even become *abuse* when it is extreme. Helen Creighton reports such a case.

> CASE EXAMPLE.   Bill Pederson . . . was manning a machine gun on a moving jeep that hit a land mine north of Hue in South Vietnam. He is now almost entirely paralyzed, so that special aides must clothe him, feed him, and swing him in and out of bed on a special lift. Pederson says that one aide who had idly ignored his repeated calls for help at the Hines (Ill.) VA Hospital finally put him in the lift and whispered, "You ever say a word or complain, and I'll let let your ass fall from this thing one day."[67]

Would it have been morally worse for an RN to have done this than an aide?

Sex is an important area of emotional expression with potential for exploitation. Professionals are concerned to establish an appropriate boundary between meeting the health needs of clients, which may involve sensitive emotional support with regard to sexual problems, and inappropriate sexual involvement.[68] The concern with limits on expressions of sexuality goes beyond a simple concern with reputation or symbolic professional purity: The professional principle of patient good limits areas for expressing deep emotional contact with patients. It is easy to imagine circumstances where deep discussions of death with dying patients would be appropriate, or where crying with patients would be acceptable, but sex with patients is more implausible. Justifying these kinds of deep contact requires showing that they serve the good of the patient, or at least that they are consistent with patient good.

The ways nurses, physicians, and patients use flirtation and sexual and non-sexual touching provide a deep psychological texture to professional-client interac-

[66]Philip Blaiberg, *Looking at My Heart* (New York: Stein & Day Publishers, 1968), pp. 56–57, 65–66, 69.

[67]Helen Creighton, "Law for the Nurse Supervisor: Abuse of Patients," *Supervisor Nurse* (June 1976), p. 14.

[68]Kathleen M. Fenner, *Ethics and Law in Nursing* (New York: D. Van Nostrand Company, 1980), p. 155; Charles Clay Dahlberg, "Sexual Contact between Patient and Therapist," *Medical Aspects of Human Sexuality* (July 1971), 34–56; Marion Nesbitt Blondis and Barbara E. Jackson, *Nonverbal Communication with Patients: Back to the Human Touch*, 2nd ed. (New York: John Wiley & Sons, Inc., 1982), pp. 107–19; Sydney Siemens and Rose C. Brandzel, *Sexuality: Nursing Assessment and Intervention* (Philadelphia: J.B. Lippincott Company, 1982), pp. 4–5, 410–11; Martin R. Lipp, *Respectful Treatment: The Human Side of Medical Care* (New York: Harper & Row, Publishers, Inc., 1977), pp. 119–23; David J. Withersty, "Sexual Attitudes of Hospital Personnel: A Model for Continuing Education," *American Journal of Psychiatry*, 133 (1976), 573–75; Gertrude B. Ujhely, *The Nurse and Her Problem Patients* (New York: Springer Publishing Co., Inc., 1963), p. 36; W.H. Masters, V.E. Johnson, and R.C. Kolodny, eds., *Ethical Issues in Sex Therapy and Research*, vols. I and II (Boston: Little, Brown, & Company, 1977 and 1980).

tions. Such exchanges can be empowering and reassuring for both clinicians and patients, but they can also express deeply ingrained sex roles, put people in their place, cause hostile or humiliating feelings, and obtain cooperation manipulatively. Customary ways of handling sexual contact *among* professionals is equally important to defining the emotional character of professional life. The "marriage" of nurses and physicians fundamental to the Victorian birth of the nursing profession (see text p. 40) has been expressed during this century in the fantasies and customs of sex relations among nurses and doctors. For example, in a recent pulp nursing novel directed at an adolescent audience, the young nurse and handsome physician work together to rescue a very sick little girl. Later in the book, the nurse and physician fall in love, marry, and adopt the child from her uncaring mother. Such innocent fantasies, however, must be compared with less beneficent expression of sexual feelings. For instance, a female physician tells this story:

> As a resident, I initiated a brief sex act with another resident in one of the empty hospital rooms. Some nurses saw us leaving the room. I felt a flush of power. As a physician, I could do such a thing with impunity, while the nurses would be penalized for such impropriety.

A nurse educated in a hospital nursing school during the 1930s remembers that the nursing students, who lived in a dormitory, were allowed *only* to date medical interns and residents. To take another case, psychiatrists sometimes develop complex theories justifying sex with their patients, but most such theories can be seen as self-deceived accounts by powerful men rationalizing exploitation of women patients.[69]

Sex between nurses and patients is apparently rare. The *Nursing '74* survey respondents reported on whether patients made seductive or sexual advances toward them. Seventy-three percent reported that patients did so only occasionally or once or twice. Only 2 percent of nurses reported frequent advances, and 25 percent reported that patients never made advances. *Nursing '74* also asked how nurses responded to patients who made advances. Sixty-six percent of female nurses and 44 percent of male nurses reported that they never responded to advances, while 0.3 percent of female and 2 percent of male nurses reported intercourse with patients.[70] Physicians report slightly higher rates of sexual contact with patients in the few studies that have been done. In one study, for example, 5 percent to 7.2 percent of male physicians reported having had intercourse with patients.[71]

The general presumption against sex with patients has an important exception—one's spouse or lover. Here the ethical issues take a different turn because the important relationship to protect may be the personal relationship rather than the professional one. Ethical problems arise from undertaking professional relations with family and friends. Should you charge your spouse for the week of care you gave at home? Can you show good professional judgment in coping with serious

[69]Phyllis Chesler, *Women and Madness* (New York: Avon Books, 1972), pp. 148–68.

[70]"Nursing Ethics: The Admirable Professional Standards of Nurses: A Survey Report," Part I, *Nursing '74*, 4, 9 (September 1974), 43.

[71]Sheldon H. Kardener, Marielle Fuller, and Ivan N. Mensh, "A Survey of Physicians' Attitudes and Practices Regarding Erotic and Nonerotic Contact with Patients," *American Journal of Psychiatry*, 130 (1973), 1077–81.

health problems of those close to you? Are you using your professional role to dominate or exploit your spouse?

The conventional view on exploitation of patients' feelings might be summarized as follows: It is expected that nurses receive emotional rewards from their work. These rewards should be derived from acts for the good of the patient. Seeking emotional satisfaction by exploiting the emotional vulnerabilities of clients or by abusing their feelings is unprofessional. What remains problematic is the depth and range of emotional involvement. Is it important to maintain a cool detachment or simply to reserve a small center of balance? Is this an issue about behavioral presentations of oneself to clients or about one's deeper feelings? Do these questions mainly address one's efficacy as a healer or one's self-protection in emotionally difficult work?

Hospital Routine

I have tried to separate issues of patient good from those of exploitation. Not all issues can be easily divided. Some ethical problems of nurses involve both. For example, hospital routine is sometimes inconvenient or harmful to patients. Common complaints include sleep loss from frequent nocturnal taking of vital signs and rising early for medications and baths. On one hand, this results from the efforts of nurses to allocate care to many patients, that is, from their sense of justice in patient care. On the other hand, it arises from short resources, inappropriate institutional design, and staff interest in making work more convenient and less stressful for themselves. Such problems require a multi-level approach from What can I do for this patient now? to What sort of health care institution would I like to be working in ten years from now?

Summary

The structure of nursing practice creates occasions on which nurses participate in exploiting patients. Patients are exploited when they involuntarily give more than they get. Many areas of practice provide occasions for possible exploitation.

Nurses who accept *gifts or tips* must be careful that they express genuine reciprocity and not patients' self-abnegation or dependency. Excessive *salaries and profits* in health care are eventually paid by patients and the public. Historically, both nurses and patients have been exploited for the profit of others. *Theft* from patients is so obviously exploitive that it is not mentioned in nursing codes, and nurses can lose their licenses for it.

Experimentation on human subjects creates risks for patients. It is important that nurses conduct or participate only in experimentation that is worthwhile, does not impose undue risks on patients, and to which subjects give fully informed and voluntary consent. It is important to distinguish possible benefits to subjects from possible benefits to future patients.

Since new nurses must be *educated,* inexperienced nurses must work with patients. This can threaten patients' good, and solutions to this conflict with patient welfare require good supervision and roles for students designed to improve overall care for patients.

Since health care work is intimate and arouses strong feelings, *emotional,* and more rarely *sexual,* exploitation are hazards of the nurse-patient relationship. Fostering dependency, abusing patients, and glorying in power over patients are ways in which health professionals sometimes emotionally exploit patients.

Hospital routine expresses problems both of patient good and exploitation.

FURTHER READINGS

Accepting Money from Patients

CROSS, YVONNE, "Rogue Nurses: Tipping," *Nursing Mirror,* 134, 10 (March 10, 1972), 18–19.

ROTHMAN, NANCY LLOYD, AND DANIEL A. ROTHMAN, "Equal Pay for Comparable Work," *Nursing Outlook* (December 1980), 728–29.

Experimentation and Teaching

BARBER, BERNARD, ET AL., *Research on Human Subjects: Problems of Social Control in Medical Experimentation.* New York: Russell Sage Foundation, 1973.

BARNES, H. VERDAIN, MARK ALBANESE, AND JUDY SCHROEDER, "Informed Consent: The Use of Inpatients as Teaching-Patients for Sophomore Medical Students," *Journal of Medical Education,* 55 (August 1980), 698–703.

BEECHER, HENRY K., *Research and the Individual: Human Studies.* Boston: Little, Brown & Company, 1970.

BISHOP, V.A., "A Nurse's View of Ethical Problems in Intensive Care and Clinical Research," *British Journal of Anaesthesia,* 50 (1978), 515–18.

FREUND, PAUL A., ED., *Experimentation with Human Subjects.* New York: George Braziller, Inc., 1970.

FRIED, CHARLES, *Medical Experimentation: Personal Integrity and Social Policy.* New York: American Elsevier Publishing Co., Inc., 1974.

GRAY, BRADFORD H., ROBERT A. COOKE, AND ARNOLD S. TANNENBAUM, "Research Involving Human Subjects," *Science,* 201 (September 22, 1978), 1094–1101.

HAYTER, JEAN, "Issues Related to Human Subjects," in *Issues in Nursing Research,* eds. Florence S. Downs and Juanita W. Fleming, pp. 107–47. Englewood Cliffs, N.J.: Prentice-Hall, Inc., 1978.

LEBACQZ, KAREN, AND ROBERT J. LEVINE, "Respect for Persons and Informed Consent to Participate in Research," *Clinical Research,* 25, 3 (1977), 101–7.

MACKAY, R., ET AL., "Nurses As Investigators: Some Ethical and Legal Issues," *Nursing Digest,* 5 (Spring 1977), 7–9.

RENAUD, MARC, ET AL., "Practice Settings and Prescribing Profiles: The Simulation of Tension Headaches to General Practitioners Working in Different Practice Settings in the Montreal Area," *American Journal of Public Health,* 70 (1980), 1068–73.

RIECKEN, HENRY W., AND RUTH RAVICH, "Informed Consent to Biomedical Research in Veterans Administration Hospitals," *Journal of the American Medical Association,* 248, 3 (July 16, 1982), 344–48.

SCHAFER, ARTHUR, "The Ethics of the Randomized Clinical Trial," *The New England Journal of Medicine,* 307, 12 (September 16, 1982), 719–24.

CHAPTER 9

Loyalty:

Nurses
Should Be Loyal
to Each Other

Loyalty among professionals is often slighted in modern treatments of ethics.[1] If relations among practitioners are discussed at all, they tend to be treated as issues of *etiquette,* to contrast them with true issues of *ethics* having to do with patient care,[2] or they are treated merely as obstacles to the good of the patient.

Yet loyalty is fundamental to professionalism. Through identification with each other, cooperation, and mutual support, nurses gain power to work competently toward the good of the patient. Loyalty also grows naturally from daily acquaintance and close working relationships with others. *Loyalty* is an imprecise concept that includes showing sympathy, care, and reciprocity to those with whom we appropriately identify; working closely with others toward shared goals; keeping promises; making mutual concerns a priority; sacrificing personal interests to the relationship; and giving attention to these over a substantial period of time. Far from being a vice, loyalty expresses traditionally valued feelings among human beings. This traditional view is justified partly by the good that comes in the long run from focusing our energies on those who are closest to us and whom we therefore affect the most. It supports showing respect for persons. And it resolves potential conflicts in autonomy by making values and goals that I see as my own more like values and goals of those who work with me (see p. 50).

Strong statements of loyalty can be found in the ethical traditions of nursing. Isabel Hampton Robb expressed beautifully an idealization of the human atmosphere bonding nurses:

---

[1]See, for example, Robert M. Veatch in "Coping with Today's Ethical Dilemmas: Part 2," *Medical Economics* (December 12, 1977), p. 84: "It must not be easy to squeal on one's friends. But the duty to be nice to your friend doesn't seem comparable at all to the duty to prevent a dangerous surgeon from practicing for additional years."

[2]Isabel Hampton Robb distinguishes ethics from etiquette in *Nursing Ethics: For Hospital and Private Use* (Cleveland: J.B. Savage, 1900), pp. 13–15.

. . . she must remember that, for the time being, she is a member of a large family and its privacy and internal affairs should be as loyally guarded as those of her own home circle. The individuality of each member of the family should be respected; the shortcomings or mishaps of any nurse should never be made a topic of conversation outside, either to friends in the city or to doctors. . . . The principle of loyalty must be maintained, irrespective of personal feelings.[3]

The Hippocratic Oath, which has affected the ideology of health care for so long, makes loyalty the first order of business after an oath to the gods:

To hold my teacher in this art equal to my own parents; to make him partner in my livelihood; when he is in need of money to share mine with him; to consider his family as my own brothers, and to teach them this art, if they want to learn it, without fee or indenture; . . .[4]

Although loyalty to colleagues is a virtue, it has been and continues to be a hazard to clients because feelings of loyalty to co-workers and to clients may conflict. Moreover, in comparison with co-workers, hospitalized patients are often strangers to the nurse. It is difficult to be loyal to a stranger when conflicting demands are being made by friends and colleagues. This conflict is expressed in several common problem areas.

First, loyalty to co-workers has led to keeping important information from patients. Sometimes, a patient should be told about mistakes nurses or others have made. It may be the case that the patient should be told because she or he is entitled to compensation for an injury or because further procedures are needed. Nurses rightly approach such occasions with dread. If the nurse speaks to the patient without agreement from involved staff, the act is likely to be seen as disloyal. Although the nurse may sense personal hazards here, she or he may be primarily concerned for the welfare of fellow workers.

In the past, this reluctance to share bad news about health professionals has sometimes been stated explicitly in codes of ethics. A striking example can be found in the 1900 Philadelphia College of Pharmacy "Revised Code of Ethics."

As medical practitioners occasionally commit errors in their prescriptions, which may or may not involve ill consequences to the patient if dispensed, and be injurious to the character of the prescriber, it is held to be the duty of the apothecary in all such cases to protect the physician and to have the corrections made, if possible, without the knowledge of the patient, so that the physician may be screened from censure. . . . Apothecaries, likewise, are liable to commit errors in compounding prescriptions, and we hold that in all such cases it is the duty of the physician to protect the interests of the dispenser and to stand between him and the patient as far as possible.[5]

[3]Ibid., p. 139.

[4]"Selections from the Hippocratic Corpus: Oath," in *Ethics in Medicine: Historical Perspectives and Contemporary Concerns,* eds. Stanley Joel Reiser, Arthur J. Dyck, and William J. Curran (Cambridge, Mass.: The MIT Press, 1977), p. 5.

[5]C.H. Lawall, "Pharmaceutical Ethics," *Journal of the American Pharmaceutical Association,* 10 (1921), 899.

Second, since professions hold dedication to a socially valued good as primary to their association, expressions of loyalty among them should be limited and organized by cooperation for the good of clients. But professions may lose sight of this limitation and become directed primarily to the self-interest of the group or its members. In these circumstances, self-sacrifice and sympathy for other professionals ceases to express idealism and becomes indistinguishable from personal self-interest. Sociobiologists, for instance, have argued that altruism, that is, sacrificing personal interests for the sake of others, has survival value because it contributes to the survival of the group as a whole.[6] Similarly, professionals dedicating themselves to group interests may find themselves doing very well in spite of their sacrifices. The sense of common enterprise thus needs continuing scrutiny to see whether it serves the good of clients and does not exploit them.

Third, the split between professional identity and one's private self (see p. 29) invites confused loyalties. In reporting mistakes, for example, it is easier to place patient good first when one's loyalty is strictly professional and explicitly directed to professional goals. But when one's co-worker is also a close friend, potential expressions of loyalty are much broader and less well defined. Friendship involves wide-ranging promises including those of mutual protection. Where an incompetent co-worker is also a friend, tragic conflicts of loyalty are possible. I am not suggesting that professionals avoid friendships; quite the contrary, but some discussion of views on the welfare of clients would be prudent among friends.

Fourth, loyalty to other professionals is often used mistakenly as a mode of assessment of the overall moral competence of practitioners. Since supervisors and teachers do not often directly observe students caring for patients and because they observe students in relationship to themselves, they sometimes assess the overall ethical competence of students in terms of their treatment of supervisors and teachers. A student who is uncooperative with a supervisor or who expresses a negative attitude may be evaluated as a "bad" nurse, when this apparent disloyalty in fact arises from loyalty to patients in a setting where supervisors and teachers fail to heed the interests of patients.[7]

Recent codes of professional ethics make it clear that loyalty to other professionals must be limited by the good of the patient. The ANA code states:

> Point 3: The nurse acts to safeguard the client and the public when health care and safety are affected by the incompetent, unethical, or illegal practice of any person. (ANA, 1976)

The ICN code states:

> The nurse takes appropriate action to safeguard the individual when his care is endangered by a co-worker or any other person. (ICN, 1973)

In spite of these clear statements, it continues to be difficult to organize loyalty around patient good. This is partly because health care institutions place additional strains on the loyalty of nurses.

[6]Edward O. Wilson, *Sociobiology: The New Synthesis* (Cambridge, Mass.: Harvard University Press, 1975), pp. 120–29.

[7]This has been well described in surgical education. See Charles L. Bosk, *Forgive and Remember: Managing Medical Failure* (Chicago: University of Chicago Press, 1979).

Hospitals tend to be sharply hierarchical and bureaucratic institutions. They are primarily interested in the loyalty of subordinates to the institution. This is sometimes expressed in demands from supervisors and administrators for loyalty to them. Normally this is an inequitable demand; institutions rarely reciprocate with any similar loyalty to subordinates. For example, hospitals would much prefer that nurses file *incident reports* about mistakes rather than talk to patients about them. An incident report can be kept on file and used in the hospital's legal defense, in firing or disciplining incompetent or irresponsible workers, or in reorganizing services to make incidents less likely. Supervisors and administrators often react negatively to cooperative and egalitarian movements of loyalty among staff, especially unionization. The loyalty of subordinates to the institution is an important mode of control; without it, supervisors and administrators cannot manage institutions. Where institutions as a whole fail to serve patients well, this demand for loyalty can interfere with the nurses' expressions of loyalty to nurses and patients.

Loyalty to higher-status professionals can conflict with loyalty to nurses and patients. Just as the traditional loyalty of women to their husbands has divided women historically, the loyalty of nurses to physicians has weakened nursing. Kay Partridge expresses this ironically.

> If woman came from Adam's rib, then nurses, I fear, must have come from the physician's rib.[8]

This struggle can be seen in a 1940 draft of a tentative American Nurses' Association ethics code.

> C. *Relation to Medical Profession.* Loyalty to the physician demands that the nurse conscientiously follow his instructions and that she build up the confidence of the patient in him. At the same time she will exercise reason and intelligence in carrying out orders. She is to avoid criticism of him to anyone but herself, and, if necessary, to the proper administrative officers in the institution or agency where both may be working, or to the local medical professional society.
>
> D. *Relation to Nurse.* The "Golden Rule" embodies all that could be written in many pages on the relation of nurse to nurse. This should be one of fine loyalty and helpfulness, and also, of appreciation for work conscientiously done. On the other hand, loyalty to the motive which inspires nursing should make the nurse fearless in bringing to light any serious violation of it.[9]

In this code, which was published but never adopted, criticism of physicians is only to be made "if necessary"; criticism of nurses can be made more readily upon violations of "the motive which inspires nursing." "She is to avoid criticism of him to anyone"; criticism of nurses involves "fearless . . . bringing to light." Nurses "build up the confidence of the patient" in the physician; they are not called upon to build up such confidence in nurses.

To redress the account somewhat, some early nursing leaders called upon the physician to be loyal to the nurse:

[8]Kay B. Partridge, "Nursing Values in a Changing Society," *Nursing Outlook* (June 1978), 356–60.

[9]Committee on Ethical Standards of the American Nurses' Association, "A Tentative Code for the Nursing Profession," *American Journal of Nursing,* 40 (1940), 979.

Above all, the honorable physician in his turn is always loyal to the nurse and by his manner will always show that he is convinced of her willingness and capability and will thus inspire the patient with confidence in her.[10]

Recent nursing codes of ethics express equality in loyalty between physicians and nurses:

> The interdependent relationship of the nursing and medical professions requires collaboration around the need of the client. The evolving role of the nurse in the health delivery system requires joint practice as colleagues, deliberations in determining functional relationships, and differentiating areas of practice between the two professions. (Point 11.4, ANA, 1976)

Unfortunately, the ANA code does not approach relationships with other health disciplines with the same strong sense of equality. It asserts,

> The complexity of the delivery of health care service demands an interdisciplinary approach to delivery of health services as well as strong support from allied health occupations. (Point 11.3, ANA, 1976)

Although the code calls for *support from* allied health occupations, it omits to mention *support for* allied health occupations.

In short, our complex organizations pull our limited ability to be loyal in many directions. The main priorities in nurses' professional loyalties could be identified as patients, nurses and the nursing profession, physicians, hospitals, other health professions, or society. Which of these should be central and organize the peripheral loyalties? The plausible candidates for a first priority are *patient, nursing, society,* while our historically developed institutions organize nursing priorities of loyalty as *hospital, physicians.*

Interdisciplinary *health care teams* potentially express loyalty among professionals for patient benefit. Within the team, group decision processes and mutual criticism can foster loyalty and patient care at the same time. However, historical patterns of organization pose problems for teams. Patients are still outsiders to health care; salary and benefits of team members continue to be grossly unequal; and teams must work within bureaucratic hierarchies.

Feelings and obligations of loyalty give people the power to work together. As Florence Nightingale commented,

> The health of the unit is the health of the community. Unless you have the health of the unit there is no community health: Competition, or each man for himself, and the devil against us all, may be necessary, we are told, but it is the enemy of health. Combination is the antidote—combined interests, recreation, combination to secure the best air, the best food, and all that makes life useful, healthy, and happy. There is no such thing as independence. As far as we are successful, our success lies in combination.[11]

[10]Robb, *Nursing Ethics,* p. 258.

[11]M. Adelaide Nutting, and Lavinia L. Dock, *A History of Nursing,* vol. II (New York: G.P. Putnam's Sons, 1907), pp. 277–78.

There are many forms of human "combination," and loyalty serves to maintain and strengthen them irrespective of their goals. When specific conflicts arise regarding the goals of a group, one faces conflicts between maintaining group solidarity and acting independently. At such moments, it may seem that there is an important philosophical question about the balance between self-interest and the good of patients or between patient good and loyalty to friends. However, resolving a specific dilemma and resolving a general philosophical question are not identical. In many cases, there may be little need to decide which value to sacrifice. Instead, one can ask how specific aspects of values can be coordinated to foster both. For instance, one can engage co-workers in efforts to protect the good of patients. More generally, one can seek organizational changes which support harmony between professional loyalty and dedication to patient care. When a forced choice is necessary, one might for various reasons sometimes favor loyalty and at other times patient good. Only over a long period of time and through many decisions will one's commitments reveal themselves. If one is reflective during this period, one will also have gained some perspective on general philosophical questions about self-interest and professionalism.

Summary

Loyalty to other nurses is an important obligation and an expression of human bonds that grow from working together and spending time together. This loyalty should not be belittled, even though it can threaten patient care. Patients are usually strangers relative to fellow professionals and are thus sometimes treated as outsiders. Loyalty to other nurses is altruistic unless it simply supports a pact for mutual self-interest. Conflicts between professional and personal loyalties to friends can give rise to tragic conflicts. In hierarchical organizations such as hospitals, the loyalty of employees to their supervisors is sometimes stronger than the loyalty of supervisors to those ranking lower in the hierarchy. Loyalties should express duties that are reciprocal and which harmonize for the good of all.

FURTHER READINGS

BERGER, PETER L., BRIGITTE BERGER, AND HANSFRIED KELLNER, *The Homeless Mind: Modernization and Consciousness,* chap. 2, "Bureaucracy and Consciousness," pp. 41–62. New York: Random House, Inc., 1973.

CROSS, YVONNE, "Rogue Nurses: Professional Loyalty," *Nursing Mirror,* 134, 13 (March 31, 1972), 14–16.

HIRSCHMAN, ALBERT O., *Exit, Voice, and Loyalty: Responses to Decline in Firms, Organizations, and States.* Cambridge, Mass.: Harvard University Press, 1970.

NAGEL, THOMAS, *The Possibility of Altruism.* Princeton, N.J.: Princeton University Press, 1970.

NOLAN, M.G., "Wanted: Colleagueship in Nursing," *Journal of Nursing Administration,* 6 (1976), 41–43.

ROSEN, GEORGE, "The Hospital: Historical Sociology of a Community Institution," in *The Hospital in Modern Society,* ed. Eliot Freidson, pp. 1–36. New York: The Free Press, 1963.

CHAPTER 10

Basic
Moral Concepts
and Theories

The last four chapters investigated major conventional ethical principles in nursing. They described where and how these principles should be applied, clarified them, and identified their limitations. Because health care is changing rapidly and nurses face new and difficult decisions, they find many areas where conventional principles are unclear, in conflict, inapplicable, or unrealized. Conventional principles fall short of resolving conflicts in loyalties, hazards of exploitation, vague and conflicting conceptions of patient good, disputed assessments of competency, and the like.

In order to investigate conventional principles more deeply and to improve on them, we need to engage in more reflective thinking about ethics. This requires going beyond conventional practices. It requires testing professional ethics in terms of considered personal judgment, using broad principles that form a conceptual bridge among conventional principles; analyzing them in terms of broader traditions; developing a more abstract and general vocabulary; and searching for solutions that look beyond the immediate situation.

Philosophical thinking becomes crucial at this level of reflection. Philosophical ethics has developed a number of concepts and theories for thinking about ethics from a broad perspective. Five such concepts are outlined in this chapter: respect for persons, justice, values, rights, and responsibility. Discussion is directed toward clarifying these concepts so that they can be used in analyzing major ethical problems in nursing. The sections of this chapter on moral concepts are followed by a brief section on moral theories. Philosophical moral theories are attempts to present integrated and general accounts of the *shoulds* and *oughts* underlying the use of these moral concepts. These theories and concepts are interesting in themselves, but it is important to consider how we would use them in improving conventional nursing principles and making judgments in professional work.

Respect for Persons

One basic moral concept from which many moral principles derive is respect for persons. When we try to explain why we should not lie or why we should not harm people, we often appeal to the principle that we should respect others. *Respect* in this context means something different from the concept of respect that we grow up with, that is, looking up to someone like parents or teachers. Such phrases as "taking people seriously," "taking others into account in making decisions," and "giving due weight to the welfare and wishes of people," come closer to its meaning.

The codes and conventions of nursing ethics express respect for persons in a variety of ways. Respect is the first principle in the American Nurses' Association code of ethics:

> Point 1: The nurse provides services with respect for human dignity and the uniqueness of the client unrestricted by considerations of social or economic status, personal attributes, or the nature of health problems. (ANA, 1976)

Nursing work directed toward the good of patients and loyalty to co-workers are both ways of showing respect for persons. Exploiting patients shows lack of respect for them.

The concept of respect for persons can be captured by two principles, one positive and the other negative:

PEOPLE SHOULD BE TREATED WITH EMPATHETIC CONSIDERATION. This includes listening to others, understanding them, and responding with appreciation of their intentions.[1] Empathy with a patient is not just a feeling; it involves an integrated emotional and intellectual awareness of his or her position. It is not simply identification with patients; the ability to put oneself in another's place requires maintaining a clear sense of oneself and the goals of the nurse-patient relationship. Empathy does not require that nurses simply accept patients' views without reservation; instead, it involves giving due weight to patients' attitudes and feelings in nursing judgments. Empathy is not identical with sympathy or compassion, although the latter may express empathy for patients who are suffering. In health care, abuses of this form of respect occur in the common disregard of patients' subjective accounts of their symptoms and reactions to medication. Another common abuse is the failure by physicians to take the reports of nurses seriously.

PEOPLE SHOULD NOT BE TREATED AS A MERE MEANS TO AN END. This says that people should not be treated as mere tools or implements to accomplish one's own or another's benefit. People should not be *exploited,* and their *autonomy* should be recognized. Slavery is the paradigm case of treating people as a means to an end. The health care practice most often thought to risk abuse of this principle is nontherapeutic human experimentation. In nontherapeutic research, one tries to find out something about a patient for the sake of potential benefits to other patients or for the progress of science. One *uses* research subjects. We can reconcile this

---

[1] R.S. Downie and Elizabeth Telfer, *Respect for Persons* (New York: Schocken Books, Inc., 1970); and Errol E. Harris, "Respect for Persons," in *Ethics and Society: Original Essays on Contemporary Moral Problems,* ed. Richard T. de George (Garden City, N.Y.: Doubleday & Co., Inc., 1966).

practice with the principle of respect for persons by asking potential subjects for their permission to use them. *Consent* to participate in research makes the subject of study a voluntary agent and not a mere tool or instrument. We no longer see such patients as manipulated, but instead as active participants in research.

The principle of respect for persons is so basic that it is hard to find anything more basic in ethics to justify it. Persons, people, or human beings are the main subject of morality and ethics. Our conceptions of ethics guide the actions of persons, express their needs and aspirations, assess relations among them, and are primarily created by them. It would be illogical to have a morality that lacked respect for persons, unless we were willing to study and create a morality that lacked respect for its main focus of interest. Moreover, it is reasonable to respect oneself only if one respects others. Our personal capacity for joy and suffering, our moderate reasonableness, our concern for the meaningfulness of our lives, our wish to have things our way, our limited capacities, our need for others, our mortality, our place in nature, and other basic conditions of life which we respect in ourselves can be found universally in humans. Since we respect these dimensions of ourselves, and since they are present in others, we should respect others as well.

Another way to approach respect is to consider what it is like not to be respected by others. Millions of people have experienced being lied to, manipulated, exploited, raped, robbed, tortured for sport, bombed, evicted, or simply ignored. Myriad incidents in hospital life display lack of respect for patients: addressing patients by first names or diminutives, using a "baby-talk" tone of voice, discussing patients in their hearing as though they were not there, leaving instruments lying on patients' bodies after procedures, leaving patients undraped in the hallways, inflexible hospital schedules, and so on.

Respect for persons can thus be seen as rooted in our desire to avoid suffering. We would like our capacity for suffering to be taken into serious account in the decisions of others. In fact, we suffer in some ways simply from lack of respect alone. Suffering is not nearly as powerful as the deafness of others to it. For example, consider the report of Shen Fa-liang, a Chinese villager who as a boy was indentured to a landlord for seven years to pay off his father's four-dollar debt.

> Any small mistake and he (the landlord) blew up. I had to carry water through the gate. There was a threshold and a sharp turn. If I spilled some water on the ground, he cursed me for messing up the courtyard. Once I tore the horse's collar. He cursed me and my ancestors. I didn't dare answer back. I think that was worse than the food and the filthy quarters—not being able to talk back.[2]

How to show respect for persons is an important problem area in ethics. For example, interfering with a suicide attempt may be seen as a respectful refusal to cooperate in an impulse grown from despair and as recognition of a client's overall welfare and a deeper wish to live. In contrast, *not* interfering with a suicide may express respect for a client's privacy, choice, or autonomy. The conflict between respect for a patient's *choices* and respect for a patient's *welfare* is fundamental to the debate over the traditional practice of *paternalism* introduced in Chapter 7 (pp. 90–91). Some see a certain amount of paternalism in clinical practice as respecting people by overriding their wishes in favor of a more professional sense of what is

[2]From p. 39 of *Fanshen: A Documentary of Revolution in a Chinese Village.* Copyright © 1966 by William Hinton. Reprinted by permission of Monthly Review Press.

good for their health and recovery. Others see paternalism as disrespectful in that it interferes with the personal self-management of patients, in other words, their autonomy.

The antipaternalist position is reflected in the patients' rights movement, the development of informed consent, and the growth of patient advocacy as a goal of nursing practice. It has its philosophical roots in a position taken by John Stuart Mill in *On Liberty* in 1859:

> . . . the only purpose for which power can be rightfully exercised over any member of a civilized community, against his will, is to prevent harm to others. His own good, either physical or moral, is not a sufficient warrant. He cannot rightfully be compelled to do or forbear because it will make him happier, or because, in the opinion of others, to do so would be wise or even right. These are good reasons for remonstrating with him or reasoning with him, or persuading him, but not for compelling him or visiting him with any evil in case he do otherwise. . . . In the part which merely concerns himself, his independence is, of right, absolute. Over himself, over his own body and mind, the individual is sovereign.[3]

Mill's position appears to imply that nurses and physicians should not override patients' refusals of treatment even if patients seem to act against their own health, and even if such choices threaten their lives. A health professional may attempt persuasion, but the tools of persuasion must be limited by respect for patients' liberty.

Criticisms of paternalism usually take one of three forms.

1. Some hold that personal liberty is a primary value in itself and an essential feature of human dignity and respect, so that personal choices may be disregarded only when they threaten the personal choices of others.
2. Others hold that respect for the welfare of people is the primary value and that personal liberty should be respected as an important, but not universal, means to that end. They argue that individuals are in the best position to know what is good for themselves. Even if they don't know what is good for themselves, certainly no one else is in a better position to decide. Such persons are often *weak paternalists*, that is, they hold that decisions by mentally competent persons should be respected, but that others should make decisions on behalf of the incompetent because the latter are unable to protect their own welfare.
3. Others hold that most so-called ''paternalistic'' acts are not really paternalistic. They believe that usually when physicians give paternalistic justifications for their acts, they are not really acting for the good of patients. Instead, they are acting primarily from their own self-interest and deceiving themselves about patients' needs. It is charged, for example, that physicians resist patients' requests to be allowed to die more from their own fear of death than from the patients' real needs.

Those who defend traditional medical paternalism generally claim that even normally competent adults are incompetent in important respects to make decisions about medical care. Knowledge of medicine is so technical as to be accessible only to specialists. They also claim that our emotional reactions to illness and death render us unable to handle issues we could cope with when healthy. They do not see

---

[3]John Stuart Mill, *On Liberty* (Indianapolis: The Bobbs-Merrill Co., Inc., 1956), p. 13.

why we should respect choices made out of ignorance or under duress. Thus, information which would be hard to handle should be withheld. Patients should be plunged into difficult but beneficial treatments when their natural fear of pain would lead them to hesitate foolishly. It is part of the task of the professional to push people in the direction they obviously, in the professional's judgment, need to go. Far from showing lack of respect for people, paternalism shows respect for people by recognizing their limitations.

Antipaternalists generally reply that the specialist's proper role can be fulfilled by confining communication to information and advice. An expert who requires coercion as a means belies his or her credibility as an expert. Antipaternalists also deny that to be emotional is to be incompetent to make decisions: People may be strengthened or enlightened by suffering.

The debate over paternalism is by no means settled. *First*, it is clear that since both values and facts are needed to make decisions, patients and experts on health need each other to arrive at sound decisions. This interdependency cannot be neatly sorted into a value component asserted by the patient and a technical component provided by the clinician. Communication with patients can thus include a persuasive defense of health-related values without constituting paternalism. *Second*, the role of emotions in decision making should be further explored. Decision making is a complex process, and the psychology of sound decisions is by no means clear. Nor is it clear how criteria related to psychological soundness (such as alertness) should be weighed in assessments of competence as compared with criteria related to logical soundness (such as whether a patient's conclusions follow from stated premises). *Third*, where patients are ignorant of their own good, it does *not* follow that clinicians are therefore knowledgeable about patient good. Particular circumstances influence who is in the best position to know, and where patients do not know their own good, it is possible that *no one* knows what is best for them.

Fourth, in settings where people are of equal power and intimately acquainted with each other, as in some families and close communities, the distinction between paternalism and autonomy breaks down. In such settings, individual self-knowledge depends on confirmation and recognition of others close by. What would, from an outsider, be an imposition becomes emotional support. Estrangement of health professionals from patients, isolation of patients from their support systems, and the great power of health care institutions make paternalism possible. Thus, changes in the professional-patient relationship may do more to resolve the problem of paternalism in health care than a philosophical determination of whether choices or welfare are more important components of respect for patients. For example, models of health care which make patients the primary managers of their care and make clinicians assistants to patients engaged in self-care give the professional less power to override patients' wishes.

Fifth, too much energy has been spent on identifying *one* person to make decisions. Group decision processes that include patients can do much to prevent paternalism. *Sixth*, merely because clinicians do not coerce patients, it does *not* follow that patients are not coerced. There may be other sources of coercion—family, law, occupational considerations, money, and ignorance. In a culture where values are usually merely asserted rather than explored and where most people get their health information from television, the newspapers, and rumor, too few people know very much about their own good. Genuine paternalism can help counterbalance sources of information more exploitive and less respectful than the health professions. The antipaternalist position in favor of individual liberty with regard to health should thus not be seen as a solution to the question of Who's to say? in health care, but only as a powerful objection to conventional paternalist answers to it.

A hard case for some nurses is the postsurgical patient who needs to breathe deeply and to get out of bed in order to avoid infection and to speed recovery. Sometimes alert and clearly mentally competent patients are reluctant to endure the pain and discomfort involved. Nurses sometimes threaten them with dire consequences or drag and push them from bed. Surely this is paternalism, but does it lack respect for persons? It may lack respect, for example, when the act is not really intended for the client's good but is intended to free up a critical care bed or to reduce national health care costs. But where the act is genuinely intended for the health of the patient, it is a morally acceptable form of paternalism. In such a case, the coercion is limited and of brief duration. Immediate pain and discomfort is well understood as an obstacle to sound action. Important patient values are not being overridden, since recovery is an important part of a project to which the patient is already committed. When these or similar criteria are met, paternalism can be justified.[4] The guiding principle for choosing in such cases between patient autonomy and welfare should be respect for the patient.

A second difficulty with the concept of respect occurs at the limits of "humanhood." Respect for *persons* does not mean exactly the same thing as respect for *human beings*. Kant left it open for us to respect nonhumans if they were sufficiently rational or like us in their mental life.[5] As it happens, we have little experience of nonhuman persons, but we can imagine living in a world where we meet such persons as angels, porpoises, sensitive computers, extraterrestrial travelers, and newts or dogs with medically enhanced mental faculties. A relationship to a transcendant God who is not human but nevertheless a person may be thought of as falling in the realm of a morality with respect for persons fundamental to it.

The criteria traditionally used to distinguish persons from nonpersons have also been challenged. It has been argued that we emphasize rationality and language too much, or employ too human-centered conceptions of rationality and language. If we were more aware of our basic kinship with the natural world, we would treat animals and the environment with more respect. The ways we use animals as research subjects and as food and the extent to which we destroy animal habitats and species would not be possible if we had more respect for them as persons, that is, more empathy for them and a reluctance to use them simply as a means to an end.[6]

These questions about nonhuman persons have significance for health care, for once a wedge is introduced between "a being worthy of respect," that is, a person, and a "human being," the converse concern can be introduced: Are there human beings who are not persons? For example, should fetuses and brain-dead patients be given fundamentally different considerations in health care decisions?

In 1973, the United States Supreme Court made two decisions establishing the

---

[4]For similar views of the conditions of justified paternalism, see Alan W. Cross and Larry R. Churchill, "Ethical and Cultural Dimensions of Informed Consent," *Annals of Internal Medicine*, 96 (1982), 110–13; Martin Benjamin and Joy Curtis, *Ethics in Nursing* (New York: Oxford University Press, 1981), p. 55; and James F. Childress, *Who Should Decide? Paternalism in Health Care* (New York: Oxford University Press, 1982).

[5]Immanuel Kant, *Foundations of the Metaphysics of Morals*, trans. Lewis White Beck (Indianapolis: The Bobbs-Merrill Co., Inc., 1959), pp. 46–47.

[6]For a discussion of respect for animals, see Peter Singer, *Animal Liberation: A New Ethics for our Treatment of Animals* (New York: Random House, Inc., 1975).

right to elective abortion during the first trimester of pregnancy.[7] The Court appealed to the constitutional right of privacy between a woman and her physician. The Court permitted states to regulate abortions after the first trimester for reasons concerning the mother's health so long as they were not "needlessly restrictive." If the Court had regarded fetuses as *persons* under the law, these decisions would have been impossible because a women's decision to have an abortion would not be a private matter and would have to take into consideration the interests of the fetus. The Court did not have to think of fetuses as persons because fetuses lack some of the important criteria for being persons. At early stages of development they lack a mental life, such as a concept of self or a capacity for suffering. They are not yet social beings; they lack language and the capacity for relationships with other human beings. They are in a state of extreme dependency and intimacy with their mothers, which prohibits status as independent persons. Lastly, they have no prior existence as identifiable persons with standing in society. These criteria and others like them have been subjected to much debate. When thinking about the morality of abortion, it is important that criteria of personhood not be offered arbitrarily simply in order to defend or attack the practice of abortion. It is important to ask what criteria we *should* in general use in distinguishing persons from nonpersons.

When a person dies, the obligations of respect change radically. Although some respect due a person remains, as for example in fulfilling a will and in appropriate treatment of the person's body and its parts, there is no longer any obligation to restore life or to maintain health. *Brain death* has developed as an important concept of death partly because it is consistent with our criteria for personhood. Without brain function, there is no possibility of mental life, sociality, or independence. Terminating life support for brain-dead patients thus does not violate the principle of respect for persons.[8]

The concept of respect for persons is basic to ethics. It is fundamental partly because it is flexible. It can be seen as demanding anything from minimal recognition of others' needs to universal love and striving for the welfare of all. Nevertheless, it is a good focal point for ethical reflection. Other concepts in ethics may be thought of as filling out in more detail what we mean by respect for persons.

Justice

Justice is an ancient concept that has accumulated a variety of root meanings over the centuries. To some, the basic concept of justice is *desert*—responding to people with what they *deserve,* whether they be rewards, burdens, or punishments. To others, justice is most closely linked to *harmony* and balance. For them, justice demands a global perspective on the concerns of a large number of people and seeks an overall harmony among these concerns. An important modern concept of harmony is the fundamental *equality* of human beings. It sees everyone as deserving fundamentally equal respect. A sense of justice and fairness is deeply rooted in our

---

[7]Roe v. Wade, 93 Supreme Court 705 (1973); and Doe v. Bolton, 93 Supreme Court 739 (1973).

[8]President's Commission for the Study of Ethical Problems in Medicine and Biomedical and Behavioral Research, *Defining Death: A Report on the Medical, Legal and Ethical Issues in the Determination of Death* (Washington, D.C.: U.S. Government Printing Office, 1981).

personal relations.[9] A system we perceive as unfair or unjust wins our allegiance only out of necessity.[10]

Justice has three primary areas of application:

Distributive justice focuses on the allocation of goods and services. For example, that some people starve to death while others consume too much food is an issue of distributive justice.

Retributive justice is primarily concerned with punishment for wrongdoing.

Procedural justice focuses on how things are done independent of final outcome. For example, a guilty person could receive a fair trial according to procedural justice and still be acquitted. Or, a contract that is fair in terms of procedure might still have ruinous consequences for one party.

Our discussion will focus on the area of justice most relevant to health care—distributive justice. Distributive justice applies to health care at three different levels of analysis:

How much of our national resources—taxes, gross national product, labor, investment, and so on—is it just to devote to health care? What other goods should we limit in order to provide adequate health care?

Given that we invest limited resources in health care, which aspects of health care should receive the most resources? Should we focus on acute care, extended care, prevention, or research? How should geography or the specialty interests of health care personnel affect access to care?

Given that we have limited equipment and staff, which patients should have access to them? For example, some hospitals have a shortage of critical care beds: Who should decide, on what principles, who is to lie in them? Since nurses often have responsibility for several patients on a ward, they must allocate their time: When staffing is short, principles of justice must be considered. Nurses prefer to give time to patients who really need help rather than to patients who complain excessively. Triage nurses in the emergency department must distinguish those who need immediate care from those who can wait.

Distribution of resources for chronic dialysis has taken an interesting turn in relationship to these levels of analysis. During the 1960s, in the early days of dialysis, the problem was to find a just way to choose patients to use the very limited number of machines. Sensing the difficulty of this decision, and having seen a patient dialyzed before its eyes, Congress allocated money under the Medicare program to cover most of the expense of end-stage renal disease. With no principle to limit this expense, the program grew so that by 1980 the program cost the federal government about $1 billion per year. This moves the problem of justice to another realm. Is $1 billion for dialysis a good investment of health care resources? Is it fair for dialysis patients and not hemophiliacs to receive federal assistance?

What features should characterize a fair distribution of health care? A good approach to this problem is to begin with the assumption of *equality* in distributive

[9]John Rawls, in "Justice as Reciprocity," in *Moral Problems in Medicine,* eds. Samuel Gorovitz et al. (Englewood Cliffs, N.J.: Prentice-Hall, Inc., 1976), develops the concept of fairness as a basis for the concept of justice. For developmental features of the concept of fairness, see Jean Piaget et al., *The Moral Judgment of the Child* (New York: The Free Press, 1965).

[10]Elaine Walster, G. William Walster, and Ellen Berscheid, *Equity: Theory and Research* (Boston: Allyn & Bacon, Inc., 1978) treats the relationships among stress, inequity, and the tendency of people to restore equity.

justice: Everyone should receive basically the same benefits and bear the same burdens unless relevant considerations justify treating someone differently. Equality in justice presupposes that people are very much alike in most important respects such as basic needs—food, health care, housing, clothing, longevity, transportation, friendship, and so on—and liberties—participation in decisions, self-expression, and the search for happiness. Equality in justice contrasts with historically older distributive conceptions based on fundamental differences among people. Feudal lords, for example, were seen as deserving very different things in life from serfs. Equality is still not universally accepted as important to justice, and some people see fundamental differences in the value of individuals. This is sometimes expressed in special treatment for high-status patients and casual treatment of low-status patients. The kind of attention patients receive in the emergency department, for example, may depend on how staff perceive their relative social worth.[11] Being of generally high status, physicians sometimes receive preferential treatment.

> CASE EXAMPLE.   A hospitalized physician who did not need or want private-duty nurses had numerous offers from four private-duty nurses, caring for other patients on his floor (Private-duty nurses have a reputation for refusing to help with any patients but their own.), to give him baths and backrubs, change his bed, and so forth. He accepted several of the offers from the private-duty nurses who sought him out. He remarked to us, "Isn't it peculiar that many patients complain that they can never get a bath in this hospital. I could get several a day either from the hospital nurses or the private-duty nurses of other patients."[12]

> CASE EXAMPLE.   A physician very late to a unit meeting apologized and justified his lateness with the explanation that "I was just on my way here when I got a call from a *physician* who was ill and wanted some advice, and of course, I could not say, 'Sorry, I have a meeting. I will call you back later.' "

Equality does not presume that people are alike in every respect. We do not worry whether some people prefer blues to classical music, eggplant to okra, knitting sweaters to repairing trucks. People do not need precisely the same things, and differences in taste and personal expression, even if arbitrary, do not worry us. There are thus *inequalities* that are not *inequities*. But when what people get or undergo is substantially different or when these differences affect a basic need like health, the principle of equality demands that we ask what *relevant differences* among people justify this unequal distribution. And where people are significantly different, justice demands that society respond appropriately to these differences.

Once proponents of equality accept the equality-modified-by-relevant-difference model, dispute centers on what the relevant differences are. Many principles have been proposed for distributing the burdens and benefits of society, for example,

---

[11]Julius A. Roth, "Some Contingencies of the Moral Evaluation and Control of Clientele: The Case of the Hospital Emergency Service," *American Journal of Sociology,* 77 (1972), 839–56.

[12]Raymond S. Duff and August B. Hollingshead, *Sickness and Society* (New York: Harper & Row, Publishers, Inc., 1968), p. 238.

1. To each equally (that is, no differences)
2. To each according to her merit
3. To each according to her past or future social contribution
4. To each according to what she can acquire in a free market
5. To each according to her need
6. To each according to her need; from each according to her ability
7. To each according to . . . (to be supplied by the reader)[13]

Principle 5 is most applicable to health care for two reasons. First, health care is a good only when needed; otherwise, it is a burden to patient or caretaker. Second, health professionals are by definition dedicated to a social good, so that they should distribute health care according to the good it does. But I have left room for a seventh principle because there are problems in using need to govern the use of health care resources. Some patient care could consume unlimited resources. To spare no effort to rescue very low-birth-weight infants, to attempt organ transplants on every dying patient, to perform coronary artery bypass surgery on every medically eligible candidate, or to provide dialysis wherever it would extend life however slightly, would be tremendously expensive and unproductive.[14] There should be some way to limit our commitment to those who are the most needy, but it is difficult to state what that limit should be.

Third, staff sometimes judge that some patients who need care do not merit it (Principle 2) because they abuse or neglect themselves. The paradigm case of this is the alcoholic GI bleeder (p. 203). When chronic kidney dialysis was scarce, committees were set up to decide who would receive this sometimes lifesaving treatment. Many of these "God committees" used what came to be called *social worth* criteria for selection. The committees considered, among other things, whether the patient worked, led a regular and respectable life, had dependents, made contributions to the community, and so on. Although need was not a sufficiently selective principle, use of these criteria was strongly criticized. It was felt that whatever additional principles of justice should be recognized in health care, they should not be the standard middle-class values that constitute "respectability."[15]

Access to health care services is strongly affected by the distribution of providers' labor and investment. The latter distribution is also subject to judgments of justice. Merit, contribution, and competition (Principles 2, 3, and 4) tend to govern the production side of health care practice. Depending on whether we regard health care from the consumer's point of view or the provider's, we tend to apply completely different principles to the same activity. Should Principles 2, 3, and 4 dominate health care practice, or should Principle 5 dominate? Or is there some more inclusive principle that can balance both sides, as hinted at in Principle 6, which mentions both ability and need?

One major problem in thinking about justice in health care is that we live in a

---

[13]Adapted from Gene Outka "Social Justice and Equal Access to Health Care," *Perspectives in Biology and Medicine,* 18 (1975), 185–203.

[14]Howard H. Hiatt, "Protecting the Medical Commons: Who Is Responsible?" *The New England Journal of Medicine,* 293 (1975), 235–41.

[15]Renée C. Fox and Judith P. Swazey, *The Courage to Fail: A Social View of Organ Transplants and Dialysis,* 2nd ed. (Chicago: University of Chicago Press, 1978) gives an excellent account of the early "God committees."

manifestly unjust world. Some people work two shifts a day; others are idle in wealth or poverty. Some people do productive labor; others destructive. Some people receive annual incomes measured in millions of dollars; others die of starvation, exposure, and neglect. Individual healthiness is not evenly distributed in the United States. Some differences are attributable to chance, age, and other factors beyond human control. Others are due to personal life-styles. But many differences in health status are attributable to social factors. Poverty is highly correlated with illness and other health problems,[16] and poverty is primarily a creation of society. Environmental pollutants that cause cancer or birth defects are social products. Some people are exposed to these risks more than others. For example, inner-city working-class people suffer more disease than their suburban counterparts. Poor elderly people eat less nutritious diets and live in less well heated homes than younger or wealthier people. The wealthiest fifth of the world's population lives twenty-two years longer on the average than the poorest fifth.[17]

Since most of us grow up with a sense of justice, we have to struggle with such inequities. Sometimes we *rationalize* these circumstances by trying to find relevant differences between the well-off and the worst-off to justify these inequalities. The history of race and sex discrimination is marked by a desperate search for reasons to treat whole classes of people differently. We may try to *dissociate* ourselves from these problems, but our own welfare is closely linked to that of others. The food we eat, the uniforms we wear at work, hospital equipment, medications, and money are all part of a worldwide flow that shapes virtually everyone's welfare.

There is no refuge in health care from problems of injustice. Health care is shaped by the same worldwide forces, and it tends to replicate the problems of injustice that exist everywhere: The poor have less access to health care than the rich. Health care enriches some professionals and investors and impoverishes some patients and their families. Women and minorities working in health care tend to receive less income than white men. Medicaid patients have trouble finding a physician. And so it goes.

In these circumstances, giving a precise philosophical characterization of justice is both extremely important and extremely difficult. And even when we have been able to give suitable expression to our sense of justice, *how* to achieve a just health care system is an equally difficult problem. Principles of justice do not define the social institutions required to express them, nor can health care be an island of justice in a sea of injustice. In spite of these forbidding realities, it is important to be clear about the need for justice in health care and not to let pervading injustices cloud our sense of justice.

Why is it so important to be just? Like respect for persons, justice is so basic as to be nearly indefensible. In some ways, justice is a minimal claim on a social order. If we are to live among others according to rules of conduct, we should at least demand that these rules be fair. Even and especially if we were all narrowly self-interested, we would still want these rules to be fair. When we choose principles to govern society, we cannot determine by them what positions we are likely to have in society. Out of self-interest, we would reject a society dedicated to glory for

[16]Harold S. Luft, *Poverty and Health: Economic Causes and Consequences of Health Problems* (Cambridge, Mass.: Ballinger Publishing Co., 1978).

[17]Ruth Leger Sivard, *World Military and Social Expenditures, 1981* (Leesburg, Va.: World Priorities, 1981), p. 5.

a few and slavery for the rest, because we would likely be slaves ourselves. Even if there were only a few slaves, it could be just our luck to end up among them. Thus, the self-interested person designing society in the abstract would want to be sure that he or she would have little chance of being unduly and permanently deprived.[18]

Like respect for persons, justice can be seen as concomitant to the basic structure of ethical thinking. If the ethics of ordinary life is to create conventional principles establishing basic expectations for people, then these rules, to be generally acceptable, need to grow out of what people have in common; they do not welcome special and arbitrary differences among people.

Values

Values are the foundation of the seriousness and importance of things. To say that we value something is to imply that we favor it or favor doing it. Where values conflict, as when a decision is likely to result in both good and bad consequences, we *weigh* the values involved, and if we are wise we judge in favor of the more serious, central, or weighty values. Thinking about values is thus part of making ethical decisions.

In thinking about values, we distinguish between things which are valuable only *as a means to an end* (instrumental values) and those which are valuable *in themselves* (final values).[19] Most of us make insurance payments, seek medical care, and get up early not because we enjoy doing these things in themselves, but in order to obtain other things which we value, such as security, health, and wealth. These, too, may be important to us only because of other valuable things that they get us. We may value wealth for what it can buy, health for its attractiveness to others, and so on. Other things we value in themselves. Regardless of what they may do for us, we value simple pleasures, meaningful rituals, and telling stories. We value some things—health, eating lunch, dancing, or fishing—both for themselves and for what they get us.

Since some things are valued because of other things, an argument based on values does not seem complete until we have reached a stopping point—things valued in themselves. Presumably, things valued in themselves are the goal toward which merely instrumental values are directed. Justification of our daily activities thus rests on being able to identify their relationship to some final value or values.[20] Traditionally, this bottom line has been thought of as having to be one value and has been termed the *summum bonum* or *highest good*. What is this highest good which we should all seek?

This question invites a second important distinction in understanding values. Sometimes we find that what we *actually* value is different from or in conflict with what we think we *should* value. I may actually value being busy and becoming famous when I suspect that I should value a simple and quiet life. I may have sexist

[18]This is a free rendering of John Rawls' development of a principle of justice in *A Theory of Justice* (Cambridge, Mass.: Harvard University Press, 1971).

[19]Aristotle, *Nicomachean Ethics,* trans. Martin Ostwald (Indianapolis: The Bobbs-Merrill Co., Inc., 1962), p. 3 (1094a).

[20]This value may be seen as a present concomitant of the activities themselves (such as pleasure) or as some future good to be achieved in some temporally distant consummation (such as salvation).

feelings and judgments although I am convinced by compelling arguments that I should not be this way. These conflicts raise questions about whether I *should* heed sound values, and if so, why? Would it be tragic if I were to miss the *summmum bonum?*

People have taken widely varying positions on this question. To indicate their breadth, two opposite positions are sketched here:

PLURALIST POSITION.   Some people hold a strictly individualist position on values. They believe that what they value themselves are those things that are "good for themselves." Thus, there is only what I actually value. No argument about what I should value can be very informative. If I care about Raymond Chandler novels, real estate, and Presbyterianism, it would be pointless for someone to suggest that I should really care for Toni Morrison novels, self-sacrifice, and transcendental meditation.

This pluralist position seems plausible because in the history of ideas all sorts of conflicting values have been placed on human activities. Wealth, salvation, marriage, and modern art have all been both worshipped and reviled. Jehovah's Witnesses believe that blood transfusions are a kind of eating blood proscribed by the Bible. They would thus choose to die rather than accept transfusions. Some political conservatives would prefer death in nuclear war to life in a socialist economy. Who, it may be asked, could justly insist they change their views? And if such positions cannot be criticized, what values can be? At this pole, one may also see values as having their roots entirely in human experience, so that if anything is to have value at all it must be relative to the experience of human beings. The importance of the natural world thus becomes its importance *to us*. What we believe becomes more important than some distant and imagined reality.

ABSOLUTIST POSITION.   Others see values as rooted in a reality independent of individual experience. The natural and social world has a value independent of its relationship to me. In one version of this view, values are reified in conceptions of a God who commands us to value certain things. When one defends these values, one sees oneself not as defending one's idiosyncratic point of view but as appreciating something objective to which one wants to be responsible. At this absolutist pole, one holds that to fail to value certain things is to fail in being moral or worthy of respect. The list of things some people have held we should all value is quite long— capitalism, communism, property, persons, Woody Allen films, love, pleasure, children, health, and so on. We cannot reject this position out of hand simply because people disagree over which values should be held absolutely, or because values have been forced on people. It could turn out that some of the positions were right and others wrong, and force might have been wrongly used in defense of a correct position.

Nurses in clinical practice experience the conflict between these two perspectives. On one hand, it is important to respect clients' values and to appreciate how their values guide their decisions. MacPherson warns "We must check ourselves constantly to be sure we are not imposing our values on our client."[21] On the other hand, commitment to professional nursing involves dedication to values like health, wellness, and care for others. It is hard to feel good about one's work unless one feels that these values are important and have reality for others as well as for oneself.

---

[21]Jennifer MacPherson, "Client-Centered Emergency Care," *Nursing Law and Ethics,* 2, 6 (June/July 1981), 4.

As long as we perceive the pluralist and absolutist positions as the only possibilities, we will probably be unable to resolve these questions about the reality and individuality of values. In attempting to find an intermediate position, people often inquire whether any values are held universally by all people. Unfortunately, the evidence on this issue is not straightforward. On one hand, it looks like there are lots of universal values: love, courage, the wrongfulness of egregious harm, good stories, food, shelter, and heat in the winter. On the other hand, different cultures give very particular meanings to these values. Outright killing for mercy of very old and debilitated people may be loving and beneficial in one culture, while in another it may be unloving and harmful. Differences can be generated as often as similarities. It is not even clear that if there were universal values, these would therefore have some reality independent of individual experience, or that they are therefore the most weighty and correct ones.[22]

John Stuart Mill attempted to resolve these questions by isolating a single and overriding value—happiness—as the *summum bonum*. He argued his position by analogy:

> The only proof capable of being given that an object is visible is that people actually see it. The only proof that a sound is audible is that people hear it; and so of the other sources of experience. In like manner, I apprehend, the sole evidence it is possible to produce that anything is desirable is that people actually desire it. . . . No reason can be given why the general happiness is desirable, except that each person, so far as he believes it to be attainable, desires his own happiness.[23]

This argument does not complete Mill's defense of the importance of happiness as the main value. He must argue not only that happiness is a value, but that all other values are included in happiness. He does so by arguing that virtue is desirable only as a means to or part of happiness, and that all other values are similarly part of or a means to happiness.

Another approach is to challenge the *summum bonum* model itself. Those things "good in themselves" need not also be good foundations for moral arguments. For example, good stories are nearly universally valued, but good stories would be poor candidates for the *summum bonum*. Instead of looking for ultimate or all-embracing values, we need to engage in research on specific values, their nature and their conflicts. For example, none of the following value conflicts is easily resolved by appeal to a single value like happiness:

1. Mr. Bailey will be healthier and live longer if he gives up alcohol, but he will suffer considerably more emotional anguish. Which should you support?
2. Baby Dolan will probably lead a life of mental defectiveness and crippling physical handicaps if you rescue her, but if you do not, she will probably die. Which is better, death or life with severe handicap?
3. Mr. Colt is a hypochondriac and has been maintained on regular placebo injections of vitamin B_{12} and a subclinical dose of thyroid hormone for his imagined conditions. Should you support his illusions, or should you urge him to confront his real problems?

---

[22]For a brief discussion of culture and ethics, see Paul W. Taylor, *Principles of Ethics: An Introduction* (Encino, Calif.: Dickenson Publishing Company, Inc., 1975), pp. 13–30.

[23]John Stuart Mill, *"Utilitarianism,"* in Gorovitz, *Moral Problems*, pp. 46–47.

4. Ms. Fenimore is giving birth to her second child. She wants to deliver at home and as free as possible from technological accouterments. Her physician argues that the child will be definitely, although slightly, safer if a fetal monitoring system is used during birth. As a nurse, whose point of view would you support?
5. Baby Pepper was born with an unusual metabolic defect. He needed a special diet containing arginine lyase succinate. This diet cost $2,000 per gram. Was this too much to pay to save Baby Pepper's life?
6. A young couple would prefer to have a boy. They want to have amniocentesis performed. If it's a girl, they would abort the child and try again. Would you help them find a counselor who will tell them the sex of the fetus?

Rather than attempt to resolve these questions by a general theory of value, it would be better to explore them individually in order to discover what sort of theory is needed. It is not necessarily an *imposition* for nurses to discuss values with patients. Clients' values need not be the bottom line of all health care decisions. Where nurses abstain from paternalistic expressions of values and avoid undue use of their authority, conflicts in values can be an opportunity for dialogue about our values and insights into life.

Where should this dialogue go? We know that in an imperfect world many people base their values on what they see as possible or on what they think is expected of them. Is there any way to talk about what is possible so that deeper values may come into play in decisions? We know that many people's values are shaped by advertising and other common but unrealistic conceptions of what will make them happy. How shall we identify illusory values in others and in ourselves? In an individualistic culture, people know much about how to represent their perceived interests, but they often know little about how to consider their interests in relation to those of others; nor do they know much about how to conduct a debate or to settle an issue by consensus. How can we learn these skills? Nurses working from the belief that it is possible to think reasonably about values can use the health care setting for thinking seriously about their own values and engaging in dialogue with others.

Rights

The concept of rights, as in a right to life or to health care, is relatively new in our moral vocabulary. Important early uses of the concept can be found in Locke's *Second Treatise of Government* published in 1690 and in the United States *Declaration of Independence* of 1776. The early notion of rights was offered as an argument against arbitrary depredations on people and property by public officials. Locke argued that even though the state had weighty concerns, sometimes backed by theological rationales, there were *limits* to what the state could justifiably do to people. It could not justly run roughshod over individuals—for instance, arbitrarily kill them, jail them, or take property from them—even for the public good. The concept of rights introduced a sphere of private and individual power intended to be impervious to public power.

Since the seventeenth century, the idea of rights has been greatly expanded.

The concept of *human rights* builds on the notion of basic protection for individuals to demand that states protect and provide basic goods, services, and liberties for people.[24] Human rights not only require that states abstain from torture and theft; they also demand that states provide citizens with such things as a clean water supply, food, and shelter.

To say that a person has a right to something means generally that other people have a responsibility not to interfere with that person's obtaining, possessing, or using it. For instance, my right to health means that others have a responsibility not to damage my health. This is sometimes called the concept of *negative* rights. Rights can also have a stronger or more *positive* meaning. That I have a right to something can also mean that others have a responsibility to provide me with it. For instance, the right to a clean water supply calls *negatively* on others not to foul common water sources, and it also requires *positively* that clean water facilities be publicly available.

The ground rules for using the concept of rights are complex. First, we must distinguish between *legal rights* and *moral rights*. *Legal rights* are established by systems of law, so that one can make a claim in a criminal or a civil proceeding. The legal right to vote, for example, can be defended with the assistance of the police power of the state. *Moral rights* may be backed by general opinion, good reasons, or both. They do not necessarily have legal backing. For example, only in the late 1970s did women begin to gain the legal right not to be raped by their husbands, although they had the moral right all along. Sometimes when people say, "We have a right to *X*," they mean "We have a moral right to *X*, and there should, morally, be a legal right to *X*." Many people who defend a right to health care claim something of this form.

Second, rights are related to *responsibilities* in two different ways: one moral, the other logical. (1) *Moral:* Some *rights* are contingent upon fulfilling certain *responsibilities*. For example, in a teaching contract, my right to collect my salary is contingent upon fulfilling my responsibility to teach the class. *Reciprocity* is reflected in this balance of rights and responsibilities: My ability to make claims on others generally rests on my fulfilling their claims on me. For example, the hospitals of the University of California, San Francisco, add to their Bill of Patients' Rights a statement on responsibilities of patients (see p. 202). (2) *Logical:* Responsibilities are also related to rights in another way. My *right* to something logically implies *responsibilities* of others. For instance, my right to life places a responsibility on others not to kill me. Such rights do not place a responsibility on anyone in particular. They place a responsibility on everyone and society in general to respect my claim. The right to health care normally demands that society provide health care, not that Nurse Ames or Doctor Manson provide health care. Yet rights sometimes place responsibilities on particular persons. For example, the patient's right to confidentiality places a responsibility not to divulge private information on particular nurses caring for the patient.

Third, there is some debate over whether or not some rights are *absolute,* that is to say, whether they can ever be overridden or not. Most rights are not. They may be lost because we no longer fulfill certain requirements; for example, I may not

[24]See, for example, General Assembly of the United Nations, "Universal Declaration of Human Rights," adopted in Paris, December 10, 1948, in *Human Rights,* ed. A. I. Melden (Belmont, Calif.: Wadsworth Publishing Co., Inc., 1970).

vote because I emigrated. A right may be overridden by a superior right, for instance, a patient's refusal of treatment may override a nurse's right to uphold her professional judgment of adequate care. The more narrowly exceptions are defined and the more a right is buffered by procedural safeguards, the more nearly it approaches "absolute" standing. The rights not to be tortured, raped, or degraded are good candidates for absolute rights.

What things do we have a right to? Can rights be itemized? Since we can create new rights by contracts and promises, rights can be indefinitely generated. Claims to rights can be inflated by loose reference to any justifiable aspiration as a right. Consider the right to die with dignity: People aspire to die well and there is no good reason to prevent them from doing so. Nevertheless, it is simpler to think of dying with dignity as an instance of the right to respect, to self-expression, or to the pursuit of happiness than as an independent right. Rights also proliferate in the polemic of legal disputes, such as a tenant's right to a pet or a neighbor's right to an unobstructed view. And rights are sometimes invented by institutional wisdom: It is more prudent for regulatory agencies to assert that patients in extended care facilities have a right to access (access defined) to a free telephone (described) in a convenient (defined) location than to assert vaguely that patients have a right to communicate with outsiders. The former is "surveyable" and enforceable; the latter is not.

Two points are essential. First, we should not lose sight of the force of calling something a *right*. Respect for persons includes both empathy and autonomy. The idea of rights attempts to protect these by allowing us to make *claims* or demands on others about our needs and interests, and by *formalizing* these claims by enforceable customs and laws.[25] Second, we can distinguish a shorter list of basic *fundamental*, constitutional, or human rights from other rights. Fundamental rights are closely related to the concept of justice. They identify basic needs we have in common, which should be fairly met.

Discussions of health care issues often refer to rights. On one hand, this reflects a growing awareness of patient autonomy and a wish to respect and encourage active participation by patients in their care. On the other, it arises from the increasing inability of health care institutions to meet basic human needs. The "Patients' Bill of Rights," for example, was published in 1973 by the American Hospital Association to address some of the common problem areas of hospital practice (see Appendix). The Bill lists such rights as confidentiality, refusal of treatment, informed consent to therapy and experimentation, knowledge of the names of those providing treatment, respectful care, explanation of the charges, and so on. The Bill does not create any new rights for patients. Instead, it lists clearly what patients are entitled to but do not always receive.

In these circumstances, many nurses have adopted the role of patient *advocate*. The concept of advocate is linked with the notion of rights in that one advocates the rights of patients. In advocacy, one becomes a partisan in conflicts and assumes responsibility for presenting the rights and interests of a client. In this way, the nurse becomes a sort of attorney for the sick, who may not be able to defend themselves because of their illness.

The language of rights also has defects: It tends to presuppose conflict. The

---

[25]For a fuller discussion, see Joel Feinberg, "The Nature and Value of Rights," in Gorovitz, *Moral Problems*, pp. 454–67.

concept of rights originates in the image of an individual threatened by outside forces. Sometimes this perspective is realistic in health care. However, the language of rights sometimes sounds unnecessarily adversarial. If a mutual and cooperative inquiry into different values is called for, introducing rights can harden positions and hinder communication.

For instance, talk of the right to death with dignity is usually employed in defense of limiting treatment of dying patients who prefer palliative care and support to heroic efforts to save their lives. In order for patients to have good palliative care and support, they may need to die in a hospice or at home with adequate visiting nursing care. In 1980, these facilities were often not available or not covered under many insurance plans. Without adequate facilities, assertion of a right to death with dignity is empty. In contrast, if facilities for hospice care were made available to hospitals, then patients would receive such care if they chose it without need to discuss their rights. The rhetoric of rights takes us an extra step away from the central consideration. We become involved in an abstract debate over patient autonomy instead of engaging in a reasonable and effective discussion of how to change institutions to better reflect the desires of patients. Although the language of rights arises from an ideology of patient autonomy, it sometimes obfuscates awareness of the need to provide services that respect autonomy.

Another problem with talk of rights is that it centers on the individual when many basic goods that ensure our welfare cannot be provided on an individual basis. A right to clean air is not simply the right to purchase an oxygen tank. The right to health is complex: It involves automobile speed limits, occupational health and safety regulations, building codes, access to health care institutions, and the like. Our needs cannot be effectively met so long as they are viewed as primarily a function of individual behavior.

Lastly, rights language tends to emphasize negative rights, that is, the *protection* of what one has, and not positive rights, or the *provision* of what one needs. This is because negative rights place fewer responsibilities on others than positive rights. It has thus tended to protect those who have a lot from those who have little. For instance, negative rights to property defend the possession and use of existing property in a world of extreme wealth and poverty, while positive rights to property argue for minimum income maintenance for those who need it. The right to access to health care as a negative right simply defends the access to those who already have it; a positive right argues that it should be *provided* for those who need it.

The concept of rights is indeed an important concept for the just expression of individual needs; however, it emphasizes individual conflict and underestimates collective human resources too much to provide a complete theory of ethics.

Responsibility

In order to make moral judgments about an event, we need to tell some kind of story or case study about what happened or was supposed to happen. This is why fiction and drama are such good vehicles for exploring moral insights. In such stories we identify the principal agents and explain what did or should occur. We say who is *responsible* for what and make judgments about their actions. The concept of responsibility provides the bare bones, the conceptual structure, of our moral drama. On this structure hangs the flesh of praise and blame, fault, heroism, lessons for the novice, and so on.

Causal Responsibility[26]

In our simplest stories, and as a first step in thinking about responsibility, we identify the main characters who *made things happen* in the story: "Head Nurse Prince assigned Ms. Lai San to inventory the drug cabinet." "Mr. Ryan gave Ms. Purtilo in Room 14A an overdose of insulin this morning." Each of these scenarios identifies an agent *causally responsible* for an event. In one, Head Nurse Prince is responsible for making an assignment. In the other, Mr. Ryan is responsible for an overdose.

Assignment of causal responsibility is not limited to people. We also assign causal responsibility to our *actions:* "Making that stupid remark caused (was responsible for) a lot of trouble." "Forgetting to turn the lights off is raising (is responsible for raising) our electric bill."

Our stories can identify other important figures: "The *threat* of nuclear war is the cause of (is responsible for) stress and anxiety." "*God* brought a great wind which piled up the waters." "*Germs* cause diseases." And so on. We give the central people, actions, events, objects, and processes in our stories causal responsibility for how the story goes.

Role Responsibility

Forgetting for a moment what actually happened, we can tell stories about what is *supposed* to happen. These stories are like those of causal responsibility, but they assign a different kind of responsibility: *role responsibility*. "It is Ms. Prince's responsibility to assign tasks on the unit." "It was Mr. Ryan's responsibility to determine the correct dose of insulin." "I am responsible for what I say." "The last person up is responsible for turning off the lights."

Since people do not always do what they are supposed to, the idea of role responsibility is less concrete than that of causal responsibility. In an abstract way, *roles* are made of sets of role responsibilities. For example, the role of staff nurse can be analyzed in terms of a complex set of responsibilities. These responsibilities tell us what anyone who fills the role of staff nurse should be doing.

Sometimes when a role is fully sketched out in responsibilities, the person who fills the role is protected from other responsibilities. A nurse responsible for patients on Ward 4B is only under special circumstances also responsible for patients on 5A. Or one may see something wrong in the hospital and lack role responsibility for doing something about it.

There are many kinds of roles, formal and informal, all of which carry responsibilities. Spouse, numbers runner, hostess, lead guitar, patient, and Director of Nursing are all roles that attach different responsibilities. Role and causal responsibility are the two simplest concepts of responsibility. Other concepts of responsi-

---

[26]The terminology of causal, role, liability, and capacity responsibility follows, H.L.A. Hart, *Punishment and Responsibility* (New York: Oxford University Press, 1968).

bility arise largely from our efforts to make judgments as we compare our stories of what actually happens with what was *supposed* to happen.

Liability Responsibility

Suppose we compare stories of causal and role responsibility: "Peter Parker was supposed to bring wine to the staff party" (role), and "Peter Parker actually brought potato salad to the staff party" (cause). Here is an invitation for a judgment of liability responsibility: "Why is there no wine at the party? It's Peter Parker's fault" (his liability responsibility).

Comparing the stories of role and cause is a delicate matter, for we may be too quick to make a judgment of liability. How we assign liability depends on how we fill out the rest of the account and explain any mismatch between the two stories. It may turn out that the hostess got mixed up and told Peter to bring the wrong thing. Maybe Peter is on a campaign to keep alcohol off the hospital floor. Maybe he drank it all. Maybe Mary Anne is bringing the wine later.

Judgments of liability are not always negative. Suppose Peter brought the wine as expected and also brought the potato salad, which the hostess overlooked. He may then deserve special praise, and this, too, is a delicate judgment. We can tell stories that rob him of his praise: Mary Anne actually made the salad and insisted he take it, but he took credit for it. Out of this process of adjusting our stories of role and causal responsibility come many subtle explanations of human action.

We tell these stories for many reasons: to find points for change in the future, to criticize our basic ways of life, to enlighten ourselves about human nature, to reduce human events to deeper causal principles, and so on. Such stories may occur as case studies to raise issues of moral uncertainty, dilemma, and distress. We often use such stories to encourage work to go according to plan. In these uses is the root of the term *responsibility: Responsibility* comes from *to respond,* which means *to answer.* To be responsible for something, good or bad, is to be *answerable* for it. Other words for *answer for* are *to account for,* and from this root we get *accountability.* In order to be principal agents in explanations, we have to act so that others can make judgments about our liability.

Capacity Responsibility

There are many ways to appear as a human being in a story and yet to have no attributed responsibilities. One can lack the *capacity* for responsibility. One may be unable to fulfill certain responsibilities because of mental disability—insanity, retardation, intoxication, coma, and so forth. In these cases, one would wrongly be judged liable for not fulfilling them. A person may not even be seen as a causal agent in a story, as when people say, "It was her *illness* speaking, not her." "Temporarily normal" people are generally presumed to have the capacity to fulfill their roles, and when we argue that they lack capacity responsibility, we have to give reasons for it. The normal presumption of capacity to be responsible is one way of showing respect for autonomy.

Another way to lack accountability is to act under *coercion.* If one is forced to do things, then one may drop out as a responsible character, and the coercing party becomes the agent on whom we focus.[27] Or one may refuse to *assume* responsibility and allow others to control events. Or one may try to be invisible, silent, maintain no record of one's actions, and credit others with one's own acts, in order to gain unaccountable power, although such avoidance of responsibility is more likely to result in powerlessness.

One great philosophical challenge to judgments of liability and capacity suggests that people should not really appear as the main characters in stories of responsibility at all. It is argued that all our actions can be reduced in principle to scientific laws. We are not freely choosing agents. Instead, the true stories of our actions are motivated by history, psychology, genetics, and physics. The principal agents controlling events are causal laws and the initial conditions under which the world began.[28]

This is an important challenge to the concept of responsibility and a source of concern to individuals who wonder what they can do to control events in the world around them. But if this determinist picture is supposed to deny responsibility by showing we are not really *free* in our actions, it does not work. Freedom is neither necessary nor sufficient for responsibility. For instance, sometimes we rightly judge people not responsible when they are coerced even though they were free to take risks by resisting. And if I wholeheartedly join an evil cause, even if I would have been forced to do it anyway and thus was not free, I would still be responsible for my choice.

We are both characters in, and narrators of, our stories of responsibility. We have many options about how we place ourselves in them. We may take or refuse responsibility, act responsibly or irresponsibly, and dispute with others over these assignments. Hospitals are a backdrop for many stories and claims regarding responsibilities. Different stories compete for the "true" picture of what is going on in the hospital, and different points of view reflect upon one another as in a hall of mirrors. In complex institutions like hospitals, many subtle versions of responsibility develop. For instance, the actual *process* of making decisions may be delegated to a subordinate while the *responsibility* for the decision stays with the supervisor. Or professional responsibility may be distinct from personal responsibility, as when one feels a professional responsibility to care for, and a personal responsibility to avoid, a vociferously racist patient. Other common phenomena of responsibility include the following:

1. *Unofficial responsibility:* It was Dr. May's responsibility to obtain informed consent from the patient, but he forgot. Nurse Corrigan took care of it. She did what had to be done and acted without authority.
2. *Out-of-title work:* Medical student Castle cleaned up after a mess. She made the bed and swept the floor. She caught hell from nursing and housekeeping.
3. *Avoiding blame:* Many strategies are used by individuals and institutions to avoid blame.
   a. *Risk-management:* Hospitals hire specialists to help them reduce the likelihood of being sued.

[27]There is disagreement among philosophers over this point. Sartre would argue for our responsibility under any circumstance. See Chapter 18 for a further discussion.

[28]For philosophical discussions, see Bernard Berofsky, *Free Will and Determinism* (New York: Harper & Row, Publishers, Inc., 1966).

b. *Stringent rules:* Sometimes safety procedures are designed to be so complex that no one can follow them properly and do his or her work. If an accident happens, workers in violation of safety rules can be blamed. Or a drug company may suggest lower than ideal dosages for medications they manufacture to place liability on physicians should appropriate prescribing produce untoward side effects.

c. *Scapegoating:* Although neither the patient's attending physician nor the surgeon showed up at the hospital, and they called in irrational orders, the patient's death was attributed at rounds to the intern's missing an indication on the x-ray. Although the staff nurses in the pediatric intensive care unit never communicated to Dr. Meier how much the infant was suffering, they blamed her for continuing aggressive therapy.

d. *Malpractice:* Although malpractice insurance and suits provide compensation to injured patients, they also invite a search for parties to blame and create risks for those who admit making errors. Three untoward consequences of malpractice suits upon telling true stories of responsibility are: (1) People avoid blame rather than admit it, (2) lawyers tend to sue those with the "deepest pocket" and increase the motive of those in power to increase their control over those who work for them, and (3) hiding and covering up mistakes results in unscientific and unethical practice.

e. *"Cover your ass":* Staff do a variety of things to avoid personal risks. For example, Nurse Drew was too busy to turn a patient in bed regularly and wrote in the chart that she turned the patient every two hours. During cardiopulmonary resuscitation, Nurse Beckwith charted some drugs not used as given, to show for the record that everything possible was done.

4. *Acquiring praise:*
   a. *Case 1:* It was clear to the visitor to the kidney unit that careful nursing follow-up was the main factor in patient survival, but the medical staff would not permit a study confirming this lest it redirect praise to less powerful participants.
   b. *Case 2:* Nurse Fosdick and Doctor Hawkins collaborated on a study. Fosdick wrote the protocol, did most of the legwork and calculations, and wrote the first draft of the report. Hawkins's name appeared as first author in the publication, since they both thought it would be easier to publish if the senior author was a physician.

5. *Collective omissions:* Nurse Anderson wanted to report an incident, but the hospital had failed to establish a procedure for receiving such reports. She did not know what to do.

6. *Collective responsibility:* The health care team and the Harrison family arrived at a consensus after long and serious discussion that Ms. Harrison's respiratory support should be discontinued. Although Dr. Brown "turned off" the machine, the team and family were collectively responsible for the action.

It may be impossible to tell what is going on in a complex institution, and moral judgments may have to be reserved for lack of a coherent picture. Since both individuals and institutions can bear responsibility, we need to look both at how people fulfill responsibilities and at how responsibilities are distributed among individuals and institutions before we can develop a comprehensive picture for making moral judgments. Care should therefore be taken to identify responsibilities carefully in the first phases of ethics decision procedures (see p. 67).

Ethical Theory

Philosophers sometimes attempt to give an account of ethical thinking that is unified and universal by forming an *ethical theory*. An ethical theory consists of a principle or coherent set of principles that help to make sense of the power that *oughts* and *shoulds* have in our thinking. Ethical theory attempts to show the rational or real foundations of moral principles and concepts or to give definitions of central moral terminology, such as *morally right* or *morally good*.

Philosophers approach moral theory differently from sociologists, anthropologists, historians, and psychologists. The latter specialists try to develop theories of how and why particular views on ethics grow out of societies, cultures, historical periods, and personalities. They look for the causal origins, explanations, or development of moral views. In contrast, philosophers are looking for theories that help us decide what to do, that *justify* moral views, or that give moral judgments a *foundation* in reason, knowledge, or deep principles of reality. The philosophical approach is thus *normative,* while the social science approach is *descriptive.* Two common types of normative ethical theory—consequentialism and formalism—are useful in sorting out what reasons one is appealing to in making ethical decisions.

Consequentialism

One major type of normative ethical theory states that the morally right thing to do is that act which produces the greatest good. Where, as is often the case, even the best choice produces both good and bad consequences, one should choose that act which produces the greatest expected balance of good over bad. But what is good and bad? The most famous formulation of this theory is *utilitarianism*. As expressed by John Stuart Mill, utilitarianism claims that the good is happiness and the bad unhappiness. In Mill's words,

> The creed which accepts as the foundation of morals "utility" or the "greatest happiness principle" holds that actions are right in proportion as they tend to promote happiness, wrong as they tend to promote the reverse of happiness.[29]

According to Mill, the happiness to be maximized is the happiness of all, oneself included. The happiness of each person counts equally.

This is a very brief sketch of a broad and important theory, of which there are many versions. Its main elements—concern for general happiness and balancing benefits and losses—can be found today in such diverse concerns as welfare economics, risk-benefit analysis, decision analysis, and game theory. In one important version of this theory, *rule utilitarianism,* the general-happiness criterion is not applied to specific actions but to general *rules*. It says that people should in general follow those moral rules which are likely to produce the greatest happiness for all.

Utilitarianism expresses a common belief that moral rules should not be arbitrary but serve a purpose. For instance, it helps to explain the general prohibition against lying and its exceptions. We should generally tell the truth even when deception has benefits, because in the long run the benefits of truth outweigh the benefits of illusion. General adherence to truth telling is important to us. Yet there is

[29]Mill, *Utilitarianism,* in Gorovitz, *Moral Problems,* p. 38.

room for lies: When the truth would be utterly disastrous for all and nothing gained from it, it would be morally better to lie, from both the point of view of utilitarianism and common moral intuition.

Formalism

The most common alternate perspective is called *formalism*. It is skeptical about our ability to look into the future and base our decisions on the consequences of our actions. Formalism is concerned instead with the *kind* of action we choose, not its outcome. This places happiness in a very different perspective. To paraphrase history's most prominent formalist, Immanuel Kant, the moral problem is not how to be happy, but how to be *worthy* of happiness.[30] This perspective reflects a common feeling that we are happiest when we feel we are doing something worthwhile and maintaining self-esteem, not when we are trying to please ourselves and everyone else.

Kant's formalist theory attempts to explain why ethical principles are compelling. He seats their power in the appeal certain moral principles have for our *rationality*. The compelling moral rules are those which can be universalized without contradiction, an important test of rationality. This test of moral rules is Kant's *categorical imperative:*

> Act only according to that maxim by which you can at the same time will that it should become a universal law.[31]

For example, Kant argues that one would have to reject false promises as an ethical means for obtaining money because to make a universal law of the principle, "Whenever anyone needs money, he or she will promise falsely to return it," would destroy the institution of making promises. Thus, the proposed convention or maxim can't be universalized. Kant also rejected suicide as moral on the grounds that a universal law stating in effect, "When I am in despair, I will kill myself," conflicts with a natural law, widely believed in his time, that any natural being, such as a human being, tends to and has an urge to remain in existence.

For Kant, legitimate ethical conventions had to pass two additional tests identified by him as formulations of the categorical imperative. The last and most important was that people should not be used merely as a means to an end:

> Act so that you treat humanity, whether in your own person or in that of another, always as an end and never as a means only.[32]

Kant held the autonomy of persons in high regard and urged us to respect the autonomy of others. He saw autonomy as the ability to be rational and appreciate the moral law. Kant's formalism helps to account for our sometimes strong sense of duty and our occasional willingness to act out of principle whatever the consequences. It urges us to consider how important being principled can be to our self-

[30]Kant, *Foundations,* p. 9.

[31]Ibid., p. 39. (To *will* is to *choose.* A *maxim* is a *conventional moral rule.*)

[32]Ibid., p. 47.

esteem, and it rests our sense of identity more on the purity of our motives than on our limited ability to make things turn out for the best.

We can use ethical theories to point out important aspects of our ethical decision processes and to help put them in an order that fosters reasonable decision making. For example, the procedure for making decisions in Chapter 4 employs utilitarian considerations at its third stage, identifying and weighing options, because utilitarianism emphasizes foresight, calculating the consequences of each possible option, and taking uncertainty and conflicting interests into account (see text p. 67). The formalist perspective is more useful at the fourth stage, thinking things through. Kant's criteria are useful in identifying the most sound principles and values and in deciding which are the most important to consider.

Both Kant's and Mill's theories help to interpret conventional ethical principles. Kant's concept of autonomy, for example, is related to the concept of professional autonomy discussed in Chapter 3. Both concepts require individuals to appeal to general principles of reason. But Kant's version of reason is very general and abstract; he generalizes to all humankind and uses the fundamental logical test of noncontradiction. When a professional appeals to the conventional principles of her profession, she is calling on a body of experience limited largely to the health care setting, and the reasoning process is more concrete and less strictly logical. Mill's balancing of harm and benefit is represented in risk-benefit assessments of therapy for patients when outcomes are uncertain, as discussed in Chapter 7.

Formalism and utilitarianism also help to provide unified but contrasting approaches to the various philosophical concepts of this chapter. For instance, Kant's last formulation of the categorical imperative, not using people as a means to an end, is the second criterion of *respect for persons*. Mill's approach, founded in experiential aspects of persons, is more congruent with the first criterion of respect, empathy. Kant provides a way to test values for soundness through reason and generalization and thus offers some objectivity for specific values, while Mill's theory tends to sweep all values under the heading of happiness and so tends to obscure the process of resolving conflicts among values. Unfortunately, neither theory is helpful in explaining *distributive justice*. Kant's theory is focused on individual worthiness for happiness, not the overall balance of happiness. Mill's theory tells us how to maximize happiness by *aggregating* it, while our sense of justice is concerned with the best way to *distribute* it. One person fully happy and one fully unhappy add up to the same as two people who are both neither happy nor unhappy. Although the second state is more just than the first, both outcomes are equivalent in terms of the total aggregate of happiness. Thus there is some question whether utilitarianism can explain justice and prevent sacrificing the rights of single individuals for the good of society as a whole.[33] Formalism, meanwhile, neglects very real concerns with human welfare, and it hazards embracing excessively rationalistic and arbitrary duties. The apparently "hard-edge" emphasis on duty is itself offensive to many who see ethics as a gentler and less determinate realm of thought.

This text is not oriented to developing general moral theories; most of the discussion makes do with an assortment of case analyses, concepts, plausible principles, and intuitions difficult to arrange into a coherent theory. A philosopher with a strong theoretical or synthetic bent will find this unsatisfying. But the experience of many philosophers working in health care has been that philosophical moral

[33]Rawls, *Theory of Justice*, pp. 22–33.

theories are too abstract and general to be applied with precision to specific decisions. In ordinary moral discussions, most people appeal to both formalist and
utilitarian considerations. Moreover, formalists and utilitarians are likely to agree
on most decisions in health care if they make similar assumptions about the world.
What is consistently universalizable and what is likely to work out for the best
usually come in specific cases to the same choice. Small groups making hard
decisions in health care usually come to a consensus in spite of theoretical differences, by using more immediate principles and specific, concrete considerations.
Although this circumstance suggests that something more is desirable in ethical
theory, the breadth and consistency of Kant's and Mill's work serves as a warning
that specific consensus on health care decisions is eventually subject to the tests of
reason and concern for humanity at large.

Summary

Some basic concepts and principles used in reflection on ethics are respect for
persons, justice, values, rights, responsibility, and theories of right and wrong.

Respect for persons involves empathy with others and not using people merely as a means to an end. It is perhaps the most basic concept in ethics.

Justice combines the notions of deserving, harmony, and equality. Distributive, retributive, and procedural justice are three basic types of justice. Distributive
justice is the most important for health care, and defining a principle for the just
distribution of health care is an important concern.

Values identify what is or should be important to us. They underlie the
specific goods and purposes which we seek in life. We often dispute about values,
wondering whether values are individual or universal and whether there is anything
we should value apart from what we actually value. Resolving conflicts over values
requires a social process involving debate and personal judgment.

There are many kinds of *rights:* legal and moral, ideal and actual, positive and
negative, fundamental and contractual. Rights are also related to responsibilities.
Basically, rights are justified discretionary claims on others not to interfere with
what we have or are doing. An expanded concept of rights, such as *human rights,*
can be used to defend the right to basic health care services.

In order to make moral judgments about events we need to ascertain who is
responsible for what. Responsibility is a complex concept involving the ideas of
cause, role, liability, and capacity. In complex organizations such as hospitals,
people dispute over responsibilities in order to acquire praise and to avoid blame.
Responsibility is not limited to individual human beings, but may be attributed to
collective or nonhuman entities such as diseases, events, and institutions.

Two major *theories* compete to explain what at bottom determines right from
wrong. *Utilitarianism* is a consequentialist account that says in effect that those acts
are right which produce the greatest overall balance of happiness over unhappiness.
Formalism focuses less on the consequences of acts and more on the nature of the
act itself and personal intentions. Kant developed a formalist theory based on the
requirement that valid moral principles be generalizable to everyone. Most people
combine elements of both formalism and consequentialism in their everyday moral
thinking.

FURTHER READINGS

General Works

BRANDT, RICHARD B., *Ethical Theory*. Englewood Cliffs, N.J.: Prentice-Hall, Inc., 1959.
BRODY, BARUCH A., *Beginning Philosophy*. Englewood Cliffs, N.J.: Prentice-Hall, Inc., 1977.
DONAGAN, ALAN, *The Theory of Morality*. Chicago: University of Chicago Press, 1976.
DOWNIE, R.S., *Roles and Values: An Introduction to Social Ethics*. London: Methuen & Co., Ltd., 1971.
FEINBERG, JOEL, *Social Philosophy*. Englewood Cliffs, N.J.: Prentice-Hall, Inc., 1973.
FELDMAN, FRED, *Introductory Ethics*. Englewood Cliffs, N.J.: Prentice-Hall, Inc., 1978.
FRANKENA, WILLIAM K., *Ethics* (2nd ed.). Englewood Cliffs, N.J.: Prentice-Hall, Inc., 1973.
MACKIE, J.L., *Ethics: Inventing Right and Wrong*. Middlesex, England: Penguin Books, 1977.
OLSON, ROBERT G., *Ethics: A Short Introduction*. New York: Random House, Inc., 1978.
SINGER, PETER, *Practical Ethics*. Cambridge: Cambridge University Press, 1979.
WARNOCK, G.J., *Contemporary Moral Philosophy*. London: Macmillan & Co., 1967.
WILLIAMS, BERNARD, *Morality*. New York: Harper & Row, Publishers, Inc., 1972.

Paternalism and Autonomy

BEAUCHAMP, TOM L., AND JAMES F. CHILDRESS, *Principles of Biomedical Ethics* (2nd ed.), chap. 3, "The Principle of Autonomy," pp. 59–105. New York: Oxford University Press, 1983.
CARTER, ROSEMARY, "Justifying Paternalism," *Canadian Journal of Philosophy*, 7 (1977), 133–45.
DWORKIN, GERALD, "Autonomy and Behavior Control," *Hastings Center Report*, 6 (February 1976), 23–28.
———, "Paternalism," *Monist*, 56 (1972), 64–84. Reprinted in *Moral Problems in Medicine*, eds. Samuel Gorovitz et al., pp. 185–200. Englewood Cliffs, N.J.: Prentice-Hall, Inc., 1976.
GAYLIN, WILLARD, "On The Borders of Persuasion: A Psychoanalytic Look at Coercion," *Psychiatry*, 37 (February 1974), 1–9.
GERT, BERNARD, AND C.M. CULVER, "Paternalistic Behavior," *Philosophy and Public Affairs*, 6 (Fall 1976), 45–57.
HODSON, JOHN D., "The Principle of Paternalism," *American Philosophical Quarterly*, 14 (1977), 61–69.

Ethics Concepts and Theories

CHRISTIANSEN, DREW, "Dignity in Aging," *Hastings Center Report*, 4, 1 (February 1974), 6–8.
COLETTA, SUZANNE SMITH, "Values Clarification in Nursing: Why?" *American Journal of Nursing*, 78 (December 1978), 2057–63.
DWORKIN, RONALD, *Taking Rights Seriously*. Cambridge, Mass.: Harvard University Press, 1971.
———, "What Is Equality: Part 1: Equality of Welfare," *Philosophy & Public Affairs*, 10 (1981), 185–246.
———, "What Is Equality: Part 2: Equality of Resources," *Philosophy & Public Affairs*, 10 (1981), 283–345.
FEINBERG, JOEL, *Doing and Deserving: Essays in the Theory of Responsibility*. Princeton, N.J.: Princeton University Press, 1970.

FRENCH, PETER A., ED., *Individual and Collective Responsibility.* Cambridge, Mass.: Schenkman Publishing Co., Inc., 1972.

FRIED, C., *An Anatomy of Values.* Cambridge, Mass.: Harvard University Press, 1970.

GLOVER, JONATHAN, *Responsibility.* London: Routledge & Kegan Paul, Ltd., 1970.

GRIFFIN, JAMES, "Are There Incommensurable Values?" *Philosophy and Public Affairs,* 7, 1 (1977), 39–59.

LYONS, DAVID, ED., *Rights.* Belmont, Calif.: Wadsworth Publishing Co., Inc., 1979.

MACINTYRE, ALASDAIR, "Can Medicine Dispense with a Theological Perspective on Human Nature?" in *Knowledge, Value and Belief,* eds. H. Tristram Engelhardt, Jr. and Daniel Callahan, pp. 25–43. Hastings-on-Hudson, N.Y.: The Hastings Center, 1977.

———, "A Crisis in Moral Philosophy: Why Is the Search for the Foundations of Ethics So Frustrating?" in *Knowing and Valuing: The Search for Common Roots,* eds. H. Tristram Engelhardt, Jr. and Daniel Callahan, pp. 18–35. Hastings-on-Hudson, N.Y.: Hastings Center, 1980.

———, "How Virtues Become Vices: Values, Medicine and Social Context," in *Evaluation and Explanation in the Biomedical Sciences,* eds. H. Tristram Engelhardt, Jr. and Stuart F. Spicker, pp. 97–111. Dordrecht, Holland: D. Reidel Publishing Co., 1975.

MELDEN, A.I. *Rights and Persons.* Berkeley, Calif.: University of California Press, 1977.

MILLER, DAVID, *Social Justice.* Oxford: Clarendon Press, 1976.

SINGER, PETER, "Famine, Affluence, and Morality," *Philosophy and Public Affairs,* 7, 3 (Spring 1972), 229–43.

SMART, J.J.C., AND B. WILLIAMS, *Utilitarianism.* Cambridge: Cambridge University Press, 1973.

SMITH, SHARON JEANNE, AND ANNE J. DAVIS, "Ethical Dilemmas: Conflicts among Rights, Duties, and Obligations," *American Journal of Nursing,* 80 (1980), 1463–66.

SOŁTAN, KAROL EDWARD, "Empirical Studies of Distributive Justice," *Ethics,* 92 (1982), 673–91.

STEELE, SHIRLEY M., AND VERA M. HARMON, *Values Clarification in Nursing* (2nd ed.). Englewood Cliffs, N.J.: Prentice-Hall, Inc., 1983.

VEATCH, HENRY B., *For an Ontology of Morals.* Evanston, Ill.: Northwestern University Press, 1971.

WACHTER-SHIKORA, NANCY, "Scapegoating among Professionals," *American Journal of Nursing,* 77 (1977), 408–9.

WILLIAMS, BERNARD, "The Idea of Equality," in *Philosophy, Politics and Society,* second series, eds. Peter Laslett and W.G. Runciman, pp. 110–131. Oxford: Blackwell, 1962.

CHAPTER 11

Reason, Reflection, and Research in Ethics

Caring for the sick and comforting the suffering are obviously morally worthy activities. Nurses frequently identify strongly with these basic commitments of their profession. Thus, raising ethical questions about them can make life harder for nurses: When nurses examine their commitments at the same time that they act upon them in clinical practice, they make their decision process more complex. And because nurses often identify personally with such goals as health, examining these goals involves nurses in self-examination. Like assessing oneself carefully in the mirror, questioning one's personal goals and commitments may seem threatening at first.

The process of ethical reflection is nevertheless well worth time and attention. It can improve the quality of professional decisions, raise the level of communication with others, increase sensitivity to patients, and give one a sense of clarity and enlightenment about one's work. Concepts like respect for persons, justice, values, rights, and responsibilities play an important role in conducting this examination in a systematic and reasonable way. Reflective reasoning, however, always takes place in the social context of conventional principles and practice. The cultural setting of ethical reflection creates the occasion for reflection and sets limits on potential solutions to ethical issues. There is an important interaction between cultural traditions and reasoned reflection on ethics.

Reflection in a Cultural Context

The main outlines of our moral views result from socialization. Our moral ideas are given to us formally and informally, intentionally and unconsciously, by our parents, other adults, peers, professions, and the media. People growing up in different cultures are more likely to have different views on ethics than people

152

growing up in the same culture, just as children speak the language of the culture in which they were raised.

According to one common view of the growth of moral beliefs, our principles are fixed early in life and are not much within our personal control. As part of our personalities, our moral views are determined by significant features of child rearing. Feelings of guilt and the commands of the superego jostle us in the direction of primitive conceptions of right and wrong beyond our powers of reason and desires to change. Many of us are familiar with the experience of feeling guilty even though we are sure we are right, or of not feeling guilty, even when we are sure we are wrong.

According to another common view of moral socialization, we play a much more active role in moral development. Early in life, we begin to reason about ethical issues, but in a style determined by our emerging cognitive capacities. These capacities include our ability to distinguish ourselves from others, to follow rules, to manipulate rules, to give causal explanations, to think about the future, and so on. Piaget, for example, described moral development as progressing gradually from a condition in which moral rules are perceived as external and very powerful, to one in which moral rules are internal and subject to mature judgment. He termed the early state *heteronomy* and saw development as approaching *autonomy*. He saw the process of moral maturation as continuing throughout life.

Piaget saw our moral development as analogous to our growing understanding in childhood of how to play games such as marbles. In the beginning, we roll marbles around in imitation of older children but are unable to understand the rules. Later, we are able to follow the rules, but regard them as permanent and unchangeable, perhaps created by adults or the gods. The eldest marble players see the rules for what they are: children's creations based on a desire for enjoyment and a sense of fairness. The most experienced marble players can thus vary the rules according to their sense of fairness and fun.[1]

Lawrence Kohlberg developed and refined Piaget's account of moral development. Kohlberg distinguished six stages of development grouped into three basic pairs of stages. In the first two stages, the *premoral* stages, we are mainly concerned with ourselves. The goodness or badness of an action is seen in terms of its good or bad consequences to ourselves. In early childhood, we are good in order to avoid punishment and to gain love and regard. In the third and fourth stages, the *conventional* stages, we reach a level of development where we accept the customs of our parents and peers uncritically and defend them fiercely. Right, wrong, and self-esteem are measured in terms of their conformity with what we see as general practice (third stage) or in terms of obedience to authority or "law and order" (fourth stage). The two highest levels, the *principled* stages, constitute the most mature levels of moral development. Like the experienced marble player, one moves beyond received views of right and wrong and tests actions and conventions by one's personal sense of right and wrong, justice, and responsibility. Self-conscious utilitarians and Kantians can be seen as exhibiting fifth and sixth stage moral reasoning.

Kohlberg's stages reflect how one *reasons* about one's choices, not the choices one is making. For example, if one holds that nurses should be competent, then at stage one or two one might reason, "I should be competent because I would

[1]Jean Piaget et al., *The Moral Judgment of the Child,* (New York: The Free Press, 1965).

be fired if I were not." At stage three or four, one would say, "I am competent because I uphold the ANA code of ethics." At stage five or six, one might say, "I maintain competence because I have considered the issues and judge that my competence best helps to maintain the welfare of patients and nurses alike." These brief samples of reasoning are of course oversimplifications. Like Piaget, Kohlberg connects moral reasoning with our overall cognitive reasoning capacities, and so each stage represents an overall style of reasoning. During the premoral period we are just learning the knack of rule following and are not yet able to think much beyond ourselves. In the conventional stages we can follow rules but cannot manipulate them. We are able to identify with others but lack a fully developed sense of our own identity. In the principled stages we have a strong sense of self and a highly developed and coherent approach to principles and values, so that we are able to place conventional ethics in perspective.[2]

It is controversial whether, as one becomes more developed in one's moral reasoning powers, one also becomes a better person who acts more rightly. Kohlberg is inclined to think so, but many doubt his position. Since his theory focuses on the development of reasoning powers, one could paint a picture of someone highly developed personally and intellectually but committed to an unusual theory of ethics. Machiavellianism, for example, is a reflective approach to ethics that many regard as evil. Or one could be a highly sophisticated skeptic about ethical thinking. Or one might decide, upon reflection, to endorse a sophisticated ethical theory modeled on earlier stages of development and thereby give mature support to traditionalism or self-interest. If so, a person in a principled stage would give reasons undistinguishable from those of earlier stages. For these reasons and others, we may not always judge the most morally developed person to be the morally best person.[3]

Like the psychologists discussed above, sociologists have also attempted to explain the origins of our conventional moral practices. The scope of their inquiry is in some respects broader than the psychologists'. They do not ask how *individuals* acquire moral beliefs and reasoning; they ask how *cultures* as a whole adopt and maintain central values and moral principles.

The *functionalists* see conventional moral principles as functioning positively in a culture to maintain its stability and benefit its members. Cultures in different natural and historical contexts would be expected to need different principles to maintain stability in different settings. Ritual euthanasia of the elderly among Eskimos, for example, has been interpreted as necessary for a small population in a harsh environment. The work ethic of Protestantism can be seen as supporting the development of capitalism in Western Europe. To understand a moral principle, a functionalist tries to find the role it plays in maintaining the culture as a whole.

The *social conflict* theorists have a bleaker view. They tend to see dominant moral values as benefiting a small portion of a culture—the *elite*—and as being used by the elite to maintain their domination over everyone else in the culture. The

[2]Lawrence Kohlberg, *The Philosophy of Moral Development* (San Francisco: Harper & Row Publishers, Inc., 1981). Kohlberg's concept of principled thinking and my concept of reflection are not identical. Reflection, as I use the concept in this work, is an *activity* that one may or may not choose to engage in. The principled stages label a set of human *capacities* generated by maturational processes.

[3]For further development and critique of Kohlberg, see Carol Gilligan, *In a Different Voice: Psychological Theory and Women's Development* (Cambridge, Mass.: Harvard University Press, 1982).

widely held work ethic, for example, can be seen as primarily benefiting those who own the factories and offices in which people work so hard. Submissiveness in women can be seen as serving the interests and dominance of men.

How we explain the origins of accepted moral beliefs thus depends in part on how we judge their value upon reflection. At the same time, what we reflect upon and what we perceive as problematic in ethics depends in part on our received cultural views. In the United States, many views of ethics are represented. We grow up exposed to ideas about ethics from different sources, and these ideas do not always fit well together. For example, our ideas of personal achievement sometimes clash with our ideas of equality. Our ideas of fun may conflict with our ideas of health. In order to mature in our moral views, we need to reflect reasonably on these conflicts and seek ways to resolve them.

But to be fully satisfactory, answers to moral problems must satisfy the tests of both reflective reason and cultural acceptability. The second is important because a significant dimension of resolving moral problems is the creation of new and more reasonable practices and because conventional moral principles require the acceptance and support of those who use them. We thus find ourselves in a cycle of reasoning, moving back and forth between reflection and cultural practice. The result of this process is gradual change in our views and practices. For instance, reflection by women on their traditional roles has resulted in changes in conventional practices by and in relation to women, and these new practices have led to new reflection as new issues were perceived, and so on. By thinking as reasonably as possible about ethical issues, we hope to improve the positions given us by our culture. By developing a viewpoint that meets the test of one's conscience and the reasoned scrutiny of others, we participate in the development of new cultural practices.

The Role of Reasoning in Reflection

When confronted with concepts, principles, and issues in ethics, health professionals may worry that new, special, and mysterious thinking is needed. This is not so. It is best for nurses to start with problem-solving skills they are accustomed to use in professional practice. The decision process of Chapter 4 (pp. 66–68) is based on typical clinical decision methods.

But reasoning does not mean highly intellectual cognition. Instead, reasoning in ethics requires bringing all one's faculties in a balanced way to bear on the sincere concern for human well-being in general and the meaning of human experience. Being reasonable in ethics is more like having integrity than like being smart. Available are such resources as

1. Being systematic and thorough
2. Using available evidence and thinking things through soundly
3. Maintaining a high level of consciousness and attentiveness, and keeping one's concepts and principles as clear as possible
4. Consulting with others
5. Being sensitive to one's own feelings and examining their significance
6. Appreciating the value and power of dreams, images, and symbols

In short, a *holistic* approach to ethical reasoning is in order. No one mode of reasoning will solve all issues in ethical reflection, and most basic issues are of such breadth as to demand all of our talents. One should avoid a few things in thinking about ethics:

First, reasoning in ethics is not merely a personal or individual enterprise. Although some of our moral thinking centers on the personal meaning of our lives, the ethical thinking that touches upon conventional and professional practice must meet standard tests of reasonableness, because the actions we are considering involve the practices of our profession and have consequences for patients and co-workers. Positions such as that of one physician: "I will only consent to abort potentially mentally retarded fetuses, never fetuses with mere physical handicaps such as dwarfism," may express a personal devotion to intelligence as the sole measure of human value, but such views are not likely to withstand the balanced consideration of all the issues of patient autonomy and values. Or the position that "One should *always* discuss death openly with dying patients," fails to respect reasons for exceptions to this principle. Even when such positions are sincerely held, they are still open to reasonable criticism from others.

Second, existing conventions deserve scrutiny and should not necessarily be accepted. This applies to existing conceptions of authority and official positions on the nature of health and health care. But one should not reject all conventional practices in favor of extremely general philosophical theories. Such theories cannot be applied without the mediation of conventions, cases, and intuitions.

Finally, one should not make such idealistic claims on oneself that one goes around feeling like a failure most of the time. The image of the "ideal nurse" can be destructive to good practice and mental health. Ideas about what we should do need to be rooted in the potential for change in our real situation. These potentials and realities may be very uncertain. For example, "Can I fruitfully take a stand on this issue?" may only be answered by taking a stand. At the same time, one should not rationalize the status quo.

The main point to keep in mind is the important place of reason in the study of ethics. Progress in human reasoning does not depend on our ability to cast answers at one another, but in our ability to find the sources of our disagreements. *At the heart of our ethical judgments are our reasons for them.* People have proposed many answers to questions in ethics. Plans for world peace, sure routes to health and happiness, and roads to salvation abound. What so many answers lack is a clear account of the *reasons* behind them. To illustrate this, Darwin was not famous for discovering evolution. Many people had postulated evolution long before, and many have since improved on his theory. But he presented overwhelming and convincing *reasons* for believing the evolutionary thesis. Saint Thomas Aquinas was not famous for his answer to the question of whether God exists. Many people before and since have given the same answer. His tremendous influence on the history of thought resulted from the way he approached the problem and the reasons he used to defend his position.[4]

In spite of this plea for reason in ethics, some students will continue to have a nagging feeling that reasoning in ethics is just not on a par with reasoning in science or clinical practice. Ethics just does not seem as solid and productive. This is a common feeling and a common mistake.

[4]Baruch A. Brody, *Beginning Philosophy* (Englewood Cliffs, N.J.: Prentice-Hall, Inc., 1977), p. 7.

Misconceptions about the Nature of Moral Reasoning

The rapid increase in studies of ethics in the health sciences during the 1970s can be traced to burgeoning *uncertainties, distress,* and *dilemmas* arising in clinical practice during that period. Experts in health care ethics sometimes reinforce this confusion by focusing their attention primarily on the *dilemmas.* This is because they rightly see dilemmas as pointers to the appropriate issues to study, and because posing the most puzzling problems is a way to challenge us to look at reasons, not answers. Moreover, practitioners tend to be aware of ethics only when problems arise, not when things are going well according to our moral commitments. These tendencies have the unfortunate side effects of making ethics sometimes seem directed entirely to the study of dilemmas and leading students to wonder whether there is any order in the chaos of human values at all.

In fact, there are many features of ethical thinking that we are justified in feeling sure about and for which we can give good reasons. For example, the reader should have no trouble sorting the following list of conditions and acts into categories like *good* (or *right*) and *evil* (*bad* or *wrong*):

1. Thousands of people die each day of starvation.
2. Nurses and physicians care for plague victims in a medieval town.
3. Someone inflicts pain on another for cruel and selfish reasons.
4. A judge knowingly imprisons an innocent person.
5. A physician gives placebo birth control pills to patients without their consent.
6. A fireman pulls a drowning child from the river.
7. A soldier throws a baby on his bayonet.
8. A stranger gives you directions on where you want to go.
9. A stranger donates a kidney.
10. A person comforts a grieving friend.
11. An anesthetist sexually molests his unconscious patients.

Cautious readers will be able to create stories which controvert one's immediate intuitions: The heroines and heroes harbor secret ambitions; the villains suffer pitiful and uncontrollable compulsions; the evil conditions deter worse ones; and the good ones prevent better ones. But to generate such stories is to miss the point of the examples. We *can* generate stories in which our judgment is confirmed in an ordinary way: The heroine acted generously and courageously; the villain voluntarily rejoiced in evil for its own sake.

Since science and ethics are taught in professional schools with different objectives, students are sometimes misled about ethics. Science teaching tends to focus on what is orthodox and useful in the field, while ethics teaching is usually directed to opening inquiry into the goals of practice. Thus, an ingenious solution to a scientific or technical problem generates excitement; an ingenious solution to an ethical conflict seems tenuous or manipulative. Citing a telling authority on rounds can devastate an opponent and thrill an audience, while appeals to authority in ethics are regarded with justifiable suspicion. A good diagnostic "pickup" can save the day, but an eye for subtle ethical issues can make one a nuisance.

Instead of regarding ethics as a poor science, it is better to regard ethics and science as having different objectives for their inquiries. Therefore, different styles of reasoning are most suitable to each. One should not expect, for example, to resolve the debates between the consequentialists and formalists by means of a randomized, controlled clinical trial. The precise quantification central to orthodox science is out of place in ethics. Numbers can be used in resolving moral issues only after deeper ethical commitments have been made, as in risk-benefit studies or determining financial restitution in a suit. There is no accepted scale for measuring happiness or suffering. No computer program for solving ethical problems waits around the corner.

Basic differences between science and ethics with regard to reasoning style also center on the distinction between normative and descriptive theories. For the most part, inquiry in ethics is directed to making choices and is therefore focused on normative issues. Science is primarily concerned with description and technique. This does not mean that values and norms are foreign to science. Scientific method is a *norm;* objectivity is a scientific *value;* and honesty is a scientific *virtue.* Nor is description foreign to ethics. One must be able to describe a situation before one can make a decision about it, and scientific claims may have profound significance for our ethical perspectives, as did the discovery that the earth is not the center of the universe, the theory of relativity, the discovery of cultures with different practices, Marx's analysis of capitalism, and the recognition of ecological limits on economic expansion. Science and ethics entwine in complex ways. In some realms of inquiry, normative and descriptive claims may be inseparable, as in psychological and historical explanation, health policy studies, and committee recommendations.

The concepts of human freedom and choice fit awkwardly into most scientific paradigms, because most scientific work is designed to discover explanations that leave as little room as possible for uncertainty. In contrast, the study of ethics presupposes the opportunity to make choices. A perspective that sees everything we do as determined by scientific laws, even if we can't identify them all, threatens our scope of choice. Although it is natural that these conflicting interests lead us to pursue different thinking styles, we must be uncomfortable if ethics sees us as free and science sees us as determined. Some reconciliation or integration of the two perspectives is called for and is part of the continuing work of philosophers.

These differences in styles of reasoning would not arouse so much suspicion of ethics if students did not acquire *idealized* visions of science. Ethics suffers when a historically accurate account of ethics is compared with an idealized picture of science. Neither science nor ethics is immune from uncertainty and error. Medicine and nursing have a history of fads and harmful practices, many of them supported actively by honest, scientifically minded practitioners. Useless and even harmful practices doubtless continue today.[5] Modern scientific method is not the sole form of human reasonableness, and, used without perspective, it is unreasonable. Science could be taught like ethics with a focus on unanswered questions and close attention to the great theoretical debates. And ethics could be taught more like science, as it is in law school, where knowing a body of material and decisions with regard to professional legal practice is required of students.

It is useful to remember periods in history such as the Middle Ages when the study of ethics and theology was the queen of the sciences, and the study of nature was in disrepute. To be good at reasoning in ethics and theology was to be at the cutting edge of intellectual achievement, and studies of the natural world were labeled heresy and witchcraft. Today, ethics and science have traded places. The

[5]A good historical study showing some of the pitfalls of modern medical injury is Herbert Benson and David P. McCallie, Jr., "Angina Pectoris and the Placebo Effect," *The New England Journal of Medicine,* 300 (1979), 1424–29.

sciences appear to many as jewels in the crown of reason, while the humanities lurk in the shadows of conflict. But to be skeptical about ethics and to have faith in science is rather like blaming the poor and praising the rich: Their defects and advantages are not intrinsic but are products of their relationship. It is fortunate that the dark times are past when human reason was crippled by rejecting the study of nature, but human reason is equally defective if it studies nature to the exclusion of the humanities. We need to be able to conduct factual and value inquiry in an integrated way and to invest our energies in both forms of study, lest we continue to build with half our resources.

Decision Making, Reflection, and Research in Ethics

Nurses can play an important role in the development of ethics. They of course have a central role in the development of ethics in nursing, but they can also contribute significantly to the development of medical ethics, ethics in the health sciences, bioethics, and ethics generally. Many nurses have strong scientific training, especially in interdisciplinary scientific studies. If nurses have a weakness with regard to the study of ethics, it is their lack of background in the humanities, a feature of clinicians in all health fields. However, there is nothing to prevent nurses from strengthening their studies in the humanities.

Nurses have the opportunity to develop concepts of reasoning in ethics at three different levels: decision making in the clinical setting, personal reflection, and research on ethics. Each level requires a different set of approaches directed to a different set of goals.

Decision Making

The decision process outlined in Chapter 4 (pp. 65–68) leaves many details open. With more consciousness of decision-making methods suited to nursing practice and of values expressed by series of decisions, important values and issues can be clarified. Moreover, the accumulated decisions of nurses constitute nursing practice and have an impact on health care delivery as a whole.

Personal Reflection

This is the first step in learning about ethics from clinical experience. When one gets outside of the work setting and begins to look at broader issues than the decisions at hand, one becomes involved in personal reflection. This process may be directed toward any number of objectives:

1. Gaining perspective on the work setting
2. Appreciating the meaning of one's experiences
3. Analyzing and criticizing the customs and practices of health care
4. Looking for better general principles
5. Explaining such things as suffering
6. Generating new approaches to ethical issues
7. Exploring ethical dilemmas

This kind of inquiry affects one's decisions at work and how one feels about those decisions.

Research

When the thinking through of broad ethical issues involves highly systematic study and the collection of evidence, we engage in research on ethics. By *research,* we usually mean *scientific research* and often think of laboratory or quantitative studies, but *research* can include collecting qualitative evidence and arguments carefully garnered to answer basic questions in ethics, whether normative or descriptive.

One of the earliest examples we have of research in ethics is the work of Socrates, who conducted interviews with Athenians as a basis for developing his critique of conventional Athenian values. More recently, anthropologists, sociologists, and biologists have approached basic issues in philosophical ethics. Some philosophers have conducted cross-cultural studies in order to develop their positions in ethics.[6] Research in ethics can be used to identify common moral questions, widely held values, prevalent attitudes, methods for resolving moral questions, and so on. Research can also help interpret the history and functions of conventional moral principles so that philosophical inquiry can be brought more accurately to bear on professional issues.

Many different models of research are possible in the study of ethics. The model one chooses depends on the objectives of one's inquiry. A few important ones can be described briefly.

CASE COLLECTION. If an ethical issue recurs on a service, it is worthwhile to collect brief descriptions of the incidents. This gives one an opportunity to review past experiences when new cases arise. One can study factors that varied among cases, the different decisions that were made, issues that arose, and outcomes. (In keeping records, be sure to protect confidentiality.) Careful review of a unit's past experience can help to improve future decisions and to create policies. Also, if nurses who make and use such studies report their research in journals, their experience and judgment can help nurses in different settings improve their practice. We all profit more when clinicians account for their experiences than when professional ethics faculty, isolated by their offices and classrooms, make recommendations from a distance.

Systematic case collection is not a new mode of research. It is common to clinical studies and teaching in nursing and medicine. The study of cases is also an old tradition in philosophical ethics. This tradition of *casuistry* was important in traditional Catholic ethical philosophy until it fell into very refined and corrupt positions. Despite casuistry's bad name, the systematic study of cases deserves more attention in ethics.[7]

[6]See Richard B. Brandt, *Hopi Ethics: A Theoretical Analysis* (Chicago: University of Chicago Press, 1954); and John Ladd, *The Structure of a Moral Code* (Cambridge, Mass.: Harvard University Press, 1957).

[7]Some recent efforts at casuistry in the health care literature include Anthony Shaw, "Dilemmas of 'Informed Consent' in Children," *The New England Journal of Medicine,* 289 (1973), 885–90; Derry Ann Moritz, "Understanding Anger," *American Journal of Nursing,* 78 (1978), 81–83; David L. Jackson and Stuart Youngner, "Patient Autonomy and 'Death with Dignity': Some Clinical Caveats" *The New England Journal of Medicine,* 301 (1979), 404–8; and Loretta Sue Bermosk and Raymond J. Corsini, eds., *Critical Incidents in Nursing* (Philadelphia: W.B. Saunders Company, 1973).

GROUP DECISION PROCESS.   Ethical problems are a natural subject for committee efforts. The solo performance in ethics neglects the advantages of consultation and the autonomous participation of those affected by a decision. An *ad hoc* committee to study an ethics problem in the hospital is better regarded as a *research effort* than as a judicial proceeding, because the aim of ethics study is to assist people in solving problems, not to solve problems for them.

Care in composing such committees is important. Members should be involved in or concerned with the issues, whatever their status. Patients and concerned housekeeping staff may be involved. Clarity with regard to objectives is important. Everyone should be heard. A consensus decision procedure is preferable to majority rule, and compromise should be avoided. The aim of meetings on ethics is to create a setting in which people can discuss their views honestly, express their differences intelligibly, stick close to the truth of the matter, identify the appropriate issues, and articulate as a group a justified or reasoned position. A group that has authority on the basis of its wisdom, not the offices of its members, has the appropriate power for research in ethics. Among the many good topics for ethics committees are policies for decisions about dying patients and disclosure of medical information to patients.

During 1974–1977, the National Commission for the Protection of Human Subjects of Biomedical and Behavioral Research appointed by the president, made a set of recommendations for research policy to the Department of Health, Education, and Welfare.[8] Its recommendations, although open to criticism, are noteworthy for their thoughtfulness, judgment, and clear reasoning. The work of the Commission can be seen as a good example of committee research in ethics. The committee employed a large research staff, which conducted a variety of studies on the conditions of research. The Commission also collected statements by philosophers on pertinent ethical considerations and attempted to make explicit the moral principles it used in its deliberations.

MORE STANDARD RESEARCH MODELS.   Sociologists, anthropologists, psychologists, historians, and other social scientists have done much interesting work on ethics. Their research objectives have generally been related closely to the development of theories in their own disciplines. Their techniques, however, are useful in developing normative positions on ethics. For example, such sociological studies as Renée Fox and Judith Swazey's work on heart and kidney transplantation and Charles Bosk's work on ethical issues in the training of surgical residents are extremely valuable resources of information about decision making and values in clinical settings.[9]

There are many questions with ethical dimensions that warrant research that combines both normative and descriptive considerations. Consider the following:

---

[8]The National Commission for the Protection of Human Subjects of Biomedical and Behavioral Research published nine *Reports and Recommendations* with *Appendices* containing all background studies: *Research on the Fetus* (Bethesda, Md.: Department of Health, Education, and Welfare, 1976); *Research Involving Prisoners* (1976); *Psychosurgery* (1977); *Research Involving Children* (1977); *Research Involving the Mentally Infirm* (1978); *Disclosure of Research Information* (1977); *Institutional Review Boards* (1978); *Ethical Guidelines for Delivery of Health Services* (1978); *The Belmont Report: Ethical Principles and Guidelines for the Protection of Human Subjects of Research* (1978).

[9]Renée C. Fox and Judith P. Swazey, *The Courage to Fail: A Social View of Organ Transplants and Dialysis,* 2nd ed. (Chicago: University of Chicago Press, 1978); and Charles L. Bosk, *Forgive and Remember: Managing Medical Failure* (Chicago: University of Chicago Press, 1979).

1. What moral problems arise most often in hospitals?
2. How are placebos actually used in hospitals?
3. How does one tell what a patient really wants?
4. Are demented patients competent to make some decisions about their care?
5. Are consent forms comprehensible to patients?
6. What are the attitudes of nurses and physicians toward smokers?
7. How do ethics committees conduct their work?
8. Are health personnel good at predicting treatment outcomes for seriously ill patients?
9. How was the debate over medical treatment of the poor resolved at the turn of the century?
10. How was the debate over contraception conducted and resolved?

Some of these questions have been studied; others need further work. Many of these issues involve highly subjective and individual phenomena which can challenge the researcher. Nurses interested in research will find problems like these worthy of study.

Research on ethics should not be rejected because it is value laden. Instead, the fact that research involves values should be taken into account, and the values should be dealt with as explicitly and reasonably as possible. The objective of research on ethics is not to resolve ethical issues by proving something from the facts alone, or to shape facts to fit our values. The objective is to find useful ways to integrate both factual and normative material in order to develop a coherent perspective for professional decision making in clinical settings.

Research on ethics is worthwhile because there are reasonable ways to learn about human morality. We can learn about ourselves and how to live through careful and systematic inquiry into ethical issues. Since nurses are accustomed to interdisciplinary work and integrative thought, they are well qualified to undertake these sorts of inquiries.

We can point to progress in the study of ethics and morality. At the level of conventional practice there has been increasing recognition of wider categories of human beings as deserving full respect and justice. Progress has also occurred in moral theory, as in the early discovery of the distinction between means and ends and in the more recent discovery of the distinction between consequentialist and formalist approaches to ethics. Progress has been irregular, and judgments of progress can be ethnocentric, but the concept of advancement basic to our security with scientific methods is also applicable to conventional and reflective ethics: We can claim progress in ethics as long as we express the piety so popular in science that future discoveries may, of course, overturn our present judgments.

Case Considerations

The next part of this text covers clinical problem areas in ethics that frequently come to the attention of nurses. In keeping with the varied role of reflection in ethics and an eclectic approach to ethical theory, the material presented on these areas serves a variety of purposes.

The main function of each chapter is to present a variety of *case considerations* relevant to, and sometimes crucial in, resolving problems in each area. Important conceptual distinctions, areas of dispute, and easily overlooked but important factors are identified and discussed briefly.

Where possible, discussion distinguishes between issues on which there has developed or is developing a consensus on appropriate practice and those issues still in dispute. I have not attempted to offer complete answers to issues in dispute, although I have sometimes argued more strongly for one view than another.

The material is intended not only to aid decision making, but also to identify problems deserving further ethics research. Nor is all of the discussion addressed to answering moral problems. Sometimes philosophical reflection serves simply to set existing problems in a broader and more meaningful context.

Summary

Ethical reflection is conducted with reference to the received views of morality we have grown up with. Our personal moral commitments result from a process of socialization in which we actively participate. Reasoning about ethics increases in generality and sophistication as we grow more mature.

The answers we give to ethical questions are not as important as the *reasons* we give for them. Our ability to *reason* and to *give reasons* is central to personal maturity and social progress in ethics. Reasoning in ethics is not merely intellectual. It begins with the same processes used in clinical thinking and includes broad intellectual and emotional resources. Being reasonable in ethics is more like having integrity than being rational.

We tend to become conscious of ethics only when problems arise, and we tend to be unaware of many ethical assumptions. Thus, we tend to underrate our potential to reach conclusions in ethics. Moreover, thinking of science as a sounder realm of reasoning than ethics is a misperception. In order to reason well, we need to integrate our knowledge of both science and ethics.

Reason plays an important role in three realms of ethics: *making decisions, reflection,* and *research*. There are many opportunities for further research in ethics. As researchers, nurses have important resources to contribute to progress in the study of ethics.

FURTHER READINGS

Social Foundations of Values

ALLPORT, GORDON W., PHILIP E. VERNON, AND GARDNER LINDZEY, *A Study of Values,* (3rd ed.). Boston: Houghton Mifflin Company, 1960.

BARNSLEY, JOHN H., *The Social Reality of Ethics: The Comparative Analysis of Moral Codes.* London: International Library of Sociology, Routledge & Kegan Paul, 1972.

BERGER, PETER L., AND THOMAS LUCKMANN, *The Social Construction of Reality: A Treatise in the Sociology of Knowledge.* New York: Doubleday & Co., Inc., 1967.

DEWEY, JOHN, *Human Nature and Conduct: An Introduction to Social Psychology.* New York: Modern Library, 1922.

EMMET, DOROTHY, *Rules, Roles and Relations.* Boston: Beacon Press, 1966; reprint ed., 1975.

KAHL, JOSEPH A., *The American Class Structure*. New York: Holt Rinehart & Winston General Book, 1957.

KLUCKHOHN, FLORENCE R., AND FRED L. STRODTBECK, *Variations in Value Orientations*. Evanston, Ill.: Row, Peterson, 1961.

PARSONS, TALCOTT, *Social Structure and Personality*. New York: The Free Press, 1964.

PEPPER, STEPHEN C., *The Sources of Value*. Berkeley, Calif.: University of California Press, 1958.

PERRY, RALPH B., *Realms of Value: A Critique of Human Civilization*. Cambridge, Mass.: Harvard University Press, 1954.

WHITE, RALPH K., *Value Analysis: The Nature and Use of the Method*. Glen Gardner, N.J.: Society for the Psychological Study of Social Issues, 1951.

Science and Ethics

EDEL, ABRAHAM, *Science and the Structure of Ethics*. Chicago: University of Chicago Press, 1961.

EDSALL, JOHN T., "Two Aspects of Scientific Responsibility," *Science*, 212 (1981), 11–14.

GRAHAM, LOREN R., "The Multiple Connections between Science and Ethics," *Hastings Center Report*, 9, 3 (June 1979), 35–40.

KÖHLER, WOLFGANG, *The Place of Value in a World of Facts*. New York: Liveright Publishing Corporation, 1938.

TOULMIN, STEPHEN, "Can Science and Ethics Be Reconnected?" *Hastings Center Report*, 9, 3 (June 1979), 27–34.

WARTOFSKY, MARX W., "The Critique of Pure Reason II: Sin, Science, and Society," *Science, Technology, and Human Values*, 6, 33 (Fall 1980), 5–23.

WHITE, LYNN, JR., "Science and the Sense of Self: The Medieval Background of a Modern Confrontation," *Daedalus*, 107, 2 (Spring 1978), 47–59.

Moral Reasoning

AIKEN, HENRY D., *Reason and Conduct*. New York: Alfred A. Knopf, Inc., 1961.

BAER, ELLEN D., "Philosophy Provides the Rationale for Nursing's Multiple Research Directions," *Image*, 11, 3 (October 1979), 72–74.

BRANDT, RICHARD B., *Value and Obligation: Systematic Readings in Ethics*, chap. 3, "The Justification of Ethical Beliefs," pp. 249–418. New York: Harcourt Brace Jovanovich, Inc., 1961.

CARLTON, WENDY, *"In Our Professional Opinion . . ." The Primacy of Clinical Judgment over Moral Choice*. Notre Dame, Ind.: University of Notre Dame Press, 1978.

CRISHAM, PATRICIA, "Measuring Moral Judgment in Nursing Dilemmas," *Nursing Research*, 30 (1981), 104–10.

CURTIN, LEAH L., "Nursing Ethics: Theories and Pragmatics," *Nursing Forum*, 17, 1 (1978), 4–11.

EDEL, ABRAHAM, *Method in Ethical Theory*. London: Routledge & Kegan Paul, 1963.

RAZ, JOSEPH, ED., *Practical Reasoning*. New York: Oxford University Press, 1978.

SEARLE, JOHN R., "How to Derive 'Ought' from 'Is,'" *Philosophical Review*, 19 (January 1964), 43–58.

SELLARS, WILFRID, AND JOHN HOSPERS, EDS., *Readings in Ethical Theory* (2nd ed.), chap. 7, "Relativism and Justification," pp. 335–84. Englewood Cliffs, N.J.: Prentice-Hall, Inc., 1970.

TOULMIN, STEPHEN, *Reason in Ethics*. Cambridge: Cambridge University Press, 1950; reprint ed., 1970.

CRISHAM, PATRICIA, "Measuring Moral Judgment in Nursing Dilemmas," *Nursing Research,* 30, 2 (March/April 1981), 104–10.

HOBHOUSE, LEONARD T., *Morals in Evolution: A Study in Comparative Ethics* (7th ed.). London: Chapman, 1906; reprint ed., 1951.

KETEFIAN, SHAKÉ, "Critical Thinking, Educational Preparation, and Development of Moral Judgment among Selected Groups of Practicing Nurses," *Nursing Research,* 30 (1981), 98–102.

———, "Moral Reasoning and Moral Behavior among Selected Groups of Practicing Nurses," *Nursing Research,* 30 (1981), 171–76.

KRAWCZYK, ROSEMARY, AND ELIZABETH KUDZMA, "Ethics: A Matter of Moral Development," *Nursing Outlook* (April 1978), 254–57.

MAHON, K., AND M. FOWLER, "Moral Development and Clinical Decision-Making," *The Nursing Clinics of North America,* 14, 1 (March 1979), 3–12.

MURPHY, C.C., "Levels of Moral Reasoning in a Selected Group of Nursing Practitioners" (Ph.D. dissertation, Teachers College, Columbia University, 1976).

REST, JAMES, "Cognitive Developmental Approach to Morality: The State of the Art," *Counseling Values,* 18, 2 (1974), 64–78.

———, ET AL., "Judging the Important Issues in Moral Dilemmas—An Objective Measure of Development," *Developmental Psychology,* 10 (July 1974), 491–501.

———, ET AL., "Levels of Moral Development as a Determinant of Preference and Comprehension of Moral Judgments Made by Others," *Journal of Personality,* 37 (June 1969), 225–52.

SMETANA, JUDITH G., *Concepts of Self and Morality: Women's Reasoning about Abortion.* New York: Praeger Publishers, 1982.

CHAPTER 12

Talking
with Clients

In 1961, Donald Oken reported a survey of physicians showing that 90 percent maintained a policy of withholding cancer diagnoses from patients.[1] In the twenty years since that survey, there has been a complete turnaround in medical opinion on disclosure. When the study was replicated in 1977, 97 percent of physicians *favored* disclosing a cancer diagnosis.[2] What brought about this radical shift in opinion?

As knowledge of cancer has become more widespread, familiarity has somewhat diminished the magical dread that the word *cancer* inspires. Moreover, it is generally easier to speak of death in health care settings because of the work of Elisabeth Kübler-Ross. Through extensive interviews with patients, she learned that discussions of dying, although painful, can be rewarding and beneficial for patients, their families, and staff. Kübler-Ross saw disclosure as essential to the support of a psychological process leading to acceptance of death.[3] Moreover, many health professionals came to realize that the paternalism of protecting patients from the pain of bad news was not really paternalism at all. It merely reflected the deep anxieties of health professionals toward the subject of death and dying.

During the same period, public pressure fostered greater disclosure in many social and political activities. For example, the Freedom of Information Acts were inspired by a desire for greater citizen control over government agencies and decision processes. Ralph Nader lobbied for increased disclosure of consumer product hazards. In health care, this trend could be seen in the growth of patients' rights groups, patient advocacy, and informed consent. There was a growing recognition that patients have a right to participate in decisions about their treatment, and

[1]Donald Oken, "What to Tell Cancer Patients: A Study of Medical Attitudes," *Journal of the American Medical Association,* 175 (1961), 86–94.

[2]Dennis H. Novack et al., "Changes in Physicians' Attitudes toward Telling the Cancer Patient," *Journal of the American Medical Association,* 241 (1979), 897–900.

[3]Elisabeth Kübler-Ross, *On Death and Dying* (New York: Macmillan, Inc., 1970).

consequently, have a need for information in order to participate effectively. For example, the American Hospital Association's statement on "A Patient's Bill of Rights" claims:

> The patient has the right to obtain from his physician complete current information concerning his diagnosis, treatment, and prognosis in terms the patient can be reasonably expected to understand. (AHA, 1973)

But the role of the *nurse* in the process of giving patients information is not clear. How much information are nurses obligated to offer patients? When patients ask for information, how much are nurses entitled to tell them? What sorts of advice should nurses give or withhold from patients? Questions like these cause nurses considerable doubt and stress.

Traditional views of the nurse-physician relationship have placed responsibility for the control of information primarily in the hands of physicians. In some hospitals, the unwritten policy has been, "Nurses shall give no medical information to patients not already given to patients by physicians." This *no-new-information* policy restricts nurses to underlining and amplifying basic information already given by the physician. A nursing text states this restriction tactfully, as follows:

> By the same token, whatever prognostications are offered by the nurse should be precisely as specific as the physician's, and no more.[4]

Nurses are increasingly reluctant to accept this definition of their role. Most nurses know much about health and disease, and hospital nurses often judge that patients have not been told by physicians all they need to know. Hospital routine creates times when it is difficult not to disclose information. For instance, a positive laboratory report of cancer may sit in the case record for more than a day before an attending physician discusses the laboratory results with the patient. Nurses are fully aware of the diagnosis in the record but are expected to fend off the patient's questions about the laboratory results.

Nurses who feel an obligation to respond to patient needs for information often feel anxious about such disclosure. Disagreement with physicians on disclosure has been costly to nurses, as the following case indicates:

> CASE EXAMPLE. Jolene Tuma (real name), a clinical nursing instructor at the College of Southern Idaho, was supervising students working at the Twin Falls, Idaho, hospital in 1976. She was interested in the care of dying patients and so asked to be assigned to the case of a 59-year-old woman recently admitted to the hospital in a leukemic crisis. She was told by her physician that she was dying of myelogenous leukemia,[5] and that her only hope of survival was chemotherapy. The physician described the possible side

---

[4]Lillian Sholtis Brunner et al., *Textbook of Medical-Surgical Nursing*, 2nd ed. (Philadelphia: J. B. Lippincott Company, 1970), p. 191.

[5]In its chronic form, myelogenous leukemia sometimes can be managed for years with little or no chemotherapy. Patients can live a long time with symptoms of weakness, infection, or abdominal pain. Patients usually die of an overwhelming infection or a *blast crisis* when the leukemic cells, in very primitive forms, suddenly appear in the blood and kill all the other blood cells in the bone marrow. Chemotherapy may help, but remission is not reliable and survival can be very brief.

effects to her—nausea, hair loss, fever, and bone marrow suppression—and obtained her consent.

When it was time to begin chemotherapy, Ms. Tuma, accompanied by a student, approached the patient. "The patient had been crying and, while I disclosed the side effects of this drug, she began to relate to me her own beliefs about God and herself. She had controlled her leukemia for 12 years with natural foods, and she felt God would perform a miracle on her behalf. She was apprehensive about the drug, but gave consent because her son wanted her to take it."[6] After some discussion of alternative forms of treatment, the patient pleaded with Ms. Tuma to return in the evening and to discuss alternatives with her family. Ms. Tuma and her student then began the chemotherapy.

Although Ms. Tuma told the patient that she was not sure that it was ethical or legal to do so, she met with the family that evening. Because of Ms. Tuma's concern about the consequences of the meeting, the patient asked her family not to tell her physician about it. But her daughter-in-law called the physician. The physician neither interfered with the meeting nor discussed the matter with the patient or Ms. Tuma. However, he ordered the chemotherapy stopped because of the patient's change in attitude.

At the meeting, Ms. Tuma discussed the treatment and its side effects, alternatives such as natural foods, herbal medicine, the need for blood transfusions, and Laetrile. Ms. Tuma indicated willingness to assist the patient in seeking alternative treatments, but she did not claim that any of the alternatives would cure her client nor did she recommend them. The conference resulted in a consensus that the patient would remain in the hospital and continue chemotherapy. Chemotherapy resumed after an hour and one-half interruption. The patient died two weeks later. The patient experienced some adverse side effects and was comatose most of the time. There was no indication or claim that Ms. Tuma's intervention hastened or caused the death of the patient.

After the patient died, her son complained to the physician about Ms. Tuma's conduct. The physician complained to the hospital. The hospital fired Ms. Tuma and complained to the Idaho State Board of Nursing. After hearing the case, the hearing officer concluded that Ms. Tuma had violated the state law governing nursing practice "by interfering with the physician-patient relationship and thereby constituting unprofessional conduct." The board approved the findings and suspended Ms. Tuma's license for six months. The Idaho Nursing Association issued a statement supporting the licensure board's decision. The INA stated that although it strongly supported the nurse's right and responsibility to do patient teaching and the patient's right to know, Ms. Tuma had erred in not consulting the physician, in "promoting therapy which is illegal" by indicating that it was possible to obtain Laetrile, in asking others not to discuss it with the physician, and in interrupting therapy.

Ms. Tuma appealed to the courts, and after a three year struggle, the decision of the state board was reversed by the Idaho Supreme Court. Ms. Tuma had hoped that the court would decide that the patient's right to know was superior to any interprofessional arrangements about communicating with the patient. It did not. Instead, the court held that her constitutional right to

6Jolene Tuma, *Nursing Outlook,* 25 (1977), 738.

due process was violated by the suspension. The court claimed that although it was proper for the state board to set standards for professional conduct, the board had not stated any standards in the area of disclosure, and so its ruling was void. Without published guidelines, the requirement of professional conduct was too vague to meet the requirements of due process of law.[7]

In terms of a traditional picture of nursing, Ms. Tuma acted incautiously. The physician had not delegated to her the responsibility of discussing these issues with the patient. In 1975, *Nursing '75* surveyed 15,430 nurses and asked, "When a patient who has a terminal illness bluntly asks you if he is dying and his physician does not want him to know, what do you usually do?" At that time, most nurses would have avoided the possibility of a direct confrontation with the physician. Eighty-one percent reported that they would have asked why the patient brought up the question and would have tried to get the patient to talk about his or her feelings. Fourteen percent would have told the patient that only the physician could answer that question. Only 1 percent said that they would have answered the patient's question directly.[8]

By 1980 the views of many nurses had shifted on this problem. For example, *R.N.* conducted a survey to which 12,500 nurses responded. *R.N.* modeled its question on the Tuma case.

> *Question:* A 54-year-old cancer patient is scheduled for surgery tomorrow morning. Extremely agitated, he tells the nurse, "I'm really scared about the operation. There *must* be other treatments, but the doctor refuses to tell me about them. Can't you help me?" The nurse fully explains the various alternatives, but avoids making any recommendations. Afterward, the patient clearly seems relieved and remarks to the nurse on her way out, "Well, that certainly gives me a lot to think about!" Do you think the nurse was right in answering the patient's question?

Forced to choose between the response "Yes, as patient advocate, the nurse did the right thing," and "No, the nurse violated the doctor-patient relationship," 83 percent of the respondents chose *yes* and only 17 percent of the respondents chose *no*.[9]

From one point of view, Ms. Tuma had a simple choice between responding to the patient's needs and showing deference to the physician. Posed this way, there is no dilemma. The patient made an urgent and emotionally compelling request which required a response from Ms. Tuma before she could talk with the physician. At worst, she acted discourteously. Charging her with "interfering with the doctor-patient relationship" did not identify any readily recognizable moral wrong on her part: Families and lawyers have interfered with doctor-patient relationships for years with impunity. Moreover, the physician failed to communicate with Ms. Tuma and was not punished for his failure. According to this picture, the hospital

---

[7]This case was reconstructed from the Supreme Court decision (Supreme Court of the State of Idaho, No. 12587, Twin Falls October 1978 Term, Filed April 17, 1979); letters to *Nursing Outlook*, 25 (1977), 738–43 and 26 (1978), 8–9; newspaper accounts; and personal communication with Ms. Tuma.

[8]David Popoff and *Nursing '75*, "What Are Your Feelings about Death and Dying? Part I," *Nursing '75*, 5, 8 (August 1975), 24.

[9]Ronni Sandroff, "Is It Right? Protect the M.D. . . . or the Patient? Nursing's Unequivocal Answer," *R.N.* (February 1981), 30.

and nursing association wrongly punished Ms. Tuma. The real failure was one of interprofessional communication. The hospital apparently had a problem in maintaining teamwork among nurses and physicians. That problem should have been dealt with by policy and personnel management, and Ms. Tuma should not have been blamed.

There is more to this case, however. Ms. Tuma went beyond what is usually asked of health professionals. Usually the patient decision process is pictured as follows: The patient brings his or her values to bear on a decision point; the health care team provides relevant information; and the patient chooses one of the treatment options acceptable to the health care team. Ms. Tuma did much more than provide information. She stayed with the patient throughout her decision process and helped her to work it through. The patient did not make her decision alone, but in dialogue with her family, Ms. Tuma, and the nursing student. Because of her active role in the decision, Ms. Tuma had some responsibility for her client's decision. This is a greater responsibility for patient decisions than health care professionals are generally regarded as obligated to bear. Moreover, some of the alternatives which the patient was considering are generally regarded as medically unacceptable. Laetrile is regarded in medical circles as pure quackery. If the patient had chosen Laetrile over chemotherapy, Ms. Tuma would have been even more vulnerable.

Thus, many questions underlie the Tuma case. First, how extensive is the right and responsibility of nurses to participate in the decisions of patients? How much requested information should they disclose? How honest must they be? What is the responsibility of nurses in relationship to nonstandard treatments such as Laetrile? How far may a nurse stray from professional orthodoxy in order to respond to a patient's conception of reality?

In the discussion that follows, I defend a general position favoring disclosure. A discussion of truth telling and deception in general introduces a discussion about nursing roles and about authority regarding disclosure. I suggest a policy on nursing disclosure and then explore problem areas of disclosure, such as discussing nonmedical alternatives, telling bad news, making recommendations, disclosing side effects, and using placebos.

In Favor of Disclosure

Although opinion on disclosure is by no means unanimous, most philosophers writing on the issue defend a general presumption in favor of openness and honesty. For instance, both Kant and Mill argue in favor of truth telling.[10] Reasons for honesty commonly offered include the following:

1. Manipulating information with the object of *controlling others* is like using coercion to control them. It keeps them from participating in decisions on an equal basis. Where this control is exercised for the benefit of the patient, it is paternalism. When it is used against their interest, it is fraud. In either case, it shows lack of respect for persons.

---

[10]Immanuel Kant, *Lectures on Ethics*, trans. Louis Infield (New York: Harper & Row, Publishers, Inc., 1963), pp. 147–54, and John Stuart Mill, "Utilitarianism," in *Moral Problems in Medicine*, eds. Samuel Gorovitz et al. (Englewood Cliffs, N.J.: Prentice-Hall, Inc., 1976), p. 46.

2. One result of lying and secrecy is *personal isolation.* In keeping many secrets, one becomes vulnerable while maintaining a personal illusion of power. For example, it is not rare for people to harbor what they believe to be shameful and dangerous secrets, only to find when they disclose them, that their problems are widely shared and easily dealt with. An "ugly" birthmark, a secret abortion, or an error of judgment are often either unimportant to others or experiences with which they can identify. A habit of secrecy puts one in a poor position to *check one's beliefs* against those of others. Removed from fact checking and reasonable discussion, one risks ignorance, illusions, and in the extreme, psychosis. This, then, is a matter of harm to oneself and of losing autonomy.

3. Communication should be a *reciprocal* process. There are duties of disclosure on both sides, and principles of *justice* apply to such exchanges. For the sake of their health, patients are charged with the responsibility of disclosing all relevant information fully and frankly. Full disclosure creates a relationship in which full disclosure is owed in return.[11]

4. Untruths damage the *language,* and thus do harm in the long run. Where letters of recommendation are consistently written in inflated language, people learn to give their terms other meanings. Where facts are often reported falsely, one must read their political intent and not their literal meaning. If parents lie to their children, children can neither learn the meaning of words nor appreciate the ways in which their experience is shared by others.

5. Where untruths are used to deceive, it is important that they deceive successfully. As experienced liars are aware, successful concealment of an important fact may require thoughtful and extensive misstatements and masquerade. Creating an alternative reality can become *costly and inefficient.*

6. Deceiving others may constitute an undue assumption of *responsibility.* When bad consequences occur because one is reporting the truth, one can attribute responsibility for those consequences to the unfortunate nature of reality. In contrast, when bad things occur out of fictions of one's own creation, one is more responsible for them.

These general considerations in favor of truth telling receive specific support in the health care setting. Kübler-Ross's work mentioned earlier interprets discussion of death as being generally healthy for patients. This makes disclosure part of the conventional principle of doing good for patients. Insofar as disclosure is necessary for informed consent, it shows respect for patient autonomy and respect for persons. The second point in the list warns that failure to disclose important information can isolate and separate people in conflict with nursing ideals of compassion and community support.

Nevertheless, exceptions are conceivable in health care. Withholding news of a terminal diagnosis has traditionally been regarded as a legitimate exception to honesty. Are there cases when information would be harmful to patients? Is there information about patients to which they may not be entitled?

To address these questions, a wide array of concepts needs to be sorted out, such as honesty, veracity, sincerity, dishonesty, lying, disclosure, truth telling, and deception. *Truth telling,* for instance, is ambiguous: "You should tell the truth" can mean "You should not lie" or it can mean "You should tell what you know."

---

[11]William S. Appleton, "The Importance of Psychiatrists' Telling Patients the Truth," *American Journal of Psychiatry,* 129 (1972), 742–45.

Table 12.1. Your Statements and Their Effect on Others

Your Statements	The Effects of Your Statements on Others
1. You make a true statement.	A. You give true beliefs (information) to others or confirm it for them.
2. You make no statement.	
3. You make a false statement.	B. You leave others ignorant or leave their uncertainty undisturbed.
	C. You tolerate and do not disturb false beliefs you know others to have.
	D. You create or confirm false beliefs in others.

NOTE: For the purposes of this table, *true* statements are those that you honestly believe to be true, and *false* statements are those you honestly believe to be false.

These are not identical. It is possible to withhold information without lying, and reasons for not lying are different from reasons for full disclosure.

Another important distinction is between the *verbal act* itself and its *effects on others*. When we speak, we produce a *statement*. The listener receives the statement and is affected by it. What the speaker says is not always the same as what the listener hears or believes. We may say true things, false things, or nothing at all, and these statements, or silences, may affect our listeners in varying ways. By our statements, we can confirm a person's belief or give new information, leave a person still ignorant or uninformed, allow others to continue to hold false beliefs, actively confirm their false beliefs, or create misapprehensions. These statements and their effects are outlined in Table 12.1.

Lying is usually understood as intentionally making false statements (point 3 on the table) in order to create or confirm false beliefs in others (D on the table). However, lies can also be used to avoid giving information (B). For example, a nurse may be tempted to reply falsely to a patient who asks, "Do I have cancer?" by saying, "I don't know" simply in order to avoid discussion of the issue, not in order to deceive. Or, in reply to a patient who wants to see the physician, a nurse may say "Dr. Jekyll has left the hospital," when he is still in the hospital, in order to avoid disclosing his presence and having to fetch him. It does not matter whether the patient believes the nurse or not, just so that the patient is silenced.

Making no statement (2) may also serve various purposes. Although normally used for B, silence may be used for A, C, or D. For example, nurses and physicians working for asbestos fabricating companies followed a policy for many years of not informing workers with radiological signs of asbestosis that they were ill. Workers were misled (D) into thinking they were healthy when they were in fact being seriously harmed by their work.[12]

Disclosure, however, involves issues of entitlement. For example, Ms. Blaise may tell Dr. Marlowe she wants to see her case record. She may argue, "This information is about me, about intimate aspects of my body and my personality, and vitally important to me. Moreover, I hired you to supply me with this information. So, this is *my* information and I am entitled to possess it." These are the claims of

[12]Daniel M. Berman, *Death on the Job: Occupational Health and Safety Struggles in the United States* (New York: Monthly Review Press, 1978), pp. 1–4.

the *known*. Dr. Marlowe may reply, "The knowledge is mine. It is a product of my training and labor. You did not hire me to supply you with this information. You hired me to provide you with treatment, and I use these records for my own purposes in providing you with the best treatment. Thus, it is my information and I am entitled to keep it if I think I should." These are the claims of the *knower*.

Ms. Blaise's right to the information, and therefore whether Dr. Marlowe should disclose it, depends partly on the strength of the claims of the "known" and partly on the nature of her contract with Dr. Marlowe. Are we, as the ones known, generally entitled to information about ourselves, especially information contained in records and reports? Respect for autonomy favors access to such information where it is needed to maintain autonomy and control over our personal lives. In regard to her contract with Dr. Marlowe, it is increasingly recognized that patients normally go to health professionals partly to obtain information about their health, and health education is increasingly regarded as part of the nursing role. Thus, in health care it should be assumed that patients are normally entitled to information about themselves.

As we read down the table, acts and their effects tend to be regarded as increasingly unacceptable by ethicists. *Lying,* a combination of 3 and D, is generally regarded as morally less defensible than simple failure to disclose, that is, omitting 1 or A. This is partly because the six philosophical points listed earlier in favor of honesty apply more strongly to lying than nondisclosure. One reason that misstatements (3) are usually regarded as worse than failure to make statements (1) is that the former involve much more *active* participation in the consequences to one's listener. For instance, there is a difference between tolerating false beliefs in others by passively omitting to correct them and actively creating false beliefs by lying to them. Most people hold some false beliefs. One cannot go around trying to get rid of them all. It is worse to add to the stock of false beliefs in the world than to tolerate what is already there. The difference is analogous to that between active and passive euthanasia. In passive euthanasia, the patient is allowed to die while nature takes its course. In active euthanasia, the health professional intercedes in the process of dying and attempts to ensure that the patient dies.

Nurses have observed that in some cases it is no worse to deceive by misstatement (3) than it is to deceive by nondisclosure (2). Similarly, there may be cases of active euthanasia that are not morally different from passive euthanasia. But the active cases are generally more problematic than the passive ones because the former add an element of control over patients.

Incentives for controlling others are common in the hospital. For example, patients' anger and grief may create work for the staff that could be avoided by keeping bad news from them. Control of other professionals and staff is also a motive. For example, staff may avoid criticizing each other's work in order to prevent conflict. But it is important to remember that the truth can also be used to control others. As one nursing student said,

> I tell my patients the truth so that they will trust me. When patients trust me, they are more likely to follow my instructions. By telling them the truth, I control them more effectively.

Since both truth telling and lies can be used to the same purpose, it is important to think in terms of respect for patients and sharing decision processes with them.

Disclosure by Nurses

So far, I have argued for honesty with patients and a high level of disclosure of material concerning patients. But I have said little about who on the health care team should take major responsibility for disclosing information to patients. There are several good reasons why nurses should consider moving beyond the no-new-information policy.

First, the nursing goal of patient education has created nursing programs which commonly provide training for communication with patients. Although medical schools teach physicians how to obtain histories from patients, their training in patient education is usually not nearly as thorough. Since nurses are likely to be better at communication with patients than physicians are, a leading nursing role in this area would support the good of patients.

Second, the amount of time patients spend with physicians is more scarce and expensive than the time spent with nurses. For example, in one large health maintenance organization, physicians can spend only fifteen minutes with each patient. In contrast, during their shifts, nurses usually have more frequent opportunities to discuss issues with patients (see p. 11).

Third, nurses are taking an increasing role in making judgments about patient care. In order to make these judgments they need to have open communication with patients. It is thus appropriate to extend the range of nurses' responsibility for disclosing information in order to facilitate their role in patient decision making.

As advocates for clients, nurses need a high level of autonomy in order to respond to patient's wishes with discretion. In order to act autonomously, nurses need to be able to decide freely what to discuss with their patients.

Despite these reasons, many have objected to nurses' assuming more responsibility for disclosure. Nurses do not know as much about medical diagnosis and therapy as physicians and are said to lack the authority of physicians. Further, it is said that increasing sources of information in the hospital will create disorganization because patients will receive conflicting views from different members of the health care team.

These are complex issues. For example, can it be said that a nurse who reads a diagnosis in a chart is less capable of reporting that diagnosis to the patient than the physician? If the nurse really has less authority than the physician, won't patients take that into account in making judgments based on information from nurses? And, where there are conflicting opinions on patient care in the hospital, shouldn't patients be aware of these conflicts in order to make better decisions? Until such issues are resolved, I propose a set of interim guidelines for disclosure of medical information to patients by nurses:[13]

1. Tell no outright lies.
2. Give patients all information relevant to their health and care which
   a. The nurse has a responsibility to give them, or
   b. The nurse judges there is good reason to give them.
3. The nurse has primary responsibility to give the following kinds of information:
   a. Information relevant to independent nursing functions, any procedures the nurse is conducting, and nursing diagnoses;

---

[13]Compare the Massachusetts Cancer Nurses' Group "Statement of Beliefs Related to Giving Cancer Patients Information" in the Appendix.

b. General patient health education, including self-care, chronic disease, normal bodily processes, diseases, and so on.

4. If the nurse judges that the patient should have any information that is the physician's primary responsibility to communicate, and the physician has failed to communicate the information, then it is the nurse's responsibility either to communicate that information to the patient or see that it is communicated to the patient.

5. Withholding information from patients requires professional judgment by nurses in consultation with others. If a physician orders information withheld, the nurse is justified in cooperating only if the order is justified in the nurse's professional judgment.

6. Communication is a cooperative staff function. Doubtful areas of disclosure should be subject to open discussion and formulation of policy.

Bad News

In spite of the reasons for disclosure in this chapter, some information may be too harmful to patients to disclose. Sometimes the risks of alienation and illusion that come from secrecy are outweighed by the despair risked by a misplaced truth. Mark Twain tells a story in which a mother and her child are both dying, and their respective conditions are concealed from each other. In the story, Twain argues plausibly that disclosure would have been excessively painful.[14] When considering withholding information from patients several cautionary points should be kept in mind:

IS THE STAFF SUCCESSFULLY HIDING THINGS? Surface and official realities often have emotional undertones that make the truth obvious to patients and their families. Patients can tell when they are being avoided, their gaze is being evaded, or their questions are being turned to other purposes. So much may be told by nondisclosure that disclosure would serve to make relations with the patient more harmonious and open.

IS THE INFORMATION REALLY HARMFUL? Having distressing feelings and expressing them is not necessarily a harmful process. Kübler-Ross, for example, suggests that to express feelings can aid an orderly process leading to emotional resolution. Others have pointed out that patients who express feelings may have better recoveries than other patients.[15] Since disclosure is sometimes just the first step in a process, it is important for nurses to think of disclosure as an opportunity to begin work with patients. Nurses sometimes express justifiable anger at physicians who drop bad news with a patient and leave immediately. The price of disclosure is a commitment on the part of health professionals to stay with patients and help them work through its consequences.

DOES THE HARM OF DISCLOSURE OUTWEIGH THE GOOD? Nondisclosure cannot be justified simply by showing that disclosure does *some* harm. One also needs to show that the harm outweighs the good. Insofar as the patient lacks

[14]Mark Twain, "Was It Heaven? Or Hell?" in *The Complete Short Stories of Mark Twain,* ed. Charles Neider (New York: Bantam Books, Inc., 1958).

[15]Leonard R. Derogatis, Martin D. Abeloff, and Nick Melisaratos, "Psychological Coping Mechanisms and Survival Time in Metastatic Breast Cancer," *Journal of the American Medical Association,* 242 (1979), 1504–08.

information or is deceived, the patient is unable to take part in the process of decision making. One must ask if the pain of disclosure ever outweighs this loss. Since the patient has both a right to participate in decisions and a right not to be harmed, this conflict can be very difficult for health professionals.

For example, the heart is sensitive to psychological factors, and anxiety can increase heart rate and blood pressure. After a myocardial infarction increased heart rate can be dangerous. Some research has indicated that *denying* patients survive better in the coronary care unit than nondenying patients. That is, patients who claimed not to be in danger were more likely to survive than those who recognized their precarious health. One study classified patients into *minimal, partial,* and *major* deniers. The major deniers in the CCU tended to renounce all danger.

> We had asked a 52-year-old longshoreman why the prospect of another cardiac arrest did not bother him. "Why worry? If the marker's got your name on it, you've got to buy it." Another, disclaiming any concern about being attached to a cardiac monitor, said, "Some people would be scared (by the machine) but not me. I'm called the 'iron man.' "[16]

This study found an inverse relation between denial and mortality. None of the major deniers died in the unit, while the minimal deniers, who were 8 percent of the total sample, represented 50 percent of the unit's mortality. This of course does not *prove* a causal relationship between denial and survival. Indeed, the minimal deniers may have been better aware of the danger they faced partly because they were more seriously ill. Yet, studies like these suggest that it is hazardous to meddle with denial in the CCU. Lee and Ball describe the effects of bad news on denying patients:

> . . . he deals with stress by putting troublesome things out of his mind and all he wants from others is for them to join him in this. When something *does* get his attention, his general impressionistic tendency and lack of perceptual sharpness lead to global, diffuse emotional outbursts that are characteristically dramatic and overreactive.[17]

The way out of this conflict is to think in terms of *how* to disclose and *when* to disclose. Since appreciating information takes time and is affected strongly by how things are said and by whom, it is possible to minimize the harmfulness of information by means of timeliness and care.

FOR WHOM IS THIS BAD NEWS?   What may seem like very bad news to the nurse may not be that harmful or painful to the patient. For example, making medication errors can be a dreadful experience for nurses. Making mistakes violates the first principle of professional ethical competence. It may be very difficult to admit incompetence to patients, but such admissions may prove useful in patient management. A patient who is feeling sick or whose treatment is not going well because of a medication error may be very relieved to know that a mistake was made. Rather than destroying confidence in the health professional, admitting errors may help to create an atmosphere of mutual openness and trust.

---

[16]Reprinted from Thomas P. Hackett, N.H. Cassem, and Howard A. Wishnie, "The Coronary-Care Unit: An Appraisal of Its Psychologic Hazards," by permission of *The New England Journal of Medicine* 279 (1968), 1365–69.

[17]Robert E. Lee and Patricia A. Ball, "Some Thoughts on the Psychology of the Coronary Care Unit Patient," *American Journal of Nursing,* 75 (1975), 1498–1501.

Advice

One can do more than give information to patients. Like Ms. Tuma, one can become involved personally in the client's process of making judgments. One can suggest new courses of action or back up some choices and discourage others. Such discussions go beyond merely stating facts to including judgments about values and the wisdom of choices.

The received view in nursing discourages giving advice and discussing options with clients. Payton argues that since nurses are part of an interdisciplinary team and do not have the primary responsibility for discussing treatment options, they should not, for example, bring up the "no-treatment" option so often overlooked by physicians.[18] Forti argues that giving advice damages patient autonomy, places too much responsibility on the adviser, and puts the adviser in a one-up position.[19]

I agree that some advice is inappropriate for the reasons given, but I disagree with any blanket prohibition on nursing advice or discussion of new options. Indeed, I believe that sharing nursing judgments and values with patients is an important expression of nursing responsibility. Blanket objections to advice are based on a false picture of the nurse-patient-physician relationship. When nurses abstain from advice, they do not thereby support patient autonomy, because physicians meanwhile give ample advice to patients. Recommending therapy is a basic part of the medical job. By not giving advice, nurses simply step out of the triangle and leave giving advice to the physician.

Giving advice or expressing one's own views is a more active form of communication than giving information. As nurses step into a more active role, it does *not* follow that patients must be in a more passive role. Both patient and nurse may be active. Patients do not have to accept advice that they receive. People are used to getting advice and finding their own ways to use it in making decisions. Where physician and nurse disagree, patients' autonomy may be increased by hearing conflicting views.

Nursing autonomy requires active expression of nursing values. Since nurses have a commitment to health values, they need to endorse these values in order to teach what the profession represents. Since nurses already bear responsibility for the outcome of care, they do not assume undue responsibility when they express professional views on the goals of treatment.

Advocacy does not necessarily involve giving advice to patients. The advocate, upon discovering unmet patient needs, represents those needs to other health professionals and struggles to get them met. In advocacy, the nurse moves from the patient to the health care system. In giving advice, the nurse moves from professional values to the patient. There are times to refrain from giving advice. Where one has a long-term role as a *counselor* with a client, a more passive stance is usually in order. Advice is more appropriate as an acute intervention in the hospital, where more prompt decisions are necessary.

Should nurses ever recommend unorthodox therapy to patients? First, we must ask Unorthodox to whom? Massage, touch, imagery, and symbolic modes of

[18]Rita Jean Payton, "Information Control and Autonomy: Does the Nurse Have a Role?" *Nursing Clinics of North America*, 14, 1 (March 1979), 23–33.

[19]Theresa J. Forti, "Advice: A Well-Intentioned Ineffectual Notion," *Nurse Practitioner* (January-February 1981), 25–27.

healing are taught more often in nursing schools than in medical schools. Advising a client to "Skip the Valium and take a hot bath instead" would be more orthodox from a nursing than a medical viewpoint. In taking seriously her patient's struggle over a decision, Ms. Tuma expressed nursing theory more strongly than medical theory. A nurse is on safe moral ground when making recommendations securely based in professional practice and theory. When a nurse makes a purely *personal* recommendation, it is important at least to make that clear: "This is merely my personal opinion, but I think you would be healthier if you read the Bible more." Such extranursing judgments must be approached with great caution.

The Power of Language: Side Effects and Placebos

What nurses tell clients can affect clients' health. This can be seen in two related phenomena: Telling patients about possible *side effects* of medications and procedures increases the probability that they will occur. Similarly, telling patients about possible benefits of medications makes it more likely that these will occur. *Placebos* are medications or procedures having no active agent with physiological effects upon the condition being treated. Yet they relieve pain, nausea, asthma, and other conditions.[20]

This is the realm of self-fulfilling prophecy. The rumor that a bank will fail can make the bank fail, and shouts of "you can do it" can help you do it. The effects of such communication are *real*. Mentioning nausea can make a patient really nauseous, or suggesting that this little red (sugar) pill will relieve pain can bring real relief from real pain. Patients who report such relief are normally neither insincere nor trying to please the clinician. Side effects and placebos rely on unconscious and deep psychosomatic processes. Cooperative and honorable patients are among the most suggestible *placebo responders*.

Our suggestibility raises a problem for truth telling. Patient autonomy requires disclosure, but disclosure of side effects may harm the patient. Lying is wrong, but a judicious lie could support recovery. Our deeper nature interferes with conscious control of our lives. "Just tell me the facts; I'll apply my values and make up my mind," does not complete the picture of human decision making about health.

Side Effects

Disclosure about side effects of medications has not received the careful attention that disclosure about surgery and risky procedures has. Consent forms are not required for prescription drugs, and patients rarely receive descriptive brochures with their medications. The argument against disclosure is a paternalistic one: "People should take their medicines. If we say too much about side effects, people are more likely to experience them, or worse, be frightened into noncompliance."

If in fact people were generally benefited by nondisclosure of side effects, we would have to reenter the debate over paternalism. However, practice with regard to

[20]For an excellent summary of placebo use, see Kenneth L. Melmon and Howard F. Morelli, *Clinical Pharmacology: Basic Principles in Therapeutics,* 2nd ed. (New York: Macmillan, Inc., 1978), pp. 1052–62.

medication is so chaotic that more widespread disclosure could only add an element of rationality. About 50 percent of all prescriptions are for conditions for which they are not indicated.[21] Treatment of viral infections with antibiotics is a typical case. The majority of patients do not take medications as prescribed, and at least 25 percent do not take them at all.[22] Although controlled studies of drug action are conducted routinely, there is little knowledge of the actual impact of drugs under real clinical conditions. In these uncertain circumstances, it is impossible to show that hiding side effects has significant benefits that would outweigh a presumption in favor of disclosure. Moreover, professionals show bad faith when they generally disdain psychological modes of healing but take very seriously the psychological effects of disclosing the drawbacks of treatment.

How to disclose side effects should displace the question of *whether* to disclose them. Are there ways to discuss risks and yet minimize suggestible responses? For example, patient teaching could include discussion of the phenomenon of suggestibility.

Placebos

The difficulty with placebos can be similarly resolved. Placebos seem to work best when there is a high level of confidence between clinicians and patients. This confidence should not be abused. One could simply say, "This pill has no active ingredients, but many people with legitimate problems are helped by it. Let's try it, and, if it doesn't work, let's try something else."

Placebos are sometimes used to supplement other medication, for example, to thin out the use of narcotics during withdrawal. Telling patients that some of the pills will be dummies in order to smooth the rough parts of withdrawal would not necessarily render them ineffective. Or using placebos to explore a symptom's psychological components might be consistent with disclosure.[23] Nurses involved in placebo therapy can thus support disclosure without interfering with the aims of therapy.

What is the nature of deception in using placebos? Giving a placebo need not involve a lie; one can omit to tell the truth. The purpose is deception, but the deception need not be achieved by misstatement. Instead clinicians use false beliefs that patients bring with them—popular faith in medication. Placebos are props in the theater of scientific health care, not outright lies.[24] Placebos gained medical legitimacy and interest when a physiological mechanism was found for the placebo response to pain. Circulating endorphins resembling morphine were found to attach to receptors in the brain and inhibit pain.[25] The discovery of endorphins made

[21]*Encyclopedia of Bioethics,* 1978 ed., s.v. "Drug Industry and Medicine," by Harris L. Coulter.

[22]Barry Blackwell, "Drug Therapy: Patient Compliance," *The New England Journal of Medicine* 289 (1973), 249–52.

[23]For discussion of specific cases, see Christine Cassel and Andrew L. Jameton, "Power of the Placebo: A Dialogue on Principles and Practice," *Art of Medication,* 1, 3 (December 1980), 22–28.

[24]On Table 12.1, placebo use is often 2C, not 3D, and so it is not the form of behavior lowest on the list.

[25]Jon D. Levine, Newton C. Gordon, and Howard L. Fields, "The Mechanism of Placebo Analgesia," *Lancet,* 2 (September 23, 1978), 654–57.

placebos seem less of a lie to physicians. The physiological activity of endorphins made placebos like other medications.[26]

The next step in this process of legitimization is to see the placebo responder with respect. One survey found that 72 percent of nurses believed that placebo responders were either faking or hypochondriac.[27] Instead, nurses and physicians should see placebo responders as people who are able to marshal their inner resources to deal with disease without the aid of outside physiological agents.

The next step is to give full recognition to what is already partially recognized: The emotional support and compassion of health professionals, the nurse-patient relationship in particular, is curative in its effects. It is not that nursing care has a *placebo effect* on patients. Placebos mislabel social support and self-healing as medication. Most studies of the efficacy of placebos compare placebo effects with those of medications—for example, saline injections are compared with morphine injections.[28] Since a third of patients who receive saline injections improve, it is argued that the saline injections produce the placebo effect. But many other situational factors could be identified as the cause of this response, for example, nursing care. Since placebos are symbols that are efficacious in a system of social support and relations, which, for all we know, do the real work of placebos, it is most important to have a good understanding of social factors in a case before thinking about using placebos.

The following rules for thinking about placebo use may therefore be helpful:

1. The power of placebo therapy is based on trust between client and healer. Placebo use therefore should be based on respect for the patient and for the power of the mind.
2. Do not participate in placebo therapy without understanding the social and medical situation: What are the motives of the therapist? What is the relationship among nurse-patient-physician? What condition is being treated?
3. Be clear about what the placebo is to do. Can this end be achieved by simple declarations of support by the therapist or by other less misleading modes of psychosomatic therapy?
4. Do not participate in the use of *impure placebos*—active agents used to treat conditions for which they are not indicated—where these agents have harmful side effects.
5. Do not use placebos punitively, to trick patients, or to reject them.
6. The patient's welfare should be the only consideration. Emotional and financial gains for providers cannot justify placebo use.
7. Placebos should not be given to clients who do not want them. Tell no outright lies and answer all questions honestly.
8. Care is no more nor less an essential ingredient of placebo therapy than it is of any other form of treatment.[29]

[26]It also damages typical definitions of *placebo* such as ". . . objectively without specific activity for the condition being treated." See Arthur K. Shapiro, "A Historical and Heuristic Definition of the Placebo," *Psychiatry*, 27 (1964), 52–58.

[27]James S. Goodwin, Jean M. Goodwin, and Albert V. Vogel, "Knowledge and Use of Placebos by House Officers and Nurses," *Annals of Internal Medicine*, 91 (1979), 106–10.

[28]See, for example, the review by Henry K. Beecher, "The Powerful Placebo," *Journal of the American Medical Association*, 159 (1955), 1602–06.

[29]Adapted from Cassel and Jameton, "Power of the Placebo."

Some Reservations and Questions

The arguments above defend a presumption favoring disclosure of information to patients and a stronger one against telling lies to them. The arguments appeal to such benefits as emotional health and maintaining social support. They also appeal to respect for patients' control over treatment, that is, their autonomy. Arguments against this presumption were not given much attention, but readers might consider the following:

1. What if full disclosure of information to patients approximately *doubled* the overall time nurses and doctors spent with patients? How would this affect national health care costs? If this would considerably increase costs, should we consider such educational alternatives as a public television channel with special health education programs for diabetics, the terminally ill, and others, even though such measures do not fill the social-support functions of communication?
2. Should nurses disclose mistakes in cases where disclosure is likely to lead to malpractice suits and thus some personal risk?
3. In some cultures, withholding information from dying patients is the normal procedure, and patients' families are expected to make decisions about therapy. Our culture was like this twenty years ago. What is going on in these cases? Do patients really know their diagnoses through nonverbal communication? Are families able to represent the patients' wishes effectively? Or is a fundamental difference in values displayed here, and if so, what is that difference? Surely in these cultures it is believed that it would be harmful and disrespectful to tell patients bad news. What support is there for these beliefs?

Many would admit exceptions to the presumption in favor of disclosure. When disclosure would be very harmful to patients and hinder their ability to make decisions, there is reason to withhold information. When disclosure would serve patient decision making but would cause great pain and distress, we have a *dilemma* and have to consider other factors in making a decision on particular cases.

Since giving advice is not disclosing information, advice can be withheld without violating the presumption in favor of disclosure. But other considerations favor nurses' giving advice. Nurses are a resource with regard to health values, and their advice is useful to patients. Investigating how patients handle advice given by different professions might provide useful information on the role of advice in patient care.

Many nursing dilemmas are not over whether patients should get information but over whether nurses should be the ones to give it. This chapter argues for an important nursing role in giving patients information. The common division of labor in hospitals suggests that nurses take primary responsibility for information closely associated with the functions they perform and the areas in which they are most skilled and knowledgeable. But since nurses have special skills in education and a special responsibility to give emotional support to patients and families, it can be argued that they can best communicate some information most closely associated with other specialties. Since hospitals are complex and patients have much to learn in them, organizing information flow to patients constitutes a major policy problem deserving further nursing research.

Summary

During the 1960s and 1970s, health professionals have become increasingly willing to give information to patients. However, the role of nurses in disclosure has remained unclear. As illustrated by the case of Jolene Tuma, active communication between nurse and patient can risk conflict with other health professionals. Yet, the disclosing of information is strongly supported by general philosophical arguments against secrecy, lying, and deception. Nurses have patient-education skills and modes of working with clients that offer them an important role in giving patients information. Nurses should feel free to communicate with patients on a wide variety of topics but should also cooperate with other staff in planning communication.

Some areas of disclosure require careful thought. For example, disclosing *bad news* is generally obligatory, and the price for such disclosure is a commitment by the nurse to follow through on the consequences of disclosure to the patient. Serious health risks to the patient may require that disclosure be postponed.

Discussing options and giving *recommendations* is also an important part of nurses' communication with patients. Although advice should be moderated by respect for the autonomy of patients, it is one of the important ways by which nurses can teach clients about health values.

Disclosing *side effects* of medications is generally obligatory even though it may increase the risk that side effects will occur. Such disclosure is needed in order to make medication practices more rational and to respect the autonomy of clients. Ways can be found to mitigate the suggestibility of patients.

Giving *placebos* to clients need not involve deceiving them and should never involve lying to them. Since the efficacy of placebos relies on the integrity of practitioner-client relationships, placebo use must be approached with careful attention to the relationship and with respect for patients.

Further research is needed on the drawbacks and costs of disclosure, as well as on the organizational consequences of more active disclosure by nurses.

FURTHER READINGS

ALTMAN, JOHN H., ET AL., "Patients Who Read Their Hospital Charts," *The New England Journal of Medicine*, 302, 3 (1980), 169–71.

APTEKAR, HERBERT H., "A Conspiracy of Silence," in *Critical Incidents in Nursing*, eds. Loretta Sue Bermosk and Raymond J. Corsini, pp. 325–33. Philadelphia: W.B. Saunders Company, 1973.

BANDMAN, ELSIE L., "How Much Dare You Tell Your Patient?" *R.N.* (August 1978), 39–41.

BOK, SISSELA, "The Ethics of Giving Placebos," *Scientific American*, 231, 5 (November 1974), 17–23.

———, *Lying: Moral Choice in Public and Private Life*. New York: Pantheon Books, Inc., 1978.

BRODY, HOWARD, "The Lie That Heals: The Ethics of Giving Placebos," *Annals of Internal Medicine*, 97 (1982), 112–18.

BROWN, MAUREEN, ET AL., "What to Tell the Patient," and "Are Medications a Secret?" in *Critical Incidents in Nursing*, eds. Loretta Sue Bermosk and Raymond J. Corsini. Philadelphia: W.B. Saunders Company, 1973.

CASSILETH, BARRIE R., ET AL., "Information and Participation Preferences among Cancer Patients," *Annals of Internal Medicine*, 92 (1980), 832–36.

CHEN, MARTIN K., "Hypothesis on Nurse Role Strain: Are Knowledgeable Patients Necessarily Pests in Hospitals?" *Medical Care,* 15, 4 (1977), 350–51.

DAVIES, E., J.A.T. ROBINSON, AND C.M. PARKES, "The Patient's Right to Know the Truth," *Proceedings of the Royal Society of Medicine,* 66 (1973), 533–38.

DAVITZ, LOIS JEAN, *Interpersonal Processes in Nursing: Case Histories,* "What I Want to Know, You Won't Tell," pp. 133–41. New York: Springer Publishing Co., Inc., 1970.

DODGE, JOAN S., "What Patients Should Be Told: Patients' and Nurses' Beliefs," *American Journal of Nursing,* 72, 10 (1972), 1852–54.

ELLIN, JOSEPH S., "The Solution to a Dilemma in Medical Ethics," *Westminster Institute Review,* 1, 2 (May 1981), 3–6.

FROESE, ARTHUR, THOMAS HACKETT, AND NED CASSEM, "Trajectories of Anxiety and Depression in Denying and Non-denying Acute Myocardial Infarction Patients during Hospitalization," *Journal of Psychosomatic Research,* 18 (1974), 413–20.

FROMER, MARGOT JOAN, "Teaching Ethics by Case Analysis," *Nursing Outlook* (October 1980), 604–9.

GLASER, BARNEY G., AND ANSELM L. STRAUSS, *Awareness of Dying.* Chicago: Aldine Publishing Co., 1965.

GOLODETZ, A., J. RUESS, AND R. MILHOUS, "The Right to Know: Giving the Patient His Medical Record," *Archives of Physical Medicine and Rehabilitation,* 57 (1976), 78–81.

GREENLAW, J., "Responding to Patients' Requests for Information," *Nursing Law and Ethics,* 1 (April 1980), 6.

HACKETT, THOMAS, AND NED CASSEM, "The Impact of Myocardial Infarction," *Rhode Island Medical Journal,* 57, 8 (August 1974), 327.

———, "White-Collar and Blue-Collar Responses to Heart Attack," *Journal of Psychosomatic Research,* 20, 2 (1976), 85–95.

HENDERSON, L.J., "Physician and Patient as a Social System," *The New England Journal of Medicine,* 212, 18 (1935), 819–23.

KELLY, LUCIE YOUNG, "The Patient's Right to Know," *Nursing Outlook,* 24 (1976), 26–32.

LOVELL, MARIANN C., "The Politics of Medical Deception: Challenging the Trajectory of History," *Advances in Nursing Science,* 2 (April 1980), 73–86.

MCCAFFREY, M., "Placebos for Pain?" *Nursing '82* (February 1982), 80–85.

MILLER, GEORGE A., "Patient Knowledge and Nurse Role Strain in Three Hospital Settings," *Medical Care,* 14, 8 (1976), 662–73.

———, "On Knowledge and Being a Pest," *Medical Care,* 15, 4 (1977), 351–53.

QUINT, JEANNE C., "Institutionalized Practices of Information Control," *Psychiatry,* 28 (1965), 119–32.

SANDROFF, R., "How the 'Patient Bill of Rights' Makes Honesty Easier," *R.N.* (August 1978), 42–47.

SHELDON, MARK, "Truth Telling Is Medicine," *Journal of the American Medical Association,* 247 (1982), 651–54.

SHENKIN, BUDD N., AND DAVID C. WARNER, "Giving the Patient His Medical Record: A Proposal to Improve the System," *The New England Journal of Medicine,* 289 (1973), 688–92.

SKLAR, CORINNE, "Unwarranted Disclosure," *Canadian Nurse* (May 1978), 6–8.

STANLEY, SISTER A. TERESA, "Is It Ethical to Give Hope to a Dying Person?" *Nursing Clinics of North America,* 14, 1 (March 1979), 69–80.

STEVENS, D.P., R. STAGG, AND I. MACKAY, "What Happens When Hospitalized Patients See Their Own Records," *Annals of Internal Medicine,* 86 (1977), 474–77.

WAITZKIN, H., AND J.D. STOECKLE, "The Communication of Information about Illness," *Advances in Psychosomatic Medicine,* 8 (1972), 180–215.

WEISS, ROBERT J., "The Use and Abuse of Deception," *American Journal of Public Health,* 70 (1980), 1097–99.

CHAPTER 13

Informed Consent

Informed consent is an important development of the movement toward clearer recognition of patients' rights in general. This movement supports both a right *to* health care and rights *in* health care. Informed consent is a central feature of patients' rights *in* health care. The American Hospital Association's "Statement on a Patient's Bill of Rights" states this right.

> The patient has the right to receive from his physician information necessary to give informed consent prior to the start of any procedure and/or treatment. Except in emergencies, such information for informed consent should include but not necessarily be limited to the specific procedure and/or treatment, the medically significant risks involved, and the probable duration of incapacitation. Where medically significant alternatives for care or treatment exist, or when the patient requests information concerning medical alternatives, the patient has the right to such information. The patient also has the right to know the name of the person responsible for the procedures and/or treatment. (AHA, 1973)

Informed consent has received considerable attention in the law. The older doctrine of *consent* required for surgery has been refined to *informed consent* and has been extended to cover a variety of nonsurgical therapeutic procedures. These changes have been made largely through court decisions on malpractice and not through legislation.

Many of the elements and issues of informed consent to therapy have been developed in relation to human experimentation. The U.S. Department of Health and Human Services oversees a system of institutional review boards which determines whether plans for experiments in institutions receiving federal funds treat human subjects ethically. The boards consider informed consent an essential condition of subjects' participation in experiments.

What Informed Consent Is

To *consent* to something usually means to *agree* voluntarily to it. A *voluntary* agreement in this context is one that a client makes *autonomously* (see the definition

184

of autonomy, p. 50). If a client voluntarily agrees to have a procedure performed, the client is said to consent to it. What does the word *informed* add to the concept of consent? Some people take it to mean that the clients have been given appropriate information, that is, have been *told* appropriate information. Others think that it goes beyond simple telling to include also that patients *understand* what they have been told.

Informed consent must take place against an appropriate background: The patient must be capable of consenting or refusing. For example, prisoners are said to live in a setting offering so little autonomy as to make the concept of informed consent to experimentation meaningless. Patients must also have the *competence* or capacity to make decisions. For example, some children and some mentally ill or retarded people lack the mental or emotional capacity to make decisions about their care. The person requesting the patient's consent must also be authorized to accept the patient's consent.

The kinds of information that should be included in an informed consent conversation include descriptions of

1. The procedure offered
2. Reasonable alternatives to the procedure
3. Possible benefits to the patient of the procedure
4. Risks, inconveniences, and discomforts of the procedure
5. Answers to all of the patient's questions

The clinician should use terms that clients can understand and give them a fair picture, so that clients can make active decisions about their care.

When to obtain informed consent raises many questions. In general, most people assume that informed consent should be sought for all procedures and treatment plans, except

1. In emergencies
2. When the client does not want the information
3. When the procedure is simple and the risks and discomforts are negligible
4. When the information would so upset a client that rational decision making would be impossible[1]

Informed consent is an important form of disclosure in general and can be distinguished from disclosure by its link to patient decision making and its extensive legal dimensions. The moral issues in informed consent arise against a complex and shifting legal background. Fear of involvement in lawsuits and lack of clarity about the nursing role in informed consent cause uneasiness about it among nurses. Yet the spirit behind this procedure is an important element in making patients full participants in health care.

The Rationale for Informed Consent

Arguments for informed consent usually take two different courses, although some writers combine them. Some see it as an expression of autonomy in contrast to paternalism. They see informed consent as a process giving power of choice to

---

[1]Based on George J. Annas, "Informed Consent," *Annual Review of Medicine*, 29 (1978), 9–14.

clients by respecting their decisions and giving them the information they need to make decisions.

The second justification arises from the view that informed consent is important to patient good and is thus an expression of an important conventional nursing principle. This perspective sees informed consent as producing better decisions by engaging the patient's personal values in the treatment process. Informed consent is also thought to encourage patient cooperation with treatment, appropriate refusals of treatment, communication, and health education.

Opponents of informed consent usually deny the appropriateness of patient autonomy in medical settings. They do not deny the value of autonomy in general, but they see it as harmful or impossible for patients. Some see expertise in medicine as essential to participation in medical decision making, and so would exclude patients and nurses from the process. Others see clients as emotionally unable to make decisions under the impact of disease, pain, or the possibility of death. The debate over informed consent thus refers back to the issues of paternalism and autonomy (see pp. 126–29).

Informed consent often involves signing forms and careful records of conversations with patients. "Obtaining consent" is thus a somewhat formal procedure, and complaints about this aspect of it are common: It is too formal. The law intrudes on the physician-patient relationship. Patients won't remember what they are told. Time is too short. The forms are too technical or too incomplete. Proponents of informed consent reply that these obstacles need to be taken seriously, but that our goal should be to improve conditions for obtaining informed consent, lest we allow this important process to evaporate.

Some claim that informed consent can give the client only an illusion of autonomy, because the clinician can always lead the patient by slanting information. One can glorify the benefits and deprecate the risks. Even if they do not do so deliberately, health professionals are committed to a picture of what is good for patients and so are likely to be blind to other points of view.

Indeed, since informed consent is defined in terms of declaring risks and benefits to the patient (see p. 185), it is committed to a specific model of decision making. Telling patients their duties to others or disclosing the impact of their decisions on overall public welfare are not required items in the informed consent process. Informed consent relies on an individual and pragmatic picture of decision making.

It is hard, even within these limits, to know exactly which risks and benefits to mention. One can focus on what *this* patient wants and needs to know, on what would foster a "rational decision process," or on what a "reasonable person would want to know." Even if one makes these choices, it is hard to know what to tell in some cases. Risks that are extremely unlikely but very serious are especially problematic. "We can treat your gout, but there is a very very slight risk that you may get aplastic anemia and die." "We can treat your lung infection, but there is a small risk that the antibiotic will also kill your kidneys." To take more flippant but real possibilities: "Risks of your admission to hospital include that you may be attacked and killed by another patient, an earthquake might knock the hospital down, or your landlord may rent out your apartment while you are away." Not only is it hard to know what risks to tell, it is also hard to know what risks, especially of this speculative kind, the health professional should cooperate with the patient in taking, especially when it is the patient who takes the risk and not the health professional.

Despite these difficulties, there is a critical difference between communication by which one attempts to be fair, circumspect, and frank, and that by which one tries to manipulate clients. Clinicians who appreciate the patient's point of view, who are reflective about health care commitments, and who strive to recognize both benefits and drawbacks of health care procedures will be better able to fulfill the requirements of informed consent than uncritical enthusiasts of the latest procedures. We may never be able to measure our degree of success in fully respecting each other's needs for information, but we can make respect our firm intention and learn how to express it better in the process.

The Nurse's Role in Informed Consent

As with many issues, the patriarchal tradition in hospitals creates problems for nurses who participate in the informed consent process. Two areas of conflict and uncertainty are *when* consent should be obtained and *who* should obtain it.

On What Occasions Should Informed Consent Be Obtained?

There are obvious occasions for obtaining informed consent, such as upon entry to the hospital or before major surgery. There are equally obvious occasions when informed consent is not necessary: bringing a toothbrush, giving a backrub, or turning on the television. There are risks and benefits to be appreciated in the latter actions, but they are usually well understood by everyone. In between these extremes there are thousands of encounters with hospitalized patients that may or may not invite considering informed consent. Medication usually does not legally require informed consent, but medication can be just as risky as surgery. Patients may want to make explicit choices about such procedures and interventions as venipunctures, diets, calling the social worker, psychiatric consultation, x-rays, nursing treatment plans, monitoring, sputum cultures, teaching rounds, and many others. Surely, we do not want a formal consent procedure for everything. Yet how shall we choose occasions for consent? Is there a principle involved?

On one unit, nurses made a list of procedures that required consent and those that did not. They thought the nearest general principle they could discern was that procedures done by residents and interns seemed to require forms, while procedures done by nurses did not. On another unit the principle seemed to be that if you put things *in* the patient (IVs, blood transfusions, medications), no consent was needed, but if you took things *out* of the patient (biopsies, bone marrow tests, thoracentesis), consent was required. In both settings riskiness and risk-benefit ratio were obviously *not* crucial.

It may be impossible to identify the significant points for informed consent in a hospital stay. Individual values affect what points are important, and there is no neat hierarchy of tasks and subtasks on which patient decisions can be pegged. Jehovah's Witnesses, for example, might consent to surgery and refuse a blood transfusion, while others might accept a transfusion and refuse surgery. Because uncomfortable postsurgical ambulation is normally part of surgery, no separate consent is required for it; yet patients sometimes must be strongly encouraged and even forced to undertake it.

Progress toward more orderly consent procedures could be made by identifying the most important and prevalent values at stake in the hospital and making sure that they are addressed by consent procedures. Health, safety, freedom from pain, and independence are obvious values to consider. For instance, hospitals could be clearer about the risks of hospitalization, particularly infections and mistakes, on their consent forms for admission. Subordinate procedures that standardly cause discomfort should receive explicit attention at the time consent to the overall procedure is sought.

If there is a general answer to the "when" question, it is that the decision process is ongoing and cannot be readily formalized into occasions for consent. The spirit of patient autonomy and recognition of common values should pervade the entire treatment process, so that communication with clients stands ready as an antidote to problems with consent. Unfortunately, this is not in the usual spirit of hospitals. Hospital procedures tend to be juggernauts that sweep patients and staff through their machinations, and the autonomous patient runs the risk of being crushed in its course. Here, nurse and patient have common cause.

Who Should Obtain Consent?

The American Hospital Association's statement and the law clearly identify the physician as the appropriate person to obtain informed consent. This is because the law sees the physician as the person primarily responsible for the treatment plan and most knowledgeable about health care. The physician is authorized to negotiate treatment plans with the patient on behalf of the hospital and staff. The consent must be obtained in conversation with the patient. This conversation is the *real* consent, as distinguished from the formality of signing the consent form. Sometimes physicians leave the forms to nurses, unit clerks, and other staff.

Getting forms signed may pose ethical problems. The nurse may not feel sure that real consent has taken place. Clients may have questions that indicate they do not fully understand what is going on. If the nurse refers the questions back to the physician, there may be delays, and the physician may feel inconvenienced. If nurses give clients further information, they do so without authority. The nurse also runs the risk of revealing information the physician wants withheld.

These problems are avoided by having one person obtain both the real and the paper consent. This person need not be the physician. Informed consent can be seen as part of the process of patient education. Indeed, it may be the most important part of patient education, as the need to make a decision is an important motive for learning. Since education is part of the nursing role, and since physicians are often untrained and unskilled in communication,[2] nurses may be the most appropriate staff members to conduct the informed consent process.

A decentralized model of informed consent might also be considered. Instead of placing all responsibility for communication on the physician or nurse, one could use the principle that "the one doing the procedure should get the consent." Thus the radiologist would discuss the x-ray; the nurse would discuss venipuncture and the nursing treatment plan; the respiratory therapist would discuss the respirator; and so on. This proximity principle is expressed in the disclosure guidelines above (p. 174). This places conversation at critical decision points, involves in commu-

[2]Frederic W. Platt and Jonathon C. McMath, "Clinical Hypocompetence: The Interview," *Annals of Internal Medicine* (1979), 898–902.

nication those who are most capable of the task at hand, and spreads verbal interactions more efficiently. In contrast, a very centralized model could also be considered. A specialist in communication, such as a nurse or psychologist, could be hired to do all of the informed consent.

If the physician-centered, nurse-centered, decentralized, and centralized models all seem awkward in the hospital setting, this may be because informed consent is an "added on" feature of the hospital. Hospitals were not originally designed to allow for patient decision making and it is hard, economically and bureaucratically, to find its place. Moreover, the availability of treatment alternatives is an important element of patient autonomy, and the lack of in-hospital alternatives for patients to choose from is the central flaw of the informed consent process. Informed consent requires a discussion of alternatives, but it does not require that hospitals make these alternatives available. So in many ways informed consent represents talk about autonomy, not autonomy itself.

Nurses cannot have an active role in informed consent unless they also have an active role in making decisions about patient care. Participation in informed consent requires nurses to negotiate with patients about treatment. If nurses must check all plans with physicians, they have little power to negotiate. There is power in communication, and supporters of the patriarchal tradition in medicine are reluctant to accept active nursing efforts at patient education.

> CASE EXAMPLE. A coronary care unit nurse spent an hour one morning teaching a patient about pacemakers to prepare him for an operation to install one scheduled for later that day. During the discussion she discovered, to her surprise, that the patient had not yet given informed consent to the operation, and in fact had heard nothing of it. Since he was apparently willing to have the operation, she completed the teaching and informed the physician that she had discussed the pacemaker with the patient. He made a spectacular scene on the unit, shouting: "You cut me off at the knees. The patient will not know who is running his therapy—the nurse or the physician."

Lack of nursing autonomy limits the ability of nurses to function as advocates for patient autonomy. Consider the presentation of alternatives. What alternatives should the nurse who advocates patient autonomy present? Like Jolene Tuma (pp. 167–69), a representative of the patient would want to present a broad set of alternatives. One would certainly want to present refusing treatment as a serious option in some cases, and nonmedical models of care such as holistic practices would need discussion with some patients. However, as informed consent is traditionally interpreted, it only requires the health practitioner to present the reasonable alternatives that the practitioner has to offer, and as informed consent is now conceived, "the practitioner" is the physician.

Mental Competence and Consent

Not everyone can give informed consent. Due to mental incapacities of one kind or another (immaturity, dementia, mental illness, retardation), some people are unable to appreciate the nature of the decisions facing them. They require the assistance, or the proxy decisions, of competent persons. Nurses, as close observers of the patients, are often in the best position to determine whether or not a patient has the capacity to consent to treatment. The story of Mrs. K. is one in which a nurse takes an active role in protecting patient autonomy in the face of charges that the patient lacks the capacity to refuse treatment.

CASE EXAMPLE. Mrs. K. was first seen by Dr. B. four years prior to admission. Diagnosis at that time included insulin-dependent diabetes mellitus of many years duration, severe arterial insufficiency of both legs, osteoarthritis, and glaucoma. At that time Mrs. K. was 82 years old and able to live at home with her son although she required frequent visits from home health aides and visiting nurses to oversee her medications and general care. Three years prior to admission she suffered a myocardial infarction. Frequent bouts of urinary incontinence prompted a urologic work-up which revealed a neurogenic bladder. Fifteen months prior to admission she fell and suffered a compression fracture of a vertebra. This injury confined her to a wheelchair. One year prior to admission her eyesight deteriorated to the point that she could no longer measure her insulin dose and peripheral neuropathy made self-injection almost impossible.

Mrs. K.'s son could no longer care for her despite daily home health aides, and she was admitted to a nursing home. Chronic Foley drainage was instituted because of total urinary incontinence. Nine months prior to admission Mrs. K. struck her left ankle on another patient's wheelchair and subsequently developed a superficial infection involving her left leg and foot. Antibiotic therapy controlled the infection, but subsequent skin sloughing required skin grafting on two occasions. Wound healing was poor, and she developed a gangrenous ulcer on the left heel. During the hospitalization the patient was alert and oriented although some recent memory loss was detected. She seemed able to comprehend the nature of her illness, although the poor prognosis was not discussed with her in detail.

Two months prior to admission she was readmitted semicomatose. The work-up revealed pneumonia and an enlarging ulcer on the left heel. After hydration and antibiotic therapy, her mental status improved somewhat, and she was described by the staff as "usually quite lethargic, but alert at times."

Dr. B., after consultation with the patient's surgeon, felt that local measures were futile and recommended amputation of the left leg below the knee. The patient steadfastly refused to grant permission for this procedure. Mrs. K.'s doctors questioned her ability to make a competent decision and therefore sought permission to operate from her only relative, her son. They explained the seriousness of his mother's condition, the futility of further local debridement, and the high probability that she would die as a result of the infection if the leg was not amputated. The son pleaded with his mother to accept the advice of her doctors, but she still refused, giving no reason other than that she would rather die than lose her foot. Finally, although he disagreed with the decision, the son agreed to respect her wishes and refused permission for surgery. Daily debridement was continued, and the patient was returned to her nursing home with a poor prognosis.

On admission, Mrs. K. was stuperous and unable to answer simple questions although she could follow some verbal commands. Dry gangrene was present on both feet. The left foot and ankle were extensively diseased and the right foot revealed ulcers over both ankles. The physical examination indicated that her condition was otherwise stable except for signs of possible pneumonia, and that her foot infection was the only reasonably possible cause of her poor mental status. Antibiotic and intravenous fluid therapy were instituted; however, the patient's mental status did not improve.

The son was again approached about surgery and informed that his mother was now unable to give informed consent. The surgeon told the son that there was a significant chance of intraoperative mortality, but that if she survived the operation (now an over-the-knee amputation) there was reasonable hope that the operative stump would heal. If all went well, Mrs. K. would probably require amputation of the right foot at a later date. The son signed the operative permit and surgery was scheduled for the ninth hospital day.

Nurse H. was concerned that the operation was to be carried out in opposition to the previously expressed wishes of the patient. She discussed the matter with the patient's son, who acknowledged that his mother had consistently opposed surgery and that he had previously supported her decision. But now, faced with her imminent death, he had changed his mind. He concluded the discussion by saying, "If she dies during the operation, it would probably be a blessing. She just can't go on like this, she suffers so much. I just can't stand to see her suffer. Please, operate." Nurse H. was acquainted with Mrs. K. from a prior admission. She was still concerned that Mrs. K.'s wishes be the main consideration. She thus persisted in attempting to arouse Mrs. K. to sufficient consciousness to discuss her operation.

The day before surgery Mrs. K. seemed a bit more alert, looking around the room but not following verbal commands. When Nurse H. visited, she told the patient that she was scheduled for surgery in the morning. Mrs. K. said, "No." "What did you say?" asked Nurse H. "I don't want no surgery." "But Mrs. K., if we don't remove that infected leg you will probably die." "I don't want surgery. I'm eighty-six years old and I'd rather die." The patient then closed her eyes and would not answer further questions. When Nurse H. reported the conversation to Dr. B. he cancelled surgery. In addition, Dr. B. ordered IV hydration, antibiotics, and insulin therapy discontinued. All laboratory work and vital signs were discontinued. Because of the stench, dressing changes and local wound care were continued except for surgical debridement.

The next morning the patient was more alert, sitting in a chair and feeding herself. She knew who she was but did not know that she was in a hospital, and was disoriented in time. She repeated her desire not to have surgery. She offered no opinion on antibiotics, insulin, or IV hydration, stating only that she wanted to go back to bed. For the next week the patient's mental status slowly deteriorated. She remained in an acute care setting because of difficulties with nursing home placement.

After twenty days, Mrs. K. was transferred to a nursing home for terminal care. However, the director of the facility refused to accept her because she was obtunded and in need of surgery for her gangrene. She was returned to the hospital via ambulance. In the emergency room her blood sugar was found to be very high, so she was placed on an intravenous insulin drip and readmitted. On the twenty-second hospital day Mrs. K. spiked a high fever and died two hours later.[3]

[3]This case was prepared by William S. Andereck, M.D.

There is insufficient space for a complete analysis of this case, but four observations leap to attention.

1. Mrs. K.'s mental capacity was not questioned until she refused treatment.
2. The nurse was able to take an active role in assessing Mrs. K.'s mental capacity and in obtaining her refusal of surgery.
3. The son was seen by many of the staff as the obvious decision maker on Mrs. K.'s behalf.
4. Mrs. K.'s decision had two important consequences for her care: (a) There was, as a result, no place for her in health care institutions; (b) the staff took her decision to refuse one form of care as a reason to withdraw all forms of care.

These remarks are preliminary. The central issue in this case is that of mental competence or capacity. Competence is important because it affects the patient's participation in decisions. Those who are against paternalistic treatment of competent patients often believe that incompetent patients may be treated without their consent. This is called *weak* paternalism. But what is competence, and how can we determine who is and is not competent?

What Is Mental Competence?

Competence has two meanings. It is a legal *status:* Everyone who has not been declared legally incompetent by a court is legally competent. Competence is also the *ability* to make reasonable or rational decisions about one's life. In this second sense, patient competence is analogous to the professional competence discussed in earlier chapters: Competent nurses are those who can do their work; competent patients are those who can take care of themselves. The *status* and *ability* senses of competence are related. We normally grant people the status of competence unless they lack the abilities of competence.

The level of capacity to understand that a patient needs to be considered competent depends on the treatment being considered. Where a treatment is very risky, a clinician would want a patient considering it to have a high capacity to understand it. Where nontreatment is very risky and treatment obviously beneficial, one is less likely to be concerned with the patient's competence.

There is a tendency, however, for some professionals to use the concept of competence selectively to identify patients who *refuse* treatment as incompetent. This is understandable because health professionals regard themselves as competent and generally favor the treatments they offer. They also expect to be trusted. Thus, it is sometimes hard for them to understand patients who refuse treatment. What they do not understand, clinicians often perceive as incompetence. If judgments of competence were applied more neutrally, health professionals would investigate the competence of a client who accepts a risky treatment just as thoroughly as they investigate the competence of a client who refuses a sound treatment. If *competent* effectively means *agrees with me* and *incompetent* means *disagrees with me,* we approach full or *strong* paternalism (p. 91). In such cases, clients' actual capacity ceases to be the controlling factor in determining whether their views are considered, and the professional picture of client welfare dominates.

How Can We Assess Competence?

Judgments of mental capacity are very difficult to make. We usually apply the concept of competence to the patient as a whole: "This patient is (or is not) competent." We also sometimes say "This decision or choice is competent." Or we may say that a patient is competent with respect to one activity, like managing financial affairs, but not another, such as cooking dinner. Using competence as a global concept does not take into consideration our ability to be competent in some areas of life and not others. But restricting competence narrowly and assessing it with regard to a single decision tends to equate competence with agreement. For instance, a surgeon could say "I am fully aware that you are a genius in managing your affairs, but since you disagree with me about the amputation, you are obviously not competent to make a judgment on this matter." Is there a useful characterization of competence that is neither too global nor too specific?

Assessment of patient competence in the hospital raises deep questions about the nature of decision processes and the relationships among values, expectations, and factual beliefs. But in judging competence, nurses can keep in mind common-sense considerations about mental capacity.

Ability to think clearly about one issue can indicate that a patient can think clearly about other issues. Similarly, if a patient is unable to accomplish simple mental tasks, the patient may be unable to make more complex judgments requiring simple abilities. A patient who cannot think clearly about numbers would be unable to use numerically expressed probabilities in making judgments, and so a clinician could substitute global images for numbers. A forgetful patient might be helped by frequent reminders of important facts. A "Mental Status Test" is sometimes used by psychiatrists to examine patients for simple mental abilities (see Appendix). The test indicates whether patients know simple things like their names and where they are, whether they can use simple descriptive and numerical terms, and whether they can remember a few simple words. Used cautiously and supplemented by observation and conversation, mental status tests can offer a rough indication of mental capacity. However, cultural factors, the disinclination of some people to take simple tests, the lack of a clearly defined passing score, and uncertainty about what mental skills are needed to think about values are among the obvious drawbacks to such simple instruments.

Many of us have certain misapprehensions about rationality that hamper our judgments of patient competency. These should be kept in mind when assessing it.

1. A rapid decision is not necessarily irrational. Kidney donors unrelated to transplant recipients reported that they typically made their decisions instantly. Many of them had been waiting for just such an opportunity to give themselves and in retrospect were very satisfied with their decisions.[4]
2. A person with strong feelings who expresses a lot of emotion is not necessarily irrational. People in a rage or weeping may have very good reasons for their condition and, moreover, be quite capable of insight and decisions. Emotionality is a common concomitant of insight, and emotional vulnerability an occasion for it.

[4]H. Harrison Sadler et al., "The Living, Genetically Unrelated, Kidney Donor," in *Psychiatric Aspects of Organ Transplantation: 3. Seminars in Psychiatry,* ed. Pietro Castelnuevo-Tedesco (New York: Grune & Stratton, Inc., 1971).

3. Dependent persons may be quite rational. Physical helplessness does not necessarily involve lack of judgment. Moreover, we can choose to depend on the judgment of another person out of reasonable considerations. "Doctor, you decide," may be a rational choice under certain conditions.
4. An inability to manage one's financial affairs does not necessarily imply an inability to make judgments about one's health care. Neither is a financial conservator or guardian necessarily suitable to make health-related decisions.
5. Age and maturity of judgment are not closely correlated.
6. The following dialogue is not evidence of irrationality:

> *A:* I don't want my leg cut off.
> *B:* But, if we don't take your leg, you will die. Do you want to die?
> *A:* I don't want to die.

It is rational to want neither to die nor to lose one's leg. Indeed, these are the epitome of undesirability. It is not irrational to have inconsistent *desires*. The patient may be well aware that limb and life are inconsistent.
7. It is rational to mistrust nurses and physicians and to question the good faith of those giving health services if the services appear, in the patient's judgment, of doubtful value.
8. Some psychotic people can make competent judgments about basic issues, as suggested by the following dialogue, in which an 18-year-old with a variety of symptoms—odd posture and affect, episodes of violence, fugues, etc.—is being considered for admission to a state mental hospital:

> *Interviewer:* Do you work on any hobbies in school?
> *Client:* I is D. I is attitude. D is determination. I is the opposite of D.
> *Interviewer:* Is there anything you are particularly interested in?
> *Client:* Commercialization vs. wear and tear.
> *Interviewer:* What is commercialization?
> *Client:* It's the car bodies. You drill holes in the car bodies to see if they will come through. Are you doing any research here on cars?
> *Interviewer:* No, we don't do any work on cars.
> *Client:* I am interested in electronics, the electronics of cars. It's got to be tested over and over again.
> *Interviewer* (after about thirty minutes of this): Would you like to stay here with us a while? We could probably help you, and you could find some pals on the ward, and do some of the things that you like to do.
> *Client:* No. This place frightens me. I want to go back to school.[5]

Judgments of competence are hampered by the hospital setting, which offers little opportunity to learn about a patient's thinking style, and there are many cases of borderline competence that are hard to evaluate. Patients may vary in their mental abilities from one day to the next. The hospital setting itself may damage the

[5]Thomas J. Scheff, *Mental Illness and Social Processes* (New York: Harper & Row, Publishers, Inc., 1967), p. 7.

patient's thinking processes. To the patient the hospital might seem like a hospital at one moment, and at the next, like a dungeon. There may be a gradual rise or decline in competence. A patient may have some mental faculties and not others. Different staff members may have different presumptions about competency. A social worker may presume that patients are competent and want what they say they want. An attending physician may presume that patients are under the sway of their disease and must prove their competence before receiving respect for their autonomy. And then there is the common dilemma: Where the disease affects mental function, shall we treat this patient so that we can obtain a competent decision as to whether to treat? This dilemma contrasts with the clearly unethical policy of waiting until a competent patient who refuses treatment becomes unconscious and then performing emergency treatment.

Who Should Determine Patient Competence?

This is not simply a medical or nursing question, for it concerns the standing of the person in a social system to participate in decision making. Sometimes a court is needed to make the judgment. Sometimes the decision can be made easily by anyone. Anyone can tell that an unconscious patient is incompetent. The greater the potential impact of a competency decision on the patient, and the more difficult the determination of competency, the greater the need for consultation and group decision processes. Nurses, physicians, psychiatrists, social workers, family, and a court officer may all have valuable information and reflections about the patient and the issues at hand. The patient may be able to reflect competently on his or her ability to make a decision, even if incompetent to make one.

How to Make Decisions on Behalf of Incompetent Patients

There are three common approaches to determining how to treat incompetent patients, whatever the source of incompetence: (1) the *rational-person* method, (2) *substituted judgment,* and (3) *durable statements of intent.*

RATIONAL-PERSON.   In this approach, one sets aside one's own and the patient's views, if any, and imagines what a rational or reasonable person would do in the patient's situation. Our idea of what a rational person would do in some of the bizarre and difficult problems that patients encounter is often incomplete, but that is what one tries to do. Favoring life over death, comfort over pain, and low over high risk are obvious rational considerations, but these often answer our questions incompletely, especially when the decision is between different and uncertain forms of disability, as in the case of very premature infants.

SUBSTITUTED JUDGMENT.   Here, one sets aside one's own views, and attempts to put oneself in the place of this *particular* patient. One asks "What would *this* individual decide in this situation if he or she were competent and able to think about his or her state?" For example, if one knows that the patient is a committed Jehovah's Witness, one would refuse blood transfusions on the patient's behalf, even if the rational-person standard supports transfusion.

If one sees respect for persons as respect for individual choice, the substituted judgment procedure takes precedence over the rational-person method. The rational-person method is for those who place respect for welfare over respect for choice in their reflective positions. However, when fewer and fewer facts are available about a patient's wishes (and it is common to be uncertain about an incompetent patient's wishes), the substituted-judgment method tends to merge with the rational-person method. One must fill out sketchy knowledge of a patient's individuality with generalizations about human rationality.

DURABLE STATEMENTS OF INTENT. This method relies, where available, on the patient's last formally declared and written wishes on the issue. It is a more formal version of substituted judgment, and it gives the health provider a stronger feeling that she or he is relying on the patient's actual wishes. In recent years, there has been an effort to encourage people to express their wishes regarding treatment in case they become incapacitated. The "Living Will" promoted by Concern for Dying and the California Natural Death Act (see Appendix) exemplify efforts to encourage foresight in managing care for incompetent dying patients.

Who Should Make Decisions for Incompetent Patients?

There are two kinds of questions we may ask about making decisions for incompetent patients. First, we may be primarily concerned with identifying the person or persons who should have the final legal and moral responsibility for authorizing the action. This would be the person or group who "takes responsibility" for the patient, for instance, a legal guardian. Or we may be wondering who is in the best position to make the right decision for the patient. Here, we are looking for a way to get the wisest and most understanding view of the incompetent patient's needs. The one who can most understandingly set aside his or her own concerns and address clearly the question "What would this patient choose in this situation?" is the best one to represent the patient. Perhaps no one person can do this well. In that case, a group of people concerned with the patient and working together to address this question might best represent the patient. A legal guardian would do well to listen to the views of such a group as well as to participate in it.

It is a common hospital practice to give conclusive weight to the family's wishes regarding the treatment of very ill patients about whom there is a question of competency. This is often done whether or not there is any legal authority vested in the family to make these decisions. This is done out of a variety of motives, for instance, the hazard the family poses for litigation. If the patient is incompetent, the family is the most likely source of suits. Even when this is not a motive, health professionals and families often confuse (1) the family as a source of information about the patient's values, wishes, and intentions; (2) the family's wishes, interests, and intentions with regard to the patient; and (3) the family as the authorized decision maker with regard to the patient.

If incompetent persons deserve the same basic respect as competent persons, then the interests of the family should have no more weight with regard to an incompetent patient than they would have with regard to a competent patient in similar circumstances. Nor would the family's wishes have any less weight. Where the family is able to address the question of what the patient would choose, the family is an appropriate source of information and an appropriate representative of the patient. Family members are also appropriate participants in a group process directed toward a decision about patient care. Incompetence of the patient, however, does not thereby make the family the authorized representative of the patient.

When to take the decision to a court should also depend on whether the court would make the morally best decision. Where the critical issues fall within the skills of health practitioners, a court would be superfluous. But where a legal issue needs to be settled or where important issues are in dispute among those responsible for the patient, a hearing may be necessary.

There is a tension in our culture between a desire to formalize moral and social issues under the protective arm of the law and a desire to entrust them to groups informally defined by the exigencies of a situation. In the case of Karen Quinlan, a young woman was apparently in a permanent coma, and yet not brain dead. Her family wanted her removed from her respirator so that she could die. Worried about the legal consequences, the hospital brought the matter to court for review. The court held that it did not need to be consulted if there was no reasonable possibility of Karen Quinlan returning to a "cognitive, sapient state." If a hospital ethics committee concurred, all involved would be free from legal liability.[6]

In contrast, when Joseph Saikewicz was being considered for chemotherapy for leukemia, a court ordered that he should not be treated, since his severe mental retardation (his IQ was about ten) would make him unable to appreciate the significance of the treatment and its distressing side effects, although it offered him a reasonable chance for a remission. In this case, the court decided it was the appropriate body to make the decision.[7] The possibility of recovery is important in distinguishing the role of the court in these two cases. The decision not to treat Karen Quinlan was justified by the hopelessness of her prognosis—a judgment clearly the responsibility of health professionals.

Refusing Treatment

If one makes it a practice to ask patients what care they will accept, it is inevitable that some will refuse care—even care wisely offered. The consequences of refusal may be death, and in some such cases there may be no valid reason to override the patient's wishes. Nurses can find comfort in knowing that it is not their job to rescue everyone and that there are worse things in life than death. For example, a patient may prefer to die of gangrene than to be maimed piecemeal by surgeons. Refusing care is not, however, the *end* of a dialogue, but the beginning of one. The patient's right to refuse is the bottom line of a relationship in which the patient is entitled to exercise power. But it is possible for patient and nurse to negotiate, discuss issues, and educate each other toward a common understanding. A new course of action unexpected by either party may be found.

In the case of Mrs. K., the staff decided to withdraw all treatment, even though she only refused some treatment. This decision would have been mistaken if it had been made to punish her for refusing treatment. It would also have been wrong to infer that refusing an amputation was equivalent to refusing all forms of life-saving treatment or that it meant that she did not value her life. Those who decided to discontinue treatment, however, were clear that she had reached a state in dying where further treatment, except for the sake of comfort, was pointless.

[6]In re Quinlan, 70 N.J. 10, A. 2d 647 (1976).

[7]Superintendent of Belchertown State School v. Saikewicz, 1977 Mass. Adv. Sh. 2461, 370 N.E. 2d 417 (1977).

Individualism and Consent

As with disclosure in general, implementing hospital informed consent policy requires a good understanding of how talking with patients can be integrated with the rest of the patient-care process. Making sure that consent forms reflect the real process of consent is also a management problem similar to ensuring that case records reflect actual patient care.

Awkward points in the process of coming to consensus with patients—refusals of care, questions of competence, the role of the family—raise broad issues regarding the extent to which individual choice should guide important health care decisions. A *self-care* model in which patients have very broad powers to guide their medical and nursing care competes with a *paternalist* model in which a professional conception of patient good dominates the decision process.

Nurses stand in an important position in negotiations over these two models of care. They can enter the debate as advocates of patient autonomy or as representatives of nursing conceptions of health or strive to unify these two goals. They can be active participants with patients and other health professionals in making patient-care decisions, organizers of the decision process, witnesses on behalf of fair procedures, and even adversaries of those who lack respect for patients' needs.

Where ethical issues are significant in making health care decisions, the social processes of these decisions need to be better understood, especially because so many people are involved in hospital teams. Similarly, the psychology, rationality, and moral significance of clients' and providers' decision processes need better understanding. What are the correctable obstacles to sound decision making in the hospital setting? When should patient say-so be sacrificed for more pressing goals? What individual values of clients can be translated into broader values and reflected in policies?

And what is the significance of individual autonomy in the hospital? Can it be respected in a large, complex organization? Can legal measures protect patient autonomy? Are there deep psychological needs for dependence and authority? If not, are we nevertheless so limited as individuals that we need others to make decisions for us at certain points? Can such help be given without creating dependency or dominance?

What would be lost, for instance, if hospitals delivered almost exactly what patients wanted but granted them no individual power? Suppose that in some science-fiction manner, nurses could instantly divine what patients wanted and needed and could deliver it before they could even suggest it. Or suppose that nurses could see even more deeply and override patients' desires in such a way that patients would always be grateful later for having their deepest needs respected. Would an important element of respect for persons be lost in such circumstances? In short, is it more important that patients choose what they want, or that they get what they need?

In the real world, of course, we lack telepathy, and people must tell us what they want. But must clients' needs and desires be expressed on an individual basis? What if clients owned hospitals and sat on policy boards with nurses and physicians to design the architecture of units, purchase equipment, and train personnel? By reflecting the collective desires of patients, could institutions do a better job of meeting individual tastes and needs?

Informed consent, and thus difficult decisions regarding patient competence, are crucial only in settings where there is some likelihood that the institution and personnel will fail to show respect for persons. The need for individual protection, especially a legally defined process, may result from the inappropriateness of hospital care for many clients, the power given to health professionals and administration in hospitals, and the distance of professional conceptions of patient good from clients' conceptions of their good. Nurses, so many of whom work deep in the fabric of hospitals, can help discern what direction these reflections should take.

Summary

Informed consent requires a description of the procedure offered; the reasonable alternatives to that procedure; the possible benefits to the client of the procedure; the risks, inconveniences, and discomforts of the procedure; and answers to all of the client's questions. Informed consent is championed by those who see it as beneficial to clients and those who see it as an expression of respect for their autonomy. Superimposed on a traditionally paternalistic form of practice, informed consent suffers from the lack of alternatives to standard therapies in hospitals and from insufficient decision-making power on the part of nurses. Although physicians are now legally responsible for obtaining informed consent, nurses' training in patient education and their opportunities for discussion with patients support more active nursing involvement in the consent process.

Mentally incompetent patients are not in a position to give consent, so decisions about their care must be made by others. Sometimes, judgments that patients lack mental capacity are used selectively in order to justify paternalistic treatment of patients who refuse procedures. Even when capacity is assessed fairly and reasonably, it is sometimes very difficult to determine.

There are three common ways of making decisions on behalf of incompetent patients: substituted judgment, rational-person, and durable statements of intent. Conferences among health professionals and families and appeals to courts may be necessary to make such decisions.

Questions can be raised about whether the emphasis on patient choice shown by informed consent offers much help in meeting clients' needs. Collective control of health care institutions by patients and provision of commonly desired options as regular hospital services may be more helpful.

FURTHER READINGS

Informed Consent

CARPENTER, WILLIAM T., JR., AND CAROL A. LANGNER, "The Nurse's Role in Informed Consent," *Nursing Times,* 71 (1975), 1049–51.

CASSILETH, BARRIE R., ET AL., "Informed Consent—Why Are Its Goals Imperfectly Realized?" *The New England Journal of Medicine,* 302 (1980), 896–902.

CREIGHTON, HELEN, "Law for the Nurse Supervisor: Recent Developments in Consent to Treatment," Part I, *Supervisor Nurse,* 12, 6 (June 1981), 12; and Part II, *Supervisor Nurse,* 12, 7 (July 1981), 70.

FORD, MAURICE DEG., "The Psychiatrist's Double Bind: The Right to Refuse Medication," *American Journal of Psychiatry,* 137 (1980), 332–39.

MARGOLIS, JOSEPH, "Conceptual Aspects of a Patients' Bill of Rights," *Connecticut Medicine,* 39 (1975), 582–87.

MORROW, G., J. GOOTNICK, AND A. SCHMALE, "A Simple Technique for Increasing Cancer Patients' Knowledge of Informed Consent to Treatment," *Cancer*, 42 (1978), 793–99.

TAIT, KAREN M., AND GERALD WINSLOW, "Beyond Consent—The Ethics of Decision-Making in Emergency Medicine (Trauma Rounds)," *Western Journal of Medicine*, 126, 2 (1977), 156–59.

WIENER, CAROLYN, ET AL., "Patient Power: Complex Issues Need Complex Answers," *Social Policy* (September/October 1980), 30–38.

Mental Competence

ANNAS, GEORGE J., "The Incompetent's Right to Die: The Case of Joseph Saikewicz," *Hastings Center Report*, 8, 1 (1978), 21–23.

———, "Reconciling Quinlan and Saikewicz: Decision Making for the Terminally Ill Incompetent," *American Journal of Law and Medicine*, 4 (1979), 367–96.

BAUMGARTEN, ELIAS, "The Concept of 'Competence' in Medical Ethics," *Journal of Medical Ethics*, 6 (1980), 180–84.

COHEN, STEPHEN, AND ELIZABETH HARRIS, "Mental Status Assessment," *American Journal of Nursing*, 81 (1981), 1493–1518.

MAKARUSHKA, JULIA LOUGHLIN, AND ROBERT D. McDONALD, "Informed Consent, Research, and Geriatric Patients: The Responsibility of Institutional Review Committees," *Gerontologist*, 19, 1 (1979), 61–66.

MEISEL, ALAN, LOREN H. ROTH, AND CHARLES W. LIDZ, "Toward a Model of the Legal Doctrine of Informed Consent," *American Journal of Psychiatry*, 134 (1977), 285–89.

ROTH, LOREN H., ALAN MEISEL, AND CHARLES W. LIDZ, "Tests of Competency to Consent to Treatment," *American Journal of Psychiatry*, 134 (1977), 279–84.

WIKLER, DANIEL, "Paternalism and the Mildly Retarded," *Philosophy and Public Affairs*, 8 (1979), 377–92.

CHAPTER 14

Difficult Clients

The ethics of the health care professions traditionally calls upon nurses to maintain compassion for their patients. This can be hard to do. Everyone has negative feelings toward some patients at least some of the time. Some nurses are so burned out that they hate all of their patients all of the time. Because nurses are traditionally expected to be caring and compassionate, it is often hard for nurses to acknowledge such negative feelings as anger, hatred, disinterest, and simple dislike of patients. Recently, there has been a growing literature on clinical problems in the care of disliked patients.[1]

Strong negative feelings toward patients also raise problems concerning respect for persons and the commitment of nurses to patient welfare. When feelings and principle conflict, one faces the classical moral problem of temptation. One is tempted to jam the needle in harder, omit pain medication, or scream what one is really thinking to the patient. There are also parallel positive temptations: One is tempted to spend too much time with that delightful old woman or to take home that neglected child. Ethical principles then emerge as part of an inner dialogue, like the cartoon angel and devil who whisper "Don't!" and "Do!" in the cartoon ear. Here, ethical principles are laid bare and separated from our inclinations and feel-

---

[1] An early nursing ethicist criticized "quarrelling between Nurses and patients," and observed that "there are patients who behave intolerably in spite of every consideration and kindness" (pp. 132–133 in Eva C.E. Lückes, *Hospital Sisters and Their Duties*, 2nd ed., London: J.A. Churchill, 1888). More recent discussions of disliked patients include Victoria George and Alan Dundes, "The Gomer: A Figure of American Hospital Folk Speech," *Journal of American Folklore*, 91 (1978), 568–81; Jean Goodwin and Robert Kellner, "Psychiatric Symptoms in Disliked Mental Patients," *Journal of the American Medical Association*, 241 (1971), 1117–20; James Groves, "Taking Care of the Hateful Patient," *The New England Journal of Medicine*, 298 (1978), 883–87; Joseph E. Hardison, "The Importance of Being Interesting," *American Journal of Medicine*, 68 (1980), 9–10; Solomon Papper, "The Undesirable Patient," *Journal of Chronic Diseases*, 22 (1970), 777–79; William D. Poe, "Marantology, A Needed Specialty," *The New England Journal of Medicine*, 286 (1972), 102–3.

ings.[2] Exposed in this way, ethical principles seem both obvious and frail: "The welfare of patients should be the nurse's primary concern," says the principle, but one's sincere feelings say, "This patient doesn't *deserve* my care."

Nurses have rights, and patients have responsibilities toward nurses. Patients have responsibilities in all the senses of *responsibility* discussed in Chapter 10. Their responsibilities include

1. Recognition of health professionals as human beings. For example, patients should not assault nurses.
2. Fulfilling their contractual responsibilities to clinicians. For example, patients may owe nurse practitioners payment for their care.
3. Taking care of their own health. For example, people should not maim themselves in order to obtain health care.[3]
4. Assisting in the process of their treatment. For example, people should not lie about their conditions and they should take medicines that are good for them.

Patients' responsibility for their care is a delicate issue. The American Medical Association included in its first code of ethics (1847) a section on "Obligations of Patients to Their Physicians." It employed such choice language as:

> The members of the medical profession, upon whom is enjoined the performance of so many important and arduous duties toward the community, and who are required to make so many sacrifices . . . certainly have a right to expect and require, that their patients should entertain a just sense of the duties which they owe to their medical attendant.

Besides requiring that patients select only physicians who have "received the regular professional education," and that patients be open and honest, the code also claimed,

> A patient should never weary his physician with a tedious detail of events or matters not appertaining to his disease. . . . The obedience of a patient to his physician should be prompt and implicit. He should never permit his own crude opinions as to their fitness, to influence his attention to them.[4]

Nowhere in the nursing ethics literature can such presumption be found. Physicians stated the duties of patients even though patients were not members of the AMA and had no role in writing the code. Thus, the code overlooked the consensual and reciprocal foundations of moral principles.

The Hospitals of the University of California, San Francisco, include with their statement of patients' rights a statement of patients' responsibilities.

> 1. Please keep your appointments with us. . . . In the long run, your health is your own responsibility.

[2]Immanuel Kant held that only actions independent of or in conflict with inclinations can be known to be morally worthy. See *Foundations of the Metaphysics of Morals,* trans. Lewis White Beck (Indianapolis: The Bobbs-Merrill Co., Inc., 1959).

[3]A graphic review of the varieties of self-damage by patients is Ivan Fras and Bonnie Coughlin, "The Treatment of Factitial Disease," *Psychosomatics,* 12 (1971), 117–22.

[4]Chauncy D. Leake, *Percival's Medical Ethics* (Huntington, N.Y.: R.E. Krieger Publishing Co., Inc., 1957), pp. 221–23.

2. It is your responsibility to tell your doctor about any changes in your health.
3. You have the responsibility to be considerate of other patients. . . .
4. You also have the responsibility to provide information necessary for insurance processing of your Hospitals and Clinics bills, and to plan for payment of your health care bills as soon as possible. . . .

Like the early AMA code, this statement was not written by patients. Since ethics endorses a reciprocal balance of rights and responsibilities, these two statements exemplify one of the most significant flaws in the concept of professionalism: Professional groups do not include patients as members. Thus, there is a fundamental split between professionals and patients. There can be clarity in the ethical principles of professionals, and where patients are organized, they can state their views on the ethics of health care. But there is no clear answer to the nurse's question, What are my duties to my patient when my patient fails in duties toward me? because there are no joint associations or organizations of patients and practitioners to develop a consensus about mutual rights and responsibilities.

In the absence of such a consensus, the professional must do the best he or she can to resolve conflicts with patients. One of the most common sources of anger toward patients is a feeling that patients are not living up to their responsibilities. A feeling of anger is thus often a judgment that a patient is morally *liable* for some failure to meet the responsibilities of his or her role. This chapter focuses on these moral judgments, not the common vulnerabilities of sick people which sometimes lead care givers to dislike them—neediness, dependency, weepiness, impatience, submissiveness, bad smells, ugly lesions, a desperate look in the eyes, hopelessness, depression, and the like. These also often pose a challenge to compassion, but they clearly require a compassionate response. Instead, this chapter focuses on ethical judgments about responsibility for health, noncompliance with health care regimens, and patients who are dangerous to nurses.

Responsibility for Health

Self-destructive patients commonly arouse strong negative feelings among nurses and physicians. Alcohol abuse is a prime example of this problem.

CASE EXAMPLE.   A 45-year-old alcoholic man was familiarly called "Old George" by members of the emergency-ward staff. They had seen him a hundred times over six years for visits ranging from acute gastrointestinal bleeds to a subdural hemotoma (after a fall that he barely survived). It became a standing joke that the more carefully Old George was tended and the more thoroughly he was worked up, the more furiously he drank. He was released from his hospitalization for the subdural hematoma on Monday, stitched up for multiple lacerations on Tuesday, allowed to "sleep it off" in the back hall on Wednesday, casted for a fractured arm on Thursday and admitted with wildly bleeding esophageal varices on Friday. The staff worked frantically through the night, pumping in whole blood as fast as it would go, but at 4 a.m. the intern pronounced Old George dead. The junior resident muttered, "Thank God," under his breath, and the senior resident said, "Amen" quite audibly.[5]

---

[5]Reprinted from James Groves, "Taking Care of the Hateful Patient," by permission of *The New England Journal of Medicine*, 298 (1978), 883–87.

All this treatment and frustration would not be necessary if Old George had ever gotten his life together. Only he could have taken control of the situation and stayed out of the emergency room, and it is tempting to blame him for not doing so. It is hard to feel compassion for persons guilty of what we see as a wrong, so we want to punish or reject them while at the same time we want to be respectful and compassionate. Drug-addicted clients arouse similar concerns:

> CASE EXAMPLE. Penny, a baccalaureate nursing student, had selected a clinical placement at a methadone clinic in the community. Despite her initial interest, she began demonstrating a pattern of absences from clinical time. When her faculty advisor discussed this observation with her, she blurted out the fact that, much to her surprise, she found she was unable to assist with the group meetings for pregnant heroin addicts. The thought of addicting babies before their birth—babies who would ultimately suffer because of their mothers' self-indulgences—was totally despicable to Penny. She found herself judging their choices constantly and avoiding interactions with them. "I feel like they should be shot instead of giving all this free support and sympathy."[6]

A more extreme example is from a large urban hospital:

> CASE EXAMPLE. A man had thrown acid into the face of a nurse and physician. He burned his own hands badly in the process. The police brought him by the emergency room on the way to jail. The staff nurses refused to provide care for him, and he was treated by supervisory staff. Some said that they refused care because their anger and distress would have made it difficult for them to provide optimum care.

To know how to feel in such situations, we need to clarify our ideas about personal responsibility for health.

In the late 1970s a consciousness emerged attributing many of our health problems to personal behavior and suggesting that individuals are personally responsible for their health. For example, Belloc and Breslow identify seven personal practices that are statistically linked with good health: eating moderately, eating regularly, eating breakfast, not smoking, using little alcohol, taking exercise, and getting a good night's sleep every night.[7] In addition, many health problems have their origins in personal behavior such as overeating, smoking, excessive sunbathing, skipping immunizations, riding motorcycles, riding motorcycles without helmets, driving over fifty-five miles per hour, climbing mountains, working for the fire department, becoming a physician, owning guns, and so on.[8] In the health care setting, nurses may be annoyed to see a lung cancer patient walking about the ward

---

[6]Holly Skodol Wilson and Carol Ren Kreisl, *Psychiatric Nursing* (Menlo Park, Calif.: Addison-Wesley Publishing Co., Inc., 1979), p. 45.

[7]Nedra B. Belloc and Lester Breslow, "Relationship of Physical Status, Health, and Health Practices," *Preventive Medicine*, 1 (1972), 409–21; Nedra B. Belloc, "Relationship of Health Practices and Mortality," *Preventive Medicine*, 2 (1973), 67–81; and Lester Breslow, "Prospects for Improving Health through Reducing Risk Factors," *Preventive Medicine*, 7 (1978), 449–58.

[8]For a good review of the issues here, see Robert M. Veatch, "Voluntary Risks to Health," *Journal of the American Medical Association*, 234 (1980), 50–55.

pushing an IV drip with one hand and smoking a cigarette with the other. Patients who use their IV tubes to inject heroin also irritate staff.

These observations give support to the *individualist thesis* with regard to responsibility for health. This thesis holds that the primary responsibility for health rests with the individual. As John H. Knowles, President of the Rockefeller Foundation, suggested,

> I believe the idea of a "right" to health care should be replaced by that of a moral obligation to preserve one's own health. . . . The next major advances in the health of the American people will be determined by what the individual is willing to do for himself and for society at large. If he is willing to follow reasonable rules for healthy living, he can extend his life and enhance his own and the nation's productivity.[9]

From this point of view, policy makers have considered creating incentives to encourage healthier lifestyles—education, fines, subsidies, taxes, regulations, and so on.[10] For example, Richard V. Ebert suggested in a *New England Journal of Medicine* editorial that cigarette taxes be substantially increased to encourage people to give up the habit:

> In view of the lethality of cigarettes and the relative unimportance of coal smoke as a cause of disease, why are billions of dollars being spent to avoid air pollution from coal while the tobacco industry is being subsidized by the government?[11]

Other suggested measures include higher health insurance rates for smokers, drivers, owners of guns, and so on. The individualist thesis is powerful, attractive, and consistent with many of our political and social traditions.

However, if we regard common feelings toward patients as indicative of our moral judgments about them, we do not apply the individualist thesis consistently. At least, if we take *responsibility* for health to mean *causal* responsibility for health, we make inconsistent judgments about people with the same level of causal responsibility for their accidents and illnesses. For instance, a policewoman wounded in the line of duty would receive devoted care even though she were *causally responsible* for risking her life in dangerous work. The president of a coffee company might receive well-appointed care even though his cardiac problems resulted from his "Type-A" behavior pattern. Skiers who knowingly take health risks for the sake of expensive pleasures seldom receive much anger for their broken limbs. In contrast, anger is often directed toward smokers and drinkers: The only notation in the social history section of a bedside chart may read "smoker," and such a patient may receive a mercilessly chilly reception from staff. But smokers and drinkers are neither more nor less causally responsible for their behavior than policewomen, aggressive business people, and skiers.

These differences in feelings are therefore not attributable to judgments about levels of causality, but to judgments about different levels of *liability* responsibility.

---

[9]From John H. Knowles, "Responsibility for Health," *Science*, 198 (1977), 1103. Copyright 1977 by the American Association for the Advancement of Science.

[10]Dan I. Wikler, "Persuasion and Coercion for Health: Ethical Issues in Government Efforts to Change Life-Styles," *Milbank Memorial Fund Quarterly*, 56 (1978), 303–38.

[11]Reprinted from Richard V. Ebert, "Coal Smoke and Cigarette Smoke," by permission of *The New England Journal of Medicine*, 304 (1981), 1486.

The differences are attributable to the judgment that the activities of the policewoman are more *worthwhile* than those of smokers. These common differences are attributable, therefore, to the different *values* we place on smoking and police work. Most health care staff regard public safety, business, and sports as more valuable than smoking and drinking. Clinicians focus on responsibility instead of values when they talk about their feelings, because it seems intolerant to make value judgments about patients' lives. Yet our anger shows that we actually make such value judgments.

Putting the individualist thesis in terms of values instead of responsibilities raises issues about respect for individual values. If clinicians think that they should respect clients' individual values, then they should strive to appreciate their clients' perspectives on their vices. Clinicians should take seriously the secondary gains of smoking and alcoholism. Despite its costs, alcoholism can help people to maintain a sense of community, avoid conflicts with others, stay alive in spite of deeply painful feelings, express concern over real problems in the world, and so on. One must enter seriously into a world where health is not the primary value, in order to appreciate an alcoholic client's conduct. This may be hard to do because it requires recognizing one's own vulnerability and despair.

A second path is to deny the individualist thesis. Health care tradition demands compassion for all, whatever the source of illness, and scientific explanation often attributes human actions to forces beyond personal control. So, nurses can simply deny or disregard the claim that we are fully responsible for our personal conduct. It is easy to see patients as victims of natural, psychological, and social forces. This *victim thesis* is expressed in the disease theory of alcoholism. Alcoholism can be seen as a powerful syndrome influenced by ethanol itself and the social setting of the patient. It is not a sin to be an alcoholic, but a stroke of fate that some people cannot control their response to alcohol while others can. Surely, by his last week, Old George's life was well out of his control.

Even simple health-related acts such as wearing a motorcycle helmet can be seen as involuntary. The cyclist can be seen as a victim of ignorance of accident statistics, machismo culture, exploitative advertising ("The Difference between a Bullet and a Slug" claims a cycle billboard), and "testosterone poisoning." Helmet use increases to above 90 percent and motorcycle accident mortality decreases by 30 percent when helmets are required by law.[12] This shows that wearing helmets is subject to external pressures, such as the law, and not simply an expression of personal choice.

Birth control is another example. Some writers who follow the individualist school have described patients who don't take birth control pills as directed as "more immature, irresponsible, and impulsive."[13] But surely this is no more than sophisticated name-calling. Recent studies of women who seek repeat abortions show that they are not more "immature, dependent, self-punishing" than other women. Instead,

---

[12]Geoffrey S. Watson, Paul L. Zador, and Alan Wilks, "The Repeal of Helmet Use Laws and Increased Motorcyclist Mortality in the United States, 1975–1978," *American Journal of Public Health,* 70 (1980), 579–85; and Andreas Muller, "Evaluation of the Costs and Benefits of Motorcycle Helmet Laws," *American Journal of Public Health,* 70 (1980), 586–92.

[13]Cornelis B. Bakker and Cameron R. Dightman, "Psychological Factors in Fertility Control," *Fertility and Sterility,* 15 (1964), 559–67.

. . . they are victims of technological, organizational, and logistical inadequacies as well as statistical probabilities rather than being motivationally deficient or indifferent to the dangers of unprotected sexual intercourse.[14]

It is an oversimplification to claim that some people are responsible and others irresponsible. All of us are responsible in some areas of life and not others. We show little stability over a period of time in our health-related behaviors. In a study by David Mechanic, for example, each individual tended to vary widely over a sixteen-year period in seat belt use, smoking, exercise, drinking, and risk taking.[15] Narcotics addicts may naturally discontinue drug use without health care interventions.[16] It is futile to try to avoid health risks altogether.

No matter how purely we eat and drink, no matter how carefully we guard the air we breathe, no matter how much we become involved with our doctors and they with us, the mortality rate will still be 100 percent. . . . The process of living wears us down as much as we wear ourselves down. . . . Ironically, we have come full circle to the notion of omnipotence in health care, only this time around it is not the physician who is omnipotent, but the patient. Somehow, if we can control enough, be disciplined enough and be powerful enough, we can prevent all that is potentially bad in our lives.[17]

We are faced with something of a paradox. We want to see our clients and ourselves as responsible and in control, but we also want to see them and ourselves as victims. What should we do? When faced with a difficult choice between two options, it is often wise to choose a third, and this we should do here.

We should seek another thesis because both individualist and victim theses play an ambiguous role in making moral judgments and do not help much to clarify our situation. Although the individualist thesis supports patients who are trying to maintain control of their health, it also turns attention from systematic social problems and blames individuals for what they can seldom control.[18] For example, poor health of black people living in the U.S. under the economic slavery of the second half of the nineteenth century was explained by physicians as due to bad personal habits:

. . . distaste for honest labor, fondness for alcohol, proclivity to crime and sexual vices, disregard for personal hygiene, ignorance of the laws of good nutrition, and total indifference to . . . health.[19]

[14]Barbara Howe, H. Roy Kaplan, Constance English, "Repeat Abortions: Blaming the Victims," *American Journal of Public Health*, 69 (1979), 1242–46.

[15]David Mechanic, "The Stability of Health and Illness Behaviors: Results from a 16-Year Follow-Up," *American Journal of Public Health*, 69 (1979), 1142–45.

[16]Dan Waldorf, "Natural Recovery from Opiate Addiction: Some Preliminary Findings," *Journal of Drug Issues*, 11, 1 (Winter 1981), 61–76.

[17]Reprinted from Johanna Shapiro and Deane H. Shapiro, Jr., "The Psychology of Responsibility: Some Second Thoughts on Holistic Medicine," by permission of *The New England Journal of Medicine*, 301 (1979), 211–12.

[18]William Ryan, *Blaming the Victim* (New York: Random House, Inc., Vintage Books, 1971); and Robert Crawford, "Healthism and the Medicalization of Everyday Life," *International Journal of Health Services*, 10 (1980), 365–88.

[19]*Encyclopedia of Bioethics*, 1978 ed., s.v. "Racism in Medicine," by James H. Jones.

A century ago, poverty and servitude were also explained in terms of personal failings. In 1893 David J. Brewer, a Supreme Court Justice, said,

> It is the unvarying law that the wealth of the community will be in the hands of the few. . . . The great majority of men are unwilling to endure that long self-denial and saving which makes accumulations possible . . . and hence it always has been, and until human nature is remodeled, always will be true, that the wealth of a nation is in the hands of a few, while the many subsist upon the proceeds of their daily toil.[20]

In the same historical period, Russell Conwell asserted in "Acres of Diamonds":

> I sympathize with the poor, but the number of poor who are to be sympathized with is very small. To sympathize with a man whom God has punished for his sins . . . is to do wrong . . . let us remember there is not a poor person in the United States who was not made poor by his own shortcomings . . .[21]

Victim-blaming can be found in many judgments about patient responsibility for health. One motive for the rising interest in the individualist thesis is the desire to cut the cost of health care. It is hoped that charging those responsible for their illnesses will reduce the expense to the rest of us. The motive here is not compassionate understanding of people, but self-interested conflict over resources.

Likewise, the victim thesis is no simple product of sympathy for clients. To see someone as a victim is to see that person as subject to a more powerful person or force. To see illness as robbing people of responsibility is to place them under the dominance of medicine. Alcoholism was labeled as an illness in part to bring it under the control of medicine, just as pregnancy and birth were brought under medical control earlier in the century. What appears to us as the power of science is often really the power of some people over others by means of science. What medicine represents as forces of biology are often historically contingent forces that could be subject to collective influence. As Oliver Wendell Holmes observed,

> . . . medicine, professedly founded on observation, is as sensitive to outside influences, political, religious, philosophical, imaginative, as is the barometer to the changes of atmospheric density.[22]

About virtually any illness we can tell a story in which the client appears either as a responsible person or a victim. Moreover, there is no person so in control of his or her fate that someone else cannot take control—by force, misinformation, fraud, or paternalism. At the same time, any effort to control others can be countered with a refusal to cooperate or submit. The truth about responsibility is complex: We are sometimes free when we accept necessity, sometimes victims when we claim freedom. What should nurses then think about to appreciate the issue of patient responsibility for health?

[20]Howard Zinn, *A People's History of the United States* (New York: Harper & Row, Publishers, Inc., 1980), p. 255.

[21]Ibid., p. 256.

[22]Oliver Wendell Holmes, *Medical Essays, 1842–1882* (Boston: Houghton, Mifflin Company, 1895), p. 177.

First, attributing responsibility to individual clients is not a morally neutral matter of scientific explanation. Issues of justice are involved. Feelings of blame toward clients reveal emotional commitments to views about the just allocation of the burdens of health care and maintenance. Some professionals are egalitarian in their compassion; others follow various conceptions of social worth.

Second, the *multicausal* nature of illness and health needs full recognition. Most illnesses, certainly chronic ones, display significant personal, physiological, and social dimensions. A treatment plan requires an analysis of all of these factors (a "biopsychosocial assessment") and responses to each. For instance, responses to alcoholism may include Valium, family therapy, reorganizing the alcohol treatment unit, home visits, legislation, new jobs, and more.[23]

Third, depending on their situation in society, people vary widely in their ability to control health risks. People with a high income have opportunities to control diet, time, environment, support, exercise, and the like. Others suffer the health consequences of involuntary poverty. Likewise, what we regard as personal "failings" affect us more as outside pressures on us increase (the rates of mental illness correlate well with unemployment)[24] and as opportunity to express them increase (alcoholism increases with the availability of alcohol).[25]

Fourth, liking and disliking patients has social and practical dimensions, not merely personal ones. For instance, dislike may arise from unconscious sexist and racist beliefs. (Are we victims of or responsible for such beliefs and feelings?) Duff and Hollingshead found that nurses were more likely to be aware of their patients' social class than their diagnoses.[26] Or a patient may seem manipulative because the social institutions in the background of the nurse–patient relationship invite manipulation. The addict who tries to get legal drugs from clinicians is a good example. Neither addicts' nor nurses' personalities made health professionals the only legal source of narcotics.

Fifth, the social forces that hinder assuming personal responsibility for health also hinder effective nursing care. Just as economic and social forces create a world where Old George has no safe place to go after leaving the hospital, these forces also create a health care system focused on acute care. Frustration with George is as much a product of the present limitations of nursing care as of the limitations on George's life. Many nurses would like to deal with health problems that can barely be addressed by them under the present system of health care financing.

Sixth, judgments about clients should be linked with judgments about oneself. It is important to remember when working with alcoholics and drug addicts that nurses are also vulnerable to these problems (see p. 236). The more strongly one paints one's clients as victims, the more strongly one should see oneself as a victim. Similarly, the more one sees clients as accomplices in disease, the more the nurse should admit complicity in the limitations of nursing practice. This is because

[23]Sylvia Tesh, "Disease Causality and Politics," *Journal of Health Politics, Policy and Law*, 6 (1981), 369–90, argues that the multicausal account is ineffective and biased against those most at risk of illness, but her argument rests too strongly on diseases not easily influenced by personal conduct.

[24]M. Harvey Brenner, *Mental Illness and the Economy* (Cambridge, Mass.: Harvard University Press, 1973), pp. 10–11.

[25]Dan E. Beauchamp, "The Alcohol Alibi: Blaming Alcoholics," *Society*, 12, 6 (September/October 1975), 17.

[26]Raymond S. Duff and August B. Hollingshead, *Sickness and Society* (New York: Harper & Row Publishers, Inc., 1968), p. 232.

principles of justice include both nurses and clients in their purview, and social constraints on health can affect nurses and clients similarly.

Seventh, there was some truth in the first AMA code: Patients and health professionals have reciprocal rights and duties. For nurses and patients to act with mutual responsibility, they need to recognize what is necessary to accept between them. But clarity about this cannot come about until nurses and patients meet to discuss common moral grounds. Making individual contracts with patients requires a background of community ground rules on what is fair. Thus, the incompleteness of professional ethics needs to be appreciated.

Noncompliance

When clients don't follow the instructions of clinicians, they are sometimes termed *noncompliant*. Since the term *noncompliant* has connotations of yielding to force and has been used judgmentally by clinicians, some prefer to use such words as *nonadherence* and *noncooperation*.[27]

Nurses have traditionally had an important role in obtaining patients' cooperation with health regimens. There are many techniques for obtaining cooperation, including trust, communication, direct administration of medications, continuing presence, and so on. Nursing is sometimes like missionary work. Nurses call upon patients to rally to the banner of health and recovery, and like missionaries, nurses must find ways to help the unbelievers, the weak of will, and the faithful who have gone astray.[28] And as in missionary work, nonadherence is a common problem. In a review of fifty studies, Blackwell reported that somewhere between one-quarter and one-half of outpatients do not take their medicines at all.[29] This fraction refers only to *complete* failure to take prescribed medications and does not include patients' errors in dosage, timing, sequence, and so on.

The difficult question facing nurses is How far should and may I go in obtaining cooperation from patients? When does support for patient autonomy slip over the line into paternalism? Because the techniques of obtaining compliance are subtle, this is a difficult question to answer. Consider the following two descriptions of nurses at work:

> Staff members will shame, scold, chide, even threaten (especially with children) to "do it anyhow." They will persuade or encourage: "Try to relax, honey, let us look at you—just a little." They will promise that it will soon be over and promise rewards (ice cream to children) for good performance. . . .
>
> A more subtle tactical mode than style is what might be termed "presence." Some nurses can, with their compassion, their concern, their flow of encouraging language, and comforting gestures, their gentle holding of a patient's body during a

[27]Mary Anne Stanitis and Josephine Ryan, "Noncompliance: An Unacceptable Diagnosis?" *American Journal of Nursing*, 82 (1982), 941–42.

[28]Albert R. Jonsen, "Ethical Issues in Compliance," in *Compliance in Health Care*, eds. R. Brian Haynes, D. Wayne Taylor, and David L. Sackett (Baltimore: Johns Hopkins University Press, 1979), p. 113.

[29]Barry Blackwell, "Drug Therapy: Patient Compliance," *The New England Journal of Medicine*, 289 (1973), 249–52.

painful procedure, help the patient find courage and suppress bodily movements and impulses to yell and moan.[30]

In the first vignette, nurses are being overtly manipulative; in the second, nurses are being compassionate and supportive.

An analysis of situations like those above may need to be devoted to ascertaining their psychological dynamics. Subtle forms of manipulation may be more powerful than more overt measures. Moreover, it is important to discern whether the good sought is that of the *patient* or that of the *staff*. Clients' expressions of pain and suffering can be burdensome to nurses. But not all clients appreciate stoicism, and some prefer or even feel obligated to be demonstrative. In Chapter 10 (p. 129), I suggested some conditions under which a degree of paternalistic manipulation would be acceptable, such as using a low level of coercion, and seeking an objective that is part of an overall project that the patient accepts and is congruent with the patient's deeper needs and values.

In analyzing paternalism with regard to nonadherence, it is important to recognize that noncompliance is a common and normal phenomenon. One should resist attributing noncompliance to bad character, lest the noncompliant patient become the undesirable and hated patient. Patients who are judged undesirable are more readily seen as objects suitable for manipulation. As suggested above, many causes affect how people care for their health. Each case requires a separate analysis that addresses the particular social context of the patient, the nature of the clinical effort, and the relationship of the health care institution to the patient. An early study of failure to take penicillin indicates the variety of causes for noncomplicance. Causes included lack of money (17 percent), lack of understanding of the treatment (19 percent), carelessness (27 percent), and the fact that the patient felt well (37 percent).[31]

How to obtain compliance should be considered only in company with the question of *whether* it is important to obtain compliance. Clients may not really want to take their medicine even if it is good for them, and it may be doubtful whether medication is beneficial. If the patient is mistrustful of the nurse's urging, this does not necessarily mean that the patient is irrational. Nurses are familiar with the need to correct and modify physicians' orders. Similarly, patients can reasonably doubt nursing advice. Patients may fail to adhere to a regimen because they are considering nonmedical alternatives. For a real decision to be made, the nurse will need to explore these possibilities with the patient.

When acting as intermediaries between physicians and clients, nurses may be conscious of the difficulty of keeping pressures on themselves from impinging on clients. If a physician wants a procedure done and the client is resistant, advocating the client's viewpoint may require conflict with the physician or a risk of seeming incompetent. The nurse's professional understanding of the balance between the patient's autonomy and significant health needs should outweigh bureaucratic custom. Where factors make patients irrational, nurses may need to take more control, but this requires a clear understanding of the patient's wishes and needs.

---

[30]Reprinted by permission from Shizuko Fagerhaugh and Anselm Strauss, pp. 91–92. *Politics of Pain Management: Staff-Patient Interaction,* Copyright© 1977 by Addison-Wesley Publishing Co., Inc.

[31]Blackwell, "Drug Therapy," p. 250.

Dangerous Clients

Some patients are dangerous to nurses. A patient may be obstreperously demented and strike out at everyone. Some clients are very angry; others use threats to get their way. Consider these two cases from a private community hospital:

CASE EXAMPLE.   A twenty-one-year-old man was admitted for psychomotor seizures. The nurse in charge felt that the patient was acting strangely. He appeared agitated and incoherent, and she feared for the safety of other patients. She called his doctor and asked if the patient could be sedated and/or transferred to County Hospital. The patient's doctor felt it best to avoid medication and not to discharge him. The patient's behavior remained about the same, and after some time elapsed, the nurse called the doctor again. He still felt it was best to withhold medication. A few hours later, the patient got out of bed, dressed, and attacked two nurses, causing significant injuries.

CASE EXAMPLE.   A twenty-two-year-old psychotic male was admitted with a diagnosis of acute renal failure due to an overdose. The patient had a history of three overdose attempts and a psychiatric disorder. At one time he had had a conservator, but one year earlier he was ordered mentally competent by the courts. The patient was verbally and physically abusive. The doctors told the nurses not to restrain him as it was too restrictive. The patient would kick and hit any personnel. A dialysis nurse, after being kicked in the head three times, called the doctor and refused to dialyze him. She was told to check her legal liability regarding this. She insisted that she would only dialyze the patient if he was restrained and sedated for her own personal safety.

Providing adequate care for violent patients raises potential conflicts between the professional principle of making patient good the primary concern and the personal right to protect oneself from harm. This section will discuss how to analyze the conflict in the case of dangerous patients. The next section will discuss the problem of balancing personal risks against professional obligations more generally.

Nurses encounter many hazards in their work. For instance, hospital infections are a common problem, and care must be taken in work with patients with hepatitis and other infections. In 1979 at a hospital with a large geriatric population, influenza swept through the hospital staff and left the patients untouched. The patients had been inoculated; the staff had not. Florence Nightingale called attention to the health hazards of nursing and kept statistics on the high death rate of nurses in some hospitals.[32] Some procedures, such as x-rays, can place nurses at risk, and staff ordinarily take precautions; for instance, radiation therapy involving placement of radioactive substances in patients' bodies may require protective nursing procedures.

Other risks of health care work may arise from the larger situation. For example, nurses have expressed dedication to patient care by working in battlefields

---

[32]Florence Nightingale, *Notes on Hospitals*, 3rd ed. (London: Longman, Green, Longman, Roberts, and Green, 1863), pp. 20–21.

and by caring for plague victims. In contrast, nurses have sometimes deserted patients in need when faced with personal danger. After a 1979 accident releasing nuclear radiation from the Three Mile Island power plant, some nearby nursing homes had to be closed because they were vacated by staff.[33] In 1982, the Emergency Department Nurses Association and the American College of Emergency Physicians discussed the problem of creating hospital procedures to handle radiation emergencies and protect staff at the same time.

When nurses take measures to defend themselves from dangerous patients, they sometimes explain the use of sedation or restraints as measures for the patient's good. Such measures may well benefit patients, but it is not necessary to benefit them in order to protect oneself. Although nurses may have to work closely with dangerous clients, it is both prudent and morally acceptable to protect oneself. Where self-protection also fosters patient care, a direct conflict in obligations can be avoided. But the right to self-protection rests on principles broader than professionalism and applies to every relationship. The principle of respect for persons applied to oneself justifies self-protection. Considering restraints or sedatives for obstreperous patients need not be confined to issues of the patient's interest. Moreover, protecting staff and other patients from physical violence is not simply a medical problem; it is a political and social one. In the first case above, the nurse kept returning to the physician for help. Although it was appropriate to call on him, other measures would also have been appropriate, such as calling hospital security staff or the police. Focusing on physicians for protection only reinforces their patriarchal dominance. As one physician tellingly remarked in regard to this case, "I look out for *my* nurses."

Clearly, the help of others is often needed. Few of us have the cool of the nurse who describes this scene from an emergency department at a county hospital:

Patient (pointing a gun at nurse): Get me a doctor now, or I'll kill you.

Nurse: If you kill me, you won't get seen at all.

Protecting people from personal violence is often regarded as the special province of the law. In judicial proceedings, the distinction between protecting someone from self-harm and protecting oneself from others is crucial, because the law carefully circumscribes paternalistic interventions. Moreover, distinguishing between medical and nonmedical causes of acts and medical and nonmedical judicial sentences is also crucial. But a dangerous situation is hardly the time to consider the niceties of these issues, and it is thus important that these issues be considered in advance. Broader issues than patient care are involved; for instance, justice and the rights of patients are also significant. Professional associations and unions concerned with the health and safety of staff can negotiate appropriate policies with hospitals and patient organizations.

Sedation is a medical technique that can be used for protecting others, for treatment, or for both. Physical restraints are basically a nonmedical means of protection. These methods have been a focus of struggle in mental hospitals, where they are used often enough to affect the lives of patients and staff. Although these measures are not as common in acute care hospitals, the issues surrounding them are

---

[33]J. Stanley Smith and James H. Fisher, "Three Mile Island: The Silent Disaster," *Journal of the American Medical Association*, 245 (1981), 1656–59.

very much the same: How are the needs and liberty of patients to be justly balanced against the needs of staff and other patients? A clear commitment to patient good requires that nurses take some risks in order to avoid interfering with treatment and autonomy by using sedation or restraints.

The social structure and architecture of hospitals place many people close together, sometimes with short staff and bureaucratic routines. These inadequacies can easily come to dominate patients' care. Moreover, in some settings staff may find an expression of power in restricting patients, or worse, punish or abuse patients in anger or from primitive conceptions of medical discipline. In restricting patients it is most important to distinguish patients who are actually physically dangerous from those who pose other inconveniences. Patients should not have to suffer undue restraints to facilitate nursing routines.

There are surely days when nurses would like to see all their patients heavily sedated. As one observer noted,

> For a time I studied the use of sedatives in hospital practice, and discussed with nurses the events that led up to each act of sedation. It ultimately became clear to me and to them that, no matter what the rationale was, a nurse would give a sedative only at the moment when she was no longer able to stand the patient's problems without anxiety, impatience, guilt, rage, or despair. A sedative would now alter the situation and produce for her a patient who, if not dead, was at least quiet and inclined to lie down, and who would cease to worry her for the time being. (It was always the patient and never the nurse who took the sedative.)[34]

Patients may be angry, boisterous, uncooperative, obnoxious, or simply inconvenient without being dangerous. Fear is not a reliable guide to actual danger, as it may arise from prejudice, surprise, demands of supervisors, threats to competence, and so on. By simply avoiding what one fears or sedating whom one fears, one risks moving to a narrow conception of nursing practice. As Purtilo and Cassel observed, "Moving against the edges of fear into the unknown is the source of learning.[35]

Risks and Personal Sacrifices

How much one should risk on behalf of patients is a very general issue in nursing ethics. In Chapter 12, Ms. Tuma risked her job in order to talk with a client, and in Chapter 18, a nurse will face uncertain risks in reporting substandard surgery. In any society, some personal risks and sacrifices are required of everyone. Avoiding harm to others, paying taxes, and the like involve setting aside some individual interests on behalf of the common good. If we did not generally make such contributions, we would all be worse off. How such risks and sacrifices should be distributed is an issue of justice. Nurses contribute to the overall public good,

[34]T.F. Main, "The Ailment," in *Psychosocial Nursing,* ed. Elizabeth Barnes (London: Tavistock Publications, 1968), p. 34.

[35]Ruth Purtilo and Christine K. Cassel, *Ethical Dimensions in the Health Professions* (Philadelphia: W.B. Saunders Company, 1981), p. 31.

partly by taking risks on behalf of patients, and out of justice they expect to be compensated for it. Nurses are not obligated to undertake more than their fair share of the risks of maintaining health.

Sacrifices throught of as *charity* or volunteer work are not usually required and are generally praised. Such activities create personal rewards, but partly through personal costs. Health care is a traditionally charitable enterprise, and it is thus honorable and ethical to make sacrifices for the health of patients. Exposing oneself to contagion in order to care for the sick is a traditional health care virtue. Similarly, it is a virtue to risk one's job in order to protect one's patient. Since health professionals place the good of the client first and are compensated for taking risks, nurses can in fairness be expected to undertake some risks where reducing them would hamper patient care.

Determining a fair level of risk is difficult. The health professions display conventional practices with regard to adequate levels of risk taking, and they characterize greater risks as beyond obligation and even foolish. For instance, a pathologist will receive support for refusing to perform an autopsy on a patient with hepatitis. Ambulance drivers may wait a safe distance from a violent incident underway until the police have done their work. Nurses may rightly refuse to care for some patients unless they are restrained. Some physicians have suggested that the public has no right to expect health professionals to provide care after a nuclear attack; they will be unable to provide care, and, like other survivors, they will have to meet personal and family needs.[36]

An interesting subject for investigation would be to assess the level of personal risk and sacrifice actually expected of nurses. Since basic issues of justice are involved, once determined, that conventional level is open to philosophical inquiry. On examination, we may find that it is too high, too low, or too ill-defined. These issues of justice are not confined to the relationship among nurses and patients. They also arise among health professionals when some undertake more risks than others. For example, nurses, less well paid than physicians, may undertake greater risks than physicians through direct contact with patients in carrying out medical instructions. Issues of justice also arise among health professionals and the public. Professionals sometimes feel burdened by unsafe public practices which give them more work than necessary.

One can extend oneself beyond conventional levels of risk and move toward *sainthood* and *heroism*. Being extremes, such actions are necessarily rare. If heroism and sainthood were required, they would then be conventional and no longer exceptional.[37] They must then be morally *optional*. At the same time, our moral ideals stand ready to praise sainthood and heroism and to make them meaningful.

Nurses in particular should be wary of the temptations of self-sacrifice. In the name of idealism, nurses have traditionally been called upon to work long hours at low wages and to show deference to physicians, to bring them chairs and charts; not to benefit patients, but to benefit physicians and hospital budgets. Self-abnegation by female nurses also perpetuates traditional gender discrimination. Self-sacrifice by nurses is thus best expressed when clearly on behalf of patients or directed

[36]Christine K. Cassel and Andrew L. Jameton, "Medical Responsibility and Thermonuclear War," *Annals of Internal Medicine,* 97 (1982), 426–32.

[37]J.O. Urmson, "Saints and Heroes," in *Moral Concepts,* ed. Joel Feinberg (New York: Oxford University Press, 1970), pp. 60–73.

toward strengthening nurses as a group. It is perhaps better to think in terms of acts of heroism than of saintliness.[38]

Polar to heroism lie the hazards of cowardice, abandoning patients, defensive medicine and nursing, and ungenerousness toward clients. I would suggest considering the following points in taking personal risks in patient care:

1. Personal sacrifice is justified only when there is some possibility that something may be achieved by it. That "something" can be taken quite broadly, such as avoiding complicity in wrongdoing (see pp. 283–84).
2. The greater the needs of the patient or future patients, the greater the obligation to make some sacrifice, if efficacious, to respond.
3. One should assess personal risk realistically. One should not frighten oneself into paralysis by tales of unlikely and horrendous consequences.
4. It is both prudent and morally acceptable to take steps to protect oneself.
5. One should discover what others are doing. Act collectively wherever possible.
6. Nursing is a profession, not a calling. It does not demand unlimited commitment.
7. Exposing oneself to risks in order to protect patients and to provide care is a well-established conventional obligation of the health professions.

Conflicts of interest between nurse and patient indicate a less than ideal state of affairs. When they occur, striving to create a community of interest and congruence of objectives is a much more hopeful course than pressing for a final resolution to the question, "Is it going to be me or you?" Second, the role of emotions in moral judgments needs to be better understood in ethics. Just as the full recognition of a fatal diagnosis involves the whole personality, so does taking new positions on ethics. A new rational realization of what is fair is only the leading edge to a process of maturation, during which one may experience conflicting feelings about patient care. It is an indication of crisis in health care when one's intuitive use of conventional principles of good patient care leaves one numb or full of conflict. Also indicative of crisis is the recognition upon reflection that a series of judgments fails to meet tests of reason, as when patients receive inconsistent treatment arising from ill-considered personal judgments by health care staff about client responsibility for health.

Responsibility and Causality

The issues discussed in this chapter—responsibility for health, adherence to regimen, and conflicts between clients' welfare and clinicians' safety—are subtle and complex. All of the reflective ethical concepts discussed in Chapter 10 are involved here: maintaining respect for clients, limits on paternalism in obtaining compliance, liability responsibility for health, the rights of clients not to be restrained, conflicts between health and other values, justice in allocating role responsibilities for health, and so on.

[38]Saintliness has stronger connotations of moral goodness than heroism; a hero or heroine can be noble without being moral. Heroism can be episodic, but saintliness generally requires a long track record. Heroism is more instrumental; saintliness more dispositional. Physicians are more often described as heroic than saintly, and they employ such language as *heroic intervention* and *heroic medicine*. Perhaps as a result of nursing's early development in religious orders, saintliness is more closely associated with nursing.

Moreover, both normative and descriptive modes of explanation are involved in identifying the causes of health and illness.[39] Descriptive modes are involved in scientific research on genetic, physiological, and psychological characteristics of individuals with health problems. But normative accounts are involved in deciding whether to attribute causal accounts only to individual characteristics or to move beyond individuals and seat explanatory causes in society and history. What we identify as a cause of a disease may depend on what we believe we can change, and what we believe we can change depends on both our scientific conceptions of causality and our ethical limits. For instance, those who adopt an individualistic orientation in ethics may be more comfortable with causal explanations that foster mechanical, biological, and individual approaches to health care. Those with more collective orientations may prefer social and political explanations.[40]

To interpret the conduct of clients correctly, it is important to recognize that the traditionally individualist view of clients makes it difficult to perceive many factors affecting their health. Moreover, individualism maintains a gulf between highly organized providers of care, who operate collectively, and separate clients, who do not communicate with each other. This gulf makes it difficult to set priorities when conflicts arise among providers and clients. Recognizing this gulf may help nurses to resist making their clients focal points of their frustration with the current limitations of health care practice.

When clinicians make judgments about the responsibility of their clients, they reflect and integrate a wide variety of philosophical considerations. Traditionally, nurses have had the role of controlling and manipulating clients in order to obtain compliance. But nurses are increasingly adopting a perspective of advocacy and teaching. This more egalitarian philosophy of care may lead nurses to judge clients differently. It may help both nurses and clients to analyze and resolve health problems more justly, more cooperatively, and more effectively.

Summary

Disliked clients are a common source of moral problems for nurses. Since we generally lack provider–client associations stating the reciprocal rights and responsibilities of providers and clients, it is difficult to resolve ethical questions posed by conflicts between them.

Patients who appear to be responsible for their health problems commonly arouse anger in nurses. Nurses who follow the *individualist thesis* with regard to health generally see individual patients as the major source of their own health problems. Nurses who follow the *victim thesis* tend to deny patients responsibility and to place power over disease in the hands of health professionals. The truth lies in understanding the historical and social setting of health, disease, and clinicians' power in relation to patients.

Noncompliance is a common phenomenon in patient care. Many patients fail to take their medicines. Nurses have a traditional role in obtaining patient com-

---

[39]Christopher Boorse teases apart evaluative and scientific conceptions of health in "On the Distinction between Disease and Illness," *Philosophy and Public Affairs,* 5 (1975), 49–68.

[40]This conflict in perspectives can be seen clearly in nature-nurture controversies, such as those over intelligence and race and aggression and gender.

pliance, but this function must be limited by an appreciation of rational non-compliance and respect for the autonomy of patients.

Dangerous patients are rare, but they sometimes pose a conflict between the principle of patient welfare and nurses' rights to protect themselves. This is not, strictly speaking, a health care problem, since nurses' rights to safety are more basic than their professional obligations. But in hospitals, legal and medical approaches to dangerous patients tend to be closely related. It is thus important to be clear whether one is restraining patients for their own good or to protect staff and other patients. It is also important to distinguish between dangerous clients and those who merely pose inconveniences and unpleasantness. How much personal risk nurses should take to meet professional obligations to clients is a difficult question. It is useful to think more in terms of heroism and cowardice than right and wrong, and the problem of self-sacrifice for the good of patients has been made more difficult because nurses have been exploited in the past because of their idealism.

FURTHER READINGS

The Health Professional

BONAPARTE, BEVERLY H., "Ego Defensiveness, Open-Closed Mindedness, and Nurses' Attitude toward Culturally Different Patients," *Nursing Research*, 28, 3 (1979), 166–172.

EDMUNDS, MARILYN W., "Non-Clinical Problems: Conflict," *Nurse Practitioner* (November/December 1979), 42.

FLEXNER, JOHN M., AND HARRY S. ABRAM, "A Hostile Patient: Fighting Ire with Ire," *Hastings Center Report*, 8, 1 (February 1978), 18–20.

GRUBER, KAREN A., AND HENRY E. SCHNIEWIND, JR., "Letting Anger Work for You," *American Journal of Nursing*, 76 (1976), 1450–52.

HALL, BEVERLY A., "The Effect of Interpersonal Attraction on the Therapeutic Relationship: A Review and Suggestions for Further Study," *Journal of Psychiatric Nursing and Mental Health Services* (September 1977), 18–23.

LIEF, HAROLD I., AND RENÉE C. FOX, "Training for 'Detached Concern' in Medical Students," in *The Psychological Basis of Medical Practice*, eds. Harold I. Lief, Victor F. Lief, and Nina R. Lief, pp. 12–35. New York: Harper & Row, Publishers, Inc., 1963.

MOONEY, JUDITH, "Attachment/Separation in the Nurse-Patient Relationship," *Nursing Forum*, 15 (1976), 259–64.

ROTH, JULIUS A., "Some Contingencies of the Moral Evaluation and Control of Clientele: The Case of the Hospital Emergency Service," *American Journal of Sociology*, 77 (1972), 839–56.

RUDITIS, SUSAN ELLIOTT, "Developing Trust in Nursing Interpersonal Relationships," *Journal of Psychiatric Nursing and Mental Health Services*, 17 (April 1979), 20–23.

SHAPIRO, B., "The Dead End of Altruism: A Note to Nurses," *Nursing Forum*, 15 (1976), 385–89.

WHITTAKER, ELVI, AND VIRGINIA OLESEN, "Faces of Florence Nightingale: Function of the Heroine Legend in the Occupational Sub-Culture," in *The Professional in the Organization*, ed. Mark Abrahamson, pp. 30–46. Chicago: Rand McNally & Company, 1967.

Responsibility for Health

ABLON, JOAN, "Stigmatized Health Conditions," *Social Science and Medicine,* 15B (1981), 5–9.

ALLEGRANTE, JOHN P., AND LAWRENCE W. GREEN, "When Health Policy Becomes Victim Blaming," *The New England Journal of Medicine,* 305 (1981), 1528–29.

CRAWFORD, ROBERT, "You Are Dangerous to Your Health: The Ideology and Politics of Victim Blaming," *International Journal of Health Services,* 7 (1977), 663–80.

HALLER, JOHN S., AND ROBIN M. HALLER, *The Physician and Sexuality in Victorian America.* New York: W.W. Norton & Co., Inc., 1974.

HOWELL, MARY G., "Pediatricians and Mothers," in *The Cultural Crisis of Modern Medicine,* ed. John Ehrenreich, pp. 201–11. New York: Monthly Review Press, 1978.

LEIFER, RONALD, "The Ethics of Drug Prohibition," *International Journal of Psychiatry in Medicine,* 10, 1 (1972), 70–76.

McGEE, ROBERT RAY, "Stop Blaming the Patient for Being Sick!" *Medical Economics* (August 10, 1981), 57–59.

MILLIS, JOHN S., "Wisdom? Health? Can Society Guarantee Them?" *The New England Journal of Medicine,* 283 (1970), 260–61.

SHUMAN, S.I., "The Right to Be Unhealthy," *Wayne Law Review,* 22 (1975), 61–85.

Problem Patients

BARSKY, ARTHUR J., III, "Hidden Reasons Some Patients Visit Doctors," *Annals of Internal Medicine,* 94 (1981), 492–98.

BRUCE, GREGORY, AND RUTH L. GOUGE, "Disfigured by a Violent Patient: A Case . . . and Comment," *R.N.,* 42, 1 (March 1979), 61.

CROSS, YVONNE, "Rogue Nurses: Nursing the Cruel," *Nursing Mirror,* 134, 11 (March 17, 1972), 9–12.

DAVITZ, LOIS JEAN, *Interpersonal Processes in Nursing: Case Histories.* New York: Springer Publishing Co., Inc., 1970.

JEFFREY, ROGER, "Normal Rubbish: Deviant Patients in Casualty Departments," *Sociology of Health and Illness: A Journal of Medical Sociology,* 1, 1 (June 1979), 90–107.

LIPP, MARTIN R., *Respectful Treatment: The Human Side of Medical Care,* Chap. 8, "Problem Patients," pp.108–23. New York: Harper & Row Publishers, Inc., 1977.

LORBER, JUDITH, "Good Patients and Problem Patients: Conformity and Deviance in a General Hospital," in *Patients, Physicians, and Illness* (3rd ed.), ed. E. Gartly Jaco, pp. 202–17. New York: The Free Press, 1979.

McMORROW, MARY ELLEN, "The Manipulative Patient," *American Journal of Nursing,* 81 (1981), 1188–90.

SCULLY, ROBERT E., JAMES J. GALDABINI, AND BETTY U. McNEELY, "Case Records of the Massachusetts General Hospital: Weekly Clinicopathological Exercises, Case 35–1979," *The New England Journal of Medicine,* 301 (1979), 488–96.

UJHELY, GERTRUD B., *The Nurse and Her Problem Patients.* New York: Springer Publishing Co., Inc., 1963.

———, "Two Types of Problem Patients and How to Deal with Them," *Nursing '76,* 6, 5 (1976), 64–67.

WALKER, JANE, ET AL., "Dealing with Rage," *Nursing '75,* 5, 10 (October 1975), 25–29.

Compliance

CARLSMITH, J.M., AND A.E. GROSS, "Some Effects of Guilt on Compliance," *Journal of Personality and Social Psychology,* 11 (1969), 232–39.

DANIELS, LINDA M., ET AL., "How You Can Improve Patient Compliance," *Nursing 78,* 8, 5 (May 1978), 40–47.

HOGUE, CAROL C., "Nursing and Compliance," in *Compliance in Health Care*, eds. R. Brian Haynes, D. Wayne Taylor, and David L. Sackett, pp. 247–59. Baltimore: Johns Hopkins University Press, 1979.

VARGIU, JAMES, AND NAOMI REMEN, "What Is Health For?—Human Priorities in Health Care," in "Orthodox Medicine, Humanistic Medicine and Holistic Health Care—A Forum," *Western Journal of Medicine*, 6 (1979), 471–72.

CHAPTER 15

Death,
Pain,
and Suffering

Coping with pain, suffering, and death is among the most ancient and persistent of human concerns. It places demands on our deepest resources. In response to pain, suffering, and death we look for more than simple healing and comfort—we look for explanations and justifications. The sufferer asks "Why me?" and when we see suffering all around us, we look for reasons to maintain hope. In a world of vast physical, intellectual, and cultural resources, a large portion of the population suffers pain, starvation, disease, fear, and oppression. Surely this chronic state of affairs demands an explanation; it has been a common inducement to the study of philosophy.[1]

Traditional religions address the experience of suffering. Church community, pastoral solace, and the mystery of God offer spiritual comfort for many forms of suffering. But a serious question has always accompanied this approach: God is supposedly both extremely good and extremely powerful; why then does God permit famines, epidemics, accidents, childhood leukemia, torture, and the like? As one nurse put it,

It makes me angry when a child dies. Why should a child die? Why should a young person die? I can't answer, and it bothers me a lot.[2]

Many different answers have been offered to this sort of question. One answer sees suffering as something not fully real, a fleeting shadow of God's creation, an infinitesimal blot on the cosmos.[3] Another justifies and interprets it as part of the

[1]The nineteenth-century German philosopher Arthur Schopenhauer wrote, "Death is the true inspiring genius, or the muse of philosophy," in *The World As Will and Idea*, trans. T.B. Haldane and J. Kemp (London: Routledge & Kegan Paul, 1883, 9th impr., 1948), p. 249.

[2]Lois J. Davitz and Joel R. Davitz, "How Do Nurses Feel When Patients Suffer?" *American Journal of Nursing*, 75 (1975), 1509.

[3]Saint Augustine outlined the basic philosophical issues in the theological problem of suffering and evil. One of his arguments was that evil is an imperfection, a lack, and thus an absence of something—nonexistent. See Saint Augustine, *The City of God*, trans. Gerald G. Walsh, ed. Vernon J. Bourke (Garden City, N.Y.: Doubleday & Co., Inc., 1958), pp. 244–50. For evil as very tiny, see C.S. Lewis, *The Great Divorce* (New York: Macmillan, Inc., 1946).

drama of God's work.[4] In a common version of the drama, suffering comes to us as punishment for our sins or those of our ancestors. In another, all will be made up to us after death by the future acts of God. Sometimes the meaningfulness of suffering is simply asserted as a hope, without an attempt at explanation.

These attempts to understand suffering seem frail in the presence of intense suffering. Children who must live on kidney dialysis or who are beaten into a coma by abusing parents and parents of children accidently drowned at picnics challenge our ability to accept traditional religious accounts. Dostoevsky, for example, was extremely troubled by the suffering of innocents.[5]

Yet, suffering is not an unequivocally bad process. Some see it as teaching us to appreciate deeper values,[6] or as a necessary condition of joy.[7] Suffering creates an opportunity to marshal one's personal resources and to grow in strength, even at risk of being destroyed.[8] Since suffering is a threat to personal identity,[9] it can be interpreted by identifying with its causes and claiming it as part of one's personal destiny.[10] It can also lead to greater identification with others, especially heroes, heroines, and others who suffer.[11] But if suffering is not unequivocally bad, what is?

A compassionate response to suffering is a central task of modern scientific health care practice. Health care treats such major sources of suffering as disease, pain, and death. This response to suffering lies at the heart of health care, and, from the point of view of ethics, it is central to nursing and medicine. It makes clinical practice a form of work for the good of humankind, displays an empathetic concern for others, and gives depth to the concept of profession in health care.

What is the relationship of health care to traditional approaches to suffering?[12] Some see health care as part of a larger religious project giving meaning to concrete relief from suffering. Early nursing and medical practice have historical roots in religious orders. Nightingale, for example, began her nursing work with the Institu-

---

[4]Many writers have tried to put suffering in its proper place in the spiritual drama; Augustine is among them, in *The City of God*, pp. 269–77.

[5]See, for example, Ivan's rebellion in Fyodor Dostoevsky, *The Brothers Karamozov* (New York: W.W. Norton & Co., Inc., 1976). For a more tepid search for the meaning of death, see Thornton Wilder, *The Bridge of San Luis Rey* (New York: Avon Books, 1927; reprint ed., 1955).

[6]Laurel Archer Copp, "The Spectrum of Suffering," *American Journal of Nursing,* 74 (1974), 492–93.

[7]Stanley Hauerwas, "Reflections on Suffering, Death and Medicine," *Ethics in Science & Medicine,* 6 (1979), 230.

[8]For an extended discussion, see David E. Boeyink, "Pain and Suffering," *Journal of Religious Ethics,* 2 (1974), 85–98. More briefly, see *Encyclopedia of Bioethics,* 1978 ed., s.v. "Pain and Suffering: Philosophical Perspectives," by Jerome A. Shaffer. See also, Martin Luther King, Jr., *Stride toward Freedom: The Montgomery Story* (New York: Harper & Row Publishers, Inc., 1958), p. 85.

[9]Daniel Day Williams, "Suffering and Being in Empirical Theology," in *The Future of Empirical Theology,* ed., Bernard E. Meland (Chicago: University of Chicago Press, 1969), p. 181.

[10]Hauerwas, "Reflections," p. 235.

[11]Copp, "Spectrum," p. 493.

[12]Medieval theologians struggled over the place of medicine in religion. For a brief historical account, see *Encyclopedia of Bioethics,* 1978 ed., "History of Medical Ethics: Medieval Europe: Fourth to Sixteenth Century: Disease and Medicine: Early Christian Attitudes," by Darrel W. Amundsen.

tion of Deaconesses at Kaiserswerth.[13] Others sense conflict with religious approaches to suffering. They see modern health care as part of scientific approaches to human problems, gradually displacing religious interpretations with more secular ones. Secular approaches straightforwardly assume that suffering, being undesired and unpleasant, is a harm or evil. Although some suffering may be inevitable due to human aggression, conflict, and discontent, there is more suffering in the world than necessary, and it is unjustly distributed. The problem with suffering is not to interpret it, but to combat it. Modern clinical practice replaces the religious denial that pain is real with pain-relieving drugs. It sees patients in a drama of medical discovery and conquest of disease and death instead of in a drama of religious salvation. Human science can be seen as challenging natural diseases and death created by God. The existentialist novelist Albert Camus illustrates this feeling of conflict between religion and health care with Christian plague victims who cast their infected robes on nurses who had the temerity to treat them.[14]

The raw quantitative judgment expressed in health care that the less pain, disease, and death we suffer the better is weakened by several countervailing tendencies. Some suffering is inevitable, but the focus on eliminating suffering sometimes leads clinicians to see suffering as pointless,[15] to deny or ignore the suffering they cannot prevent, and even to reject patients whose suffering they cannot help.[16] Staff sometimes pit themselves in unrealistic struggles against the inevitable death of a patient; and when frustrated, blame themselves or the patient. Besides leaving much suffering untouched, health care causes *additional* suffering. Many procedures—injections, medications, spinal taps, intubations, surgery—cause fear, pain, discomfort, nausea, and so on. Painful diagnostic tests fall into a broad category of "medically justified" suffering. Moreover, "half-way" technologies such as dialysis ameliorate problems but do not eliminate them, and so they rescue patients from some forms of suffering only to expose them to a host of others.

The focus on technology sometimes misleads staff into overlooking simple sources of pain and discomfort. For example, an elderly patient in an intensive care unit was cold and needed blankets, but no one thought to put a blanket on him because it would have covered some of the tubes. The atmosphere of some hospitals amplifies loneliness, despair, confusion, fear, and anger. Hospitals concentrate suffering into one place, and clinicians endure tremendous exposure to it. Hospital architecture is notoriously lacking in offices and "backstage" areas. Crying in toilet stalls is a widespread hospital experience. Nor is there much in the way of

[13]Cecil Woodham-Smith, *Florence Nightingale, 1820–1910* (London: Constable, 1950). Woodham-Smith records some of Nightingale's comments on Kaiserswerth: "The nursing there was nil, . . . the hygiene horrible. The hospital was certainly the worst part of Kaiserswerth. But never have I met with a higher tone, a purer devotion than there. There was no neglect. It was the more remarkable because many of the Deaconesses had been only peasants—none were gentlewomen (when I was there)" (p. 91).

[14]Albert Camus, *The Plague*, trans. Stuart Gilbert (New York: Random House, Inc., 1948), p. 210.

[15]Hauerwas, "Reflections," p. 234.

[16]Christine K. Cassel and Andrew L. Jameton, "Dementia in the Elderly: An Analysis of Medical Responsibility," *Annals of Internal Medicine*, 94 (1981), 802–7; Virginia George and Alan Dundes, "The Gomer: A Figure of American Hospital Folk Speech," *Journal of American Folklore*, 91 (1978), 568–81; and Solomon Papper, "The Undesirable Patient," *Journal of Chronic Diseases*, 22 (1970), 777–79.

support staff with skills in counseling health professionals about their reactions to pain and grief.

In working closely with patients on a daily basis, nurses become specialists in suffering. Appreciating the full range of human response to suffering requires of them considerable reflectiveness. How can nurses help patients to struggle with the meaning of their suffering? Is it appropriate for them to do so, or is this the special work of the chaplain or counselor? What can nurses do for themselves as witnesses to and participants in the suffering of patients?

Nurses do not merely work close to suffering. A compassionate and human response to suffering is the central value of health care work. Treatment of disease, as symbolized by highly technological medicine, is a much more speculative goal in health care. Health care delivery systems have little impact on the incidence of disease and death,[17] and cure of disease is morally important mainly as a means of alleviating suffering and pain. There is even some doubt whether an abnormality or disorder that did not cause suffering should be correctly termed a *disease* at all.[18] The *direct* services provided by health care systems are care, comfort, compassion, protection, and a humane response to the suffering caused by disease and dying.

In dealing with suffering and the cure of disease, nurses encounter a double stereotype. As *nurses,* they are associated with care over cure, even though care and cure are integrated processes provided by both nurses and physicians. As *women,* for the most part, they are associated with a humane and gentle response to suffering. Since skills in caring are labor-intensive—whether practiced by men or women, physicians or nurses—and have little economic value to investors, those who engage in caring do not receive the rewards and respect awarded those with more technologically oriented skills. Some nurses wish to escape this stereotype and become more closely identified with the highly technological theories associated with medicine.

Another approach to the historical problem of undervalued work is to embrace, endorse, and support some aspects of the stereotype. As providers of central and direct health care services, nurses can work toward a public emphasis on and proper valuation of their work. By focusing on skills in relieving suffering rather than on health care technology for its own sake, nurses can support more humane forms of health care. Although emphasizing skills in responding to suffering imposes emotional and political risks on nurses, compassion is an important element of nursing care. Some definitions of compassion see it as requiring entering into, sharing, and tasting the pain of others,[19] and maintaining a professional manner in the face of one's own strong personal reactions can be difficult. How should one balance one's own needs against those of patients without being exploited or self-sacrificing? For example, when is it acceptable to cry with or in front of patients?

---

[17]Thomas McKeown, *The Role of Medicine: Dream, Mirage, or Nemesis?* (Oxford: Basil Blackwell, Ltd., 1979).

[18]See Peter Sedgwick, "What Is Illness?" in *Contemporary Issues in Bioethics,* 1st ed., eds. Tom L. Beauchamp and LeRoy Walters (Encino, Calif.: Dickenson Publishing Co., Inc., 1978) and other articles in this collection on the concepts of health and disease.

[19]Anne J. Davis, "Compassion, Suffering, Morality: Ethical Dilemmas in Caring," *Nursing Law and Ethics,* 2, 5 (May 1981), 1. We can see how gender lurks even in responses to suffering: *compassion*—taking on suffering—is often associated with nursing; *detached concern*—keeping it at a distance—is often associated with medicine.

I know a lot of teachers in nursing school teach that it's OK to cry with a patient if that's the way you feel. There's nothing wrong with showing emotion. But I feel since I've been in practice, restraint is important. You won't do the patient or the family any good if you stand there dissolved in your own tears.[20]

One task in the educational preparation of nurses is to help them integrate durable personal satisfaction with professional techniques of delivering compassionate and humane care.

Understanding the ethical issues in the treatment of suffering is part of this process. In this chapter, we will address some of the ethical issues in suffering: decisions about dying, discontinuing therapy, cardiopulmonary resuscitation (CPR), and pain medication. Although ethical issues in such sources of suffering as aging, handicaps, and mental illness are important, we will not address them here.

Decisions about Dying

Patients, their families, and clinicians make decisions about the treatment of dying patients against a background of conflicting feelings about death, varying evaluations of death as a way of escaping pain and suffering, and great uncertainty about its timing. Most of us have strong feelings about death. It is a tremendous mystery: Where does the flame go when the candle goes out? Death can seem overwhelmingly threatening. When I die, I lose everything; when those I love die, I lose them.

Some of the terror of death can be dispelled by thinking about it and discussing it with others. During the 1970s, nurses greatly increased their attention to the needs of dying patients. Until then, recognizing that the death of a patient was inevitable meant for health professionals "There is nothing more we can do." But clinicians now recognize that dying people are still actively engaged in life. Respect for persons demands a response to their needs even if they have a brief future; care is not an investment but an ongoing human response. Experience from the hospice movement and research on dying show the kinds of supportive care that nurses can give through communication, pain management, and creation of appropriate physical and social settings in which to die.[21]

Influences on the process of dying are multiple. This disease has a powerful effect: Cancer may proceed slowly and heart disease swiftly. Similarly, suicide poses very different problems than lateral sclerosis. Culture is an important factor: The death of a fifteenth-century Native American tribal elder in North Dakota differs from the death of a twentieth-century movie star in Los Angeles. The attitudes, values, and character of the patient shape the dying process and decisions about it.

[20]Davitz and Davitz, "How Do Nurses Feel?" p. 1506.

[21]See Cicely Saunders, *Care of the Dying* (London: Nursing Times, 1976); Sandol Stoddard, *The Hospice Movement: A Better Way of Caring for the Dying* (Briarcliff Manor, N.Y.: Stein and Day Publishers, 1978); Barbara McNulty, "St. Christopher's Outpatients," *American Journal of Nursing*, 71 (1971), 2328–30; Cicely Saunders, "The Last Stages of Life," *American Journal of Nursing*, 65 (1965), 70–75; and Kenneth B. Wentzel, "Dying Are the Living: St. Christopher's Hospice, London," *American Journal of Nursing*, 76 (1976), 956–57.

Most regard death as an evil and something to avoid as long as possible. Some judge only extreme suffering as worse than death. In contrast, others see death as a natural and positive fulfillment or completion of living.[22] Since the meaning of suffering and death varies so widely among people, no simple calculus can balance suffering against death. The patient's evaluation is essential.

Disclosure is thus very important to dying patients. Honesty is both salutary and morally obligatory (see pp. 170–71). Honesty with the dying, however, means much more than mere verbal disclosure of bad news. It also involves continuity of communication and concern during the process of coming to terms with death. Hardly anyone immediately and clearly recognizes the approach of his or her own death. The whole personality must adjust. Thus, *denial* is very common. Denial consists of an intellectual but unemotional response, or an emotional response without conscious recognition of death. Denial permits patients to say, "I know I am dying, and I know that I am not dying."

Timing of communication is thus very important. It must progress according to the patient's pace. Family members, nurses, and physicians may participate in the process at different rates.

> CASE EXAMPLE. A 54-year-old Japanese gardener was admitted to the hospital with shortness of breath. During his hospital stay he deteriorated inexorably. He had an enlarged heart, signs of a possible cardiac infection, and irregular heart signs, but no diagnosis was forthcoming. The nursing staff judged that he was dying on the basis of their experience of dying patients in the unit. They wanted to treat him as a dying patient and to discuss death with him. Since they had no diagnosis, the physicians were unwilling to accept that he was dying. Instead, they energetically pursued the clinical puzzle. His sudden death from a heart attack was an emotional blow to the divided staff. A rare heart tumor was diagnosed on autopsy, and his death was a subject of staff concern long afterward.

Here, different staff perceptions of the patient's prognosis affected the rate at which staff came to terms with his death.

Setting is also an important factor. Dying does not fit well in tertiary hospitals, which are oriented to treatment and cure. Patients may need or want to die at home or in a hospice. In these settings, visiting can be better managed; pain control can become a central focus; and intrusive testing, surveillance, and treatment can be avoided.

Dying patients pose many difficulties for nurses, who work in considerable uncertainty about the timing and trajectory of dying. Death reminds them of their own mortality. As strangers to most patients, nurses only provide them with minimal community. Often patients are unable to state their own wishes with regard to dying because they are too debilitated or uncertain. Staff may feel unsure how to respond to patients' deeper spiritual needs in the crisis of dying. But overcoming these obstacles can be tremendously satisfying. One response is to meet the simple needs of patients—a sip of water, attention to bedsores, a cool washcloth, and quiet. Mystery and dread can be staved off by acts as simple as holding hands.

While a patient approaches death, questions may arise about terminating

---

[22]Carl G. Jung, "The Soul and Death," in *The Meaning of Death,* ed. Herman Feifel (New York: McGraw-Hill Book Company, 1969), pp. 3–15.

curative efforts. Such decisions are usually discussed in literature separate from the care of the dying. This division is unfortunate, because decisions to switch from curative efforts to supportive care, or vice versa, occur as part of the overall care of the dying patient. Patients in hospices may decide to change to more aggressive forms of treatment, and patients in intensive care units may want to receive only palliative care.

It may be difficult for health professionals to hold back from extensive life-saving efforts. They may accept death only when all curative attempts fail, and exhaustion becomes the decision point. Such decisions have become a typical point of conflict between nurses and physicians. In many cases, nurses appear to be more ready than physicians to accept that patients are dying and to provide palliation, support, and comfort rather than heroic measures. The case of the Japanese gardener discussed above illustrates this conflict well. Such conflicts place considerable stress on staff, especially when nurses find themselves devoting bedside care to an essentially dead body for an absent attending physician unready to make a decision.[23] Such conflicts can be resolved only when nurses take an active role in decisions about allowing patients to die.

Since patients' vital signs vary from day to day, it is difficult to make the transition from cure to support and to know when it is appropriate to discontinue treatment or not to institute it. Whether decisions to discontinue are appropriate or not can only be determined by careful study of each case. Consider, for example, the case of a child slowly dying of a progressive neurological disease:

CASE EXAMPLE. O.A. is a five-year-old girl with a diagnosis of metachromatic leukodystrophy. Her neonatal and early development were normal until about one year of age, when she stopped achieving developmental milestones. By the age of two, she had developed severe weakness, uncontrolled movements, difficulty in swallowing, and slack muscle tone. The diagnosis of MLD meant that O.A. was suffering from an incurable, progressive, and fatal disease.

Since diagnosis, O.A. has received ongoing, supportive medical and nursing treatment. About a year ago, the progress of her disease reached a plateau, leaving her in an essentially vegetative state. She lives in an extended care facility (ECF), and her mother and grandmother visit her weekly. They recognize the seriousness of her condition, seem to care for her, and seem to get something from their visits with her.

O.A. has generalized seizures that are difficult to control and require high doses of medication. These medications keep her in a heavily sedated state and contribute to her vegetative level of consciousness. The medications also have a risk of causing respiratory failure. Every few months, O.A. has a bout of pneumonia. Treatment for this involves admission to an acute care hospital to drain her lungs and administer antibiotics. The present treatment plan is to continue these kinds of support, but staff and family have agreed that she should not be resuscitated in the case of heart or respiratory failure. Accordingly, the attending physician has written a "do-not-resuscitate (DNR)" order in O.A.'s chart.

---

[23]This is a common complaint of nurses. For a vivid description of nursing care of respirator patients, see Terry Daniels, "The Nurse's Tale," *New York* (April 30, 1979), 37–41.

The staff who cared for O.A. asked themselves a number of painful questions. First, should they be treating her pneumonia, or would it be more humane to allow her to die the next time she contracts it? Second, if she were to go into respiratory failure during an injection of seizure medication, should the nurse initiate resuscitation? Third, is it wrong to cause O.A. pain by injections and suctioning? These three specific questions fall under the general headings of discontinuing treatment, hastening dying, DNR orders, and administration of pain medication. These subjects are discussed next with occasional references to O.A.'s case.

Discontinuing Therapy

In the late 1970s, a consensus developed among health professionals that it is morally acceptable and appropriate to allow people to die in certain circumstances. There were too many horror stories of moribund people tortured by futile, expensive, and painful treatment. Health professionals began to recognize more clearly the limits of their power to hinder death. A number of interacting considerations are important in deciding whether or not to discontinue treatment. Four types of considerations are presented next, in generally descending order of importance. Decisions to discontinue therapy can be aided by outlining them under these headings.[24]

Medical Indications

Can therapy be offered that can reasonably be expected to slow or ameliorate the fatal course of the disease? Since this judgment is a matter of probabilities and hardly ever certain, it requires considering the patient's condition carefully. When death appears to be inevitable and imminent, there is no obligation to provide more than palliative care. Disagreements are not for the most part over this principle, but over how small a possibility of recovery means that death is inevitable and how near death must be to count as imminent. Most would agree that O.A. has no possibility of recovery, but that her death is not yet imminent. Thus, in her case, medical indications are not decisive.

Patients' Preferences

Respect for persons demands that patients be consulted and listened to with regard to therapy. Competent patients have a legal right to withhold consent to treatment. Even when therapy may delay death significantly, competent patients may legally refuse it, and where such refusals reflect a patient's real needs and wants, they should ethically be respected in most cases. For instance, Mrs. K.'s refusal of an amputation (pp. 190–91) deserved respect although her condition was critical.

[24]This four-point schema is based on the work of Albert R. Jonsen. For a short version, see Bernard Lo and Albert R. Jonsen, ''Clinical Decisions to Limit Treatment,'' *Annals of Internal Medicine*, 93 (1980), 764–68. For a fuller version, see Albert R. Jonsen, Mark Siegler, and William J. Winslade, *Clinical Ethics: A Practical Approach to Ethical Decisions in Clinical Medicine* (New York: Macmillan, Inc., 1982).

Patients' choices and attitudes can help resolve questions about the futility of therapy and the nearness of death. Some patients prefer aggressive treatment and would like to see their care givers resist death as long as possible; others are ready to die or are unwilling to risk lengthy periods of morbidity and disability.

One may have legitimate reservations about a patient's refusal of treatment.[25] Patients can change their minds; for instance, a woman dying of breast cancer struggled for long periods over whether to accept pain medication or whether to suffer according to the dictates of her personal religious beliefs. Patients may speak metaphorically: A young man dying of a multiple immune failure said "I want to die; leave me alone," but on further discussion, it appeared that he wanted more considerate treatment and fewer uncomfortable diagnostic tests. Patients may not appreciate how painful and futile a treatment is or may have exaggerated fears of a procedure. When patients are unable to speak for themselves, nurses may be able to ascertain their wishes from their character, their prior statements, and relatives' and friends' reflections about what they would wish. Determining patients' wishes takes care, time, and consultation with family and friends. Nurses as patient advocates play a significant role in ascertaining what patients prefer.

Quality of Life

Would halting therapy be acceptable in cases where patients are too debilitated to have an opinion and where the likely outcome would involve minimal quality of life? Comparative concepts such as "high," "poor," and "minimal" quality of life are vague assessments about possible recovery from disease, level of consciousness, level of physical function, freedom from suffering, ability to relate to others, and the patient's ability to understand the course of treatment.

Some hold that to make judgments about lifesaving care on a quality-of-life basis is to show variable respect for persons depending on their qualities, and that it should thus not be considered.[26] Others hold that equal respect for persons requires taking each person's quality of life with equal seriousness, so that one can respectfully employ quality-of-life considerations to discontinue treatment. I am presently inclined to accept the latter position, partly because I am impressed with the dismal prospects of some painful and heroic treatments near death, and partly because I believe it possible to respectfully and seriously consider another's quality of life. It is crucial in such considerations to distinguish the *patient's* actual or probable assessment of quality of life from the assessment of *others* about that quality and from the patient's impact on others' quality of life. A quadriplegic artist of strong character who provides rewarding company may prefer death to life without creative work, while a brain-damaged alcoholic may find a life of staggering down halls, smoking cigarettes, and harassing nurses extremely rewarding. For instance, a court made a plausible decision in the *Saikewicz* case that Mr. Saikewicz was too mentally debilitated to make the suffering from lengthy cancer chemotherapy meaningful to him.[27]

[25]David L. Jackson and Stuart Youngner, "Patient Autonomy and 'Death with Dignity': Some Clinical Caveats," *The New England Journal of Medicine*, 301 (1979), 404–8.

[26]*Encyclopedia of Bioethics*, 1978 ed., s.v. "Quality of Life," by Warren T. Reich.

[27]Superintendent of Belchertown State School v. Saikewicz, 1977 Mass. Adv. Sh. 2461, 370 N.E. 2d 417 (1977).

The painfulness of therapy in relationship to the prospects for recovery must also be considered.[28] One aspect of the distinction between *ordinary* and *extraordinary* therapy is the pain and discomfort imposed on the patient in relationship to its goals. O.A.'s quality of life was minimal and expected to decline. Her therapy probably involved pain, but it could be minimized by medication, and the progress of the disease was expected to bring pain to an end before long.

O.A. is one of many debilitated patients living in ECFs who are referred periodically to acute care institutions to treat acute episodes such as pneumonia. Hospital staff often feel uncomfortable about treating such patients. The patients seem moribund in the hospital; they return to what the staff assume to be dismal treatment facilities; and staff are concerned that profits may dominate the motives of referring facilities and physicians. In treating such cases, it is important to resist limiting care to simple treatment of the acute condition. Staff should inquire about the patient's condition prior to the acute illness and press for improvement in the quality of care in the referring institution. Decisions to withhold care should only be made in consultation with family and ECF staff.

Nurses at the ECF might have decided not to refer O.A. for treatment. A recent study found that of 190 patients acquiring pneumonia in ECFs, eighty-nine were not referred for treatment. Nine percent of treated patients died, while 59 percent of untreated patients died. The study suggests that an implicit decision to allow patients to die was being made in these cases. The study found that patients with more serious diagnoses, lower mental status, less mobility, and more pain or those on heavier narcotic medication were more likely to be allowed to die of pneumonia.[29] In determining what to do in O.A.'s case, hospital staff consulted with ECF staff frequently and occasionally visited her there. Although allowing her to die in the ECF without referral for acute care can be reasonably defended, the staff decided to continue treatment because of *external factors*.

External Factors

External factors are the effects on others of continuing or discontinuing treatment. These may include financial costs to others. Daily charges for cancer patients in intensive care units averaged $1500 to $2000 in 1976–1977.[30] These figures do not include physicians' fees. Who pays, and at what sacrifice? Will therapy exhaust the family's savings and property? Although less quantifiable, costs can also be measured in terms of stress, staff time, burdensomeness, and inconvenience. Such factors are important where they have a large impact on the patient's family or on other patients. The distant impact of a patient's care on the public budget is normally not significant and should not be considered in the clinical decision.

Costliness to others represents the second aspect of the difference between ordinary and extraordinary means. Some modes of care, such as feeding patients,

[28]Sharon H. Imbus and Bruce E. Zawacki, "Autonomy for Burned Patients When Survival Is Unprecedented," *The New England Journal of Medicine*, 297 (1977), 308–11.

[29]Norman K. Brown and Donovan J. Thompson, "Nontreatment of Fever in Extended-Care Facilities," *The New England Journal of Medicine*, 300 (1979), 1246–50.

[30]Alan D. Turnbull et al., "The Inverse Relationship between Cost and Survival in the Critically Ill Cancer Patient," *Critical Care Medicine*, 7 (1979), 20–23.

are much less burdensome than others, such as dialysis. One needs a sense of proportion in judging the extraordinariness of care, and there is no sharp distinction between ordinary and extraordinary. Feeding some patients by mouth may take hours of staff time, and hyperalimentation may be as risky and invasive as dialysis.

In O.A.'s case, her family felt that they had rewarding communication with her and that she continued to receive something from them. Although her case is clearly a borderline one, the staff judged that this combination of external and quality-of-life factors marginally outweighed her continued suffering and that continued care was justified.

Which of these four categories are most relevant is dependent on the case, and so careful discussion of these issues is required. Decision making should be a team effort involving patient, family, friends, nurses, physicians, and other actively involved staff. When the patient is not able to participate, a guardian may be appointed, and in some cases a court hearing may be advisable.

Speeding up the Process of Dying

Discontinuing therapy and allowing patients to die can be distinguished from causing their deaths or hastening their dying. This is the standard distinction between *passive* and *active* euthanasia. Giving a lethal agent such as potassium chloride or an overdose of morphine in order to kill the patient is active euthanasia. Sigmund Freud, for example, during a long ordeal with throat cancer asked his physician to kill him with morphine, and his wish was respected.[31] There are two common positions on the ethical difference between active and passive euthanasia. According to one, there is no real difference between them: Where death is inevitable and suffering is likely to be prolonged by not allowing a patient to die, there is good reason to perform active euthanasia.[32] According to the other position, there is a deep and important difference between taking a hand in the process of death and standing back from it.

The distinction between active and passive interventions is deeply rooted in our culture. Criminal law, for example, distinguishes between allowing to die and active killing. It has rarely become involved in cases of passive euthanasia or termination of care, but overdoses of morphine to kill patients are technically murder even if well motivated.[33] Nurses who speed patients along in the night run the risk of making the headlines: "Angel of Mercy Charged in Deaths," "Three Nurses Accused of a Mercy-Killing," "Autopsies Ordered in 12 Coronary Unit Deaths," and so on.[34]

There are good reasons for defending the traditional distinction between ac-

---

[31]Max Schur, *Freud: Living and Dying* (New York: International Universities Press, 1972), pp. 408, 529.

[32]The most concise statement of this position is James Rachels, "Active and Passive Euthanasia," *The New England Journal of Medicine*, 292 (1975), 78–80.

[33]A good discussion of the legal aspects of active euthanasia is George P. Fletcher, "Prolonging Life: Some Legal Considerations," *Washington Law Review*, 42 (1967), 999–1016.

[34]Although both physicians and nurses are legally vulnerable in cases of active euthanasia, nurses who overdose patients without consulting the physician run much greater legal risks than physicians who overdose patients without consulting the nurse.

tive and passive euthanasia. The "reduction-of-suffering" argument in favor of active euthanasia rests on an oversimplified picture of the circumstances of dying. Much uncertainty accompanies the process of dying, so "speeding" death may only defeat a possible rescue. When death is so certain that its probabilities would be little affected by an active step, discontinuing therapy is normally just as effective in producing it. Even when the impact of direct intervention on the patient is small, to witness death and to take a direct hand in it are very different levels of participating in the course of nature. Especially where there is some question whether one is acting for the sake of the patient or to meet one's own needs, most regard allowing death to occur as ethically less hazardous than causing it. Consider the following case of euthanasia gone awry:

> CASE EXAMPLE.   An elderly patient was dying of cancer, and her large family was on the wards day and night waiting for her to die. The waiting period was very long, and both staff and family were tiring. It was decided to move things along a little by increasing the morphine dose. As sometimes happens with morphine, the patient recovered strength and became more alert. It would have been appropriate at this point to send her home, but the family was determined to see her die. So, the physician increased the morphine dose further until she became comatose and died.

This perhaps apocryphal story concretely illustrates a crucial distinction between the processes of active and passive euthanasia: In allowing a patient to die, one would support an unexpected recovery, but in this case the effort to cause death became an intention to ensure the patient's death.[35]

There are borderline cases between allowing patients to die and active killing. For example, removing a patient from a respirator involves a physical action, but it allows the dying process to continue rather than introducing a new assault on the patient's life. So, it is more active than simply not putting the patient on a respirator in the first place and less active than an overdose of morphine, insulin, or lidocaine. Although discontinuing therapy requires more overt activity than not instituting it and bears some of the psychological impact of active euthanasia, discontinuing therapy would be justifiable in most circumstances where not instituting therapy would be justified.[36]

Large doses of narcotics can also be used actively or passively. The distinction between the two can be fine, as the following three cases indicate:

1. Treating the patient's pain with heavy doses of narcotics, risking that the patient will die, hoping the patient will not, monitoring the patient's condition closely, and taking measures to reduce the narcotics if necessary
2. Treating pain with heavy doses of narcotics, risking that the patient will die, not minding, or even hoping that the patient dies, not monitoring the patient, and not stepping in to prevent death
3. Using morphine to kill the patient as painlessly as possible

Since large doses of morphine may be needed to control pain and can be tolerated by patients, it may be unclear what is intended. Health professionals sometimes take

---

[35]Bonnie Steinbock, "The Intentional Termination of Life," *Ethics in Science & Medicine*, 6 (1979), 59–64.

[36]Jonsen et al., *Clinical Ethics*, p. 116.

refuge from hard decisions in that unclarity, and so "snowing the patient under" can be a source of tension between nurses and physicians. This is likely to happen where nurses do not participate in treatment decisions and yet have the "hands-on" responsibility of administering morphine.

Although the distinction between active and passive euthanasia is an important one, active euthanasia is not always decisively ruled out, and nurses have in good conscience given overdoses of morphine to patients with a clear intention of killing them. Where suffering is prolonged and severe, pain uncontrollable, recovery impossible, management difficult, the patient ready to die, and everyone's motives pure, active euthanasia can be reasonably defended. Though not common, such circumstances occur. In contrast, because active euthanasia is a question worthy of serious debate, nurses who conscientiously object to it are entitled to refuse to participate. Moreover, it is morally imprudent to hasten death without appreciating the issues through active and informed participation in decisions.

Do-Not-Resuscitate (DNR) Orders

Calling a code, CPR, or *cardiopulmonary resuscitation* is a central hospital ritual. When a patient suddenly stops breathing or the heart stops, large numbers of staff can be called in to revive the patient on an emergency basis. Quick resuscitation on a strong patient can mean rescue and eventual recovery. But CPR can also mean calling patients back from death to a vegetative state or flailing an essentially dead body with extreme measures.

Since CPR is an emergency procedure, it is essential to decide *in advance* whether to call a code if a patient arrests. Normally, a code should be called. But sometimes a patient on a dying trajectory cannot be revived to any advantage and an opportunity to allow a moribund patient to die is lost. When a decision has been made to withhold emergency resuscitation, the primary physician should write a "no-code" or "do-not-resuscitate (DNR)" order in the patient's chart. A DNR order would be justified wherever terminating therapy is justified, or where therapy should be continued but where the outcome of resuscitation is likely to be poor.

Where DNR decisions are not made explicitly by the team and where code decisions are not indicated in the record, nurses are concerned about their legal liability regarding CPR emergencies. Where staff think a patient should be allowed to die and no DNR order is in the record, they may protect themselves by conducting *mini-CPR* or a *slow code*. In such cases, they respond slowly to the emergency, apply remedies half-heartedly, and hope that the patient will not revive before a physician officially halts the procedure. The practice of slow codes is vastly inferior, ethically and procedurally, to openly discussing such decisions and charting them in the case record. Slow codes usually indicate unclarity about goals of treatment, lack of communication among staff, unwillingness to acknowledge a terminal prognosis, or an attempt to create a charade of all-out effort for the family and the law. A written DNR order can be reassessed on a daily basis and changed as necessary. Such procedures provide occasions for staff to discuss decisions about limiting therapy.

Patients can be classified to indicate the overall level of treatment intended. Massachusetts General Hospital developed a classification system that has been widely modified and imitated. The MGH system indicates four levels of care, summarized as follows:

Class A: Maximal therapeutic effort without reservation.

Class B: Maximal therapeutic effort without reservation but with daily evaluation.

Class C: Selective limitation of therapeutic measures. Exact limitations should be specified carefully to foster the overall welfare of the patient. Class C patients are not considered as candidates for admission to the Intensive Care Unit. A *DNR* order is a common Class C limitation.

Class D: All therapy is to be discontinued, except measures to keep patients comfortable.[37]

Since the phrases *coding, code status,* and *code classification* refer generally to levels of treatment and specifically to CPR, nurses should be clear about how they use such terms as "code," "no code." A *DNR* order may be consistent with otherwise aggressive treatment, depending on the particular needs of the patient.

In O.A.'s case, it was not clearly consistent for the staff to have distinguished treatment for pneumonia from CPR. Although treating pneumonia is conventionally regarded as more ordinary than CPR, in O.A.'s case, both were invasive and required a major investment of time and staff. Sometimes during treatment procedures such as suctioning and injections of seizure medications, O.A.'s heart would beat irregularly or she would stop breathing. In spite of the DNR order, staff felt that it was appropriate to resuscitate her in these cases, since omitting CPR when one had just caused an arrest would be too much like active euthanasia.

Pain Medication

Traditionally, relief from pain is one of the most immediate and precious health care services. There were periods in history when opium was practically the only effective medication in the western pharmacopoeia.[38] Certainly pain medication continues to be a major therapeutic agent, reducing both the physical and psychological damage of disease. Yet pain medication is a source of conflict in the ethics of health care. Pain medication can be harmful to health. Pain itself, if not excessive, can be useful in reminding patients to restrict activity. Pain is also useful in diagnosing and monitoring symptoms. In contrast, pain medication can reduce alertness and the patient's ability to follow instructions. It can depress vital signs and cause death. Used excessively, most pain medications are addictive. In a classic medical ethics case, two physicians disputed whether to treat a painful broken leg with an aspirin/propoxyphene compound or methadone. One was for stoicism and low risk of addiction via the compound; the other for effective pain relief in spite of the risk of addiction posed by methadone.[39] The classic solution is to turn the question over to the patient, but inherent in pain medication is a conflict between the

---

[37]Adapted from the Clinical Care Committee of the Massachusetts General Hospital, "Optimum Care for Hopelessly Ill Patients," by permission of *The New England Journal of Medicine,* 295 (1976), 362–64.

[38]Oliver Wendell Holmes, *Medical Essays, 1842–1882* (Boston: Houghton Mifflin Company, 1895), pp. 202–3.

[39]Robert M. Veatch, *Case Studies in Medical Ethics* (Cambridge, Mass.: Harvard University Press, 1977), pp. 17–21.

immediate "care" motives of comfort and relief from pain, and the "cure" motives of recovery and full function. This conflict is especially sharp where diagnostic measures cause pain.

People in pain have a moral claim on others for help in relieving it. We want to respond compassionately to pain, to help those in the most severe pain first, and do not want to neglect anyone who is experiencing pain. At the same time, in spite of physiological and behavioral signs, patients are the main judges of how much pain they are experiencing. Patients vary widely in their expression of pain, from stoic to hysterical, and it is often hard to tell who is most in need. Since patients rarely discuss the issue among themselves, it is often up to nurses to determine whose pain deserves the most immediate attention. A just determination of who is most in need thus requires complex communication among nurses and patients.

Sometimes nurses suspect that patients' expressions of pain are dishonest or exaggerated:

> When I don't feel a patient is really in pain or has some kind of emotional problem and keeps calling for a nurse, I get annoyed. I mean, there are patients who really need me. Then you have one who doesn't need you but constantly puts on his light. When this happens I know I take my time to answer.[40]

Doubt can arise about such syndromes as chronic back pain, where patients are suspected of malingering or seeking narcotics. Nurses thus face a real problem of respect for persons. We teach an ethic of respect for patients' autonomy, but what if some clients exploit this trust and compassion? If nurses respond to clients with cynicism, patients who are really in pain will be neglected.

In addition to issues of justice and respect for persons, the problem of pain relief involves the problem of responsibility for health. Questions about the reality of pain sometimes get mixed up with questions about responsibility for pain, as in this case:

> I just couldn't feel anything for this woman even though she had a great deal of pain. This was her sixth operation for beauty's sake. When she complained, I couldn't see her pain as being real.[41]

In this case, it is likely that the patient was in real pain, but the nurse judged it was the patient's fault and therefore not to be taken as seriously as the pain of "real" victims.

Nurses and physicians sometimes use placebos with patients they do not trust or whom they blame for being ill. This is a misuse of placebos. Even though placebos do not contain any "real" pain medication, they can be effective in treating real pain in patients. People respond to placebos even when they are completely mentally healthy and not responsible for their illness or pain (see pp. 179–80). Yet, nurses and physicians often believe that clients who respond to placebos are not really in pain. Thus, placebos are sometimes inappropriately used to determine if a patient's pain symptoms are real. As a senior resident said,

---

[40]Davitz and Davitz, "How Do Nurses Feel?" p. 1507.

[41]Ibid., p. 1506.

Placebos are used with people you hate, not to make them suffer, but to prove them wrong.[42]

Since placebos are not "real," they are valued less than narcotics.

> The ordering of active narcotic analgesics seems to be viewed as a gift from the doctor to the patient; placebo is substituted when the physician feels too angry with the patient to bestow a "real" gift. Alcoholics are frequently seen as undeserving. One physician described the case of a 50-year-old alcoholic with reflux esophagitis and esophageal stricture. This man was given intramuscular thiamine for pain because "we didn't think the pain was worthy of 75 mg of Demerol."[43]

Although narcotics are valued more highly than placebos, they are used with suspicion. Our cultural background regards relieving pain with drugs as legitimate but views using drugs for pleasure as illegitimate. Moreover, health professionals in particular have responsibilities to discourage taking health risks for pleasure and lack a responsibility to provide the public with recreation. Using narcotics also provokes anxiety among health professionals because they are particularly vulnerable to abusing drugs themselves.[44] Thus, health professionals maintain a delicate balance between the appropriate use and abuse of narcotics. Concern for abuse sometimes leads physicians to underestimate effective dose ranges, overestimate the danger of addiction, and overestimate a drug's duration of action.[45] Some observers also report that some nurses, wishing to be cautious about pain medication, further reduce physicians' orders.

In a free market economy, addicting drugs are extremely dangerous. They are cheap to make and produce a market of dedicated purchasers. If narcotics were open to advertising and marketing, we would likely see an epidemic of addiction comparable to the widespread use of opium, morphine, and heroin in the late nineteenth and early twentieth centuries. For instance, Bayer first started marketing heroin in 1898 and billed it as a cure for morphine addiction and a treatment for minor pains and coughs.[46] The situation with regard to tobacco today is similar. Nicotine is addicting and cigarettes are dangerous to health, and yet there is a wide market for cigarettes that resists reduction.

The U.S. system for regulating narcotics involves health professionals deeply in controlling their distribution. As "gatekeepers" of the legal supply of narcotics, health professionals are under tremendous pressure to account for the use of narcot-

---

[42]James S. Goodwin, Jean M. Goodwin, and Albert V. Vogel, "Knowledge and Use of Placebos by House Officers and Nurses," *Annals of Internal Medicine,* 91 (1979), p. 108.

[43]Ibid., p. 108.

[44]Linda V. Jefferson and Barbara E. Ensor, "Help for the Helper: Confronting a Chemically-Impaired Colleague," *American Journal of Nursing,* 82 (April 1982), 574–77; Rothlyn P. Zahourek, "Even 'People Helpers' Need Help—Stress and Addictive Behavior in Nurses," *Imprint (September 28, 1981),* 30–33; Jerry Kolesar, "It Could Happen to You," *Canadian Nurse* (November 1980), 20–22; Kate Fulton, "Drug Abuse among Nurses: What Nursing Management Can Do," *Supervisor Nurse* (January 1981) 18–20; and George E. Vaillant, Jane R. Brighton, and Charles MacArthur, "Physicians' Use of Mood-Altering Drugs," *The New England Journal of Medicine,* 282 (1970), 365–70.

[45]Richard M. Marks and Edward J. Sachar, "Undertreatment of Medical Inpatients with Narcotic Analgesics," *Annals of Internal Medicine,* 78 (1973), 173–81.

[46]Michael Smith, "The Lilly Connection: Drug Abuse and the Medical Profession," *Science for the People,* 10, 1 (January/February 1978), 9–15.

ics. This circumstance invites patients to pressure health professionals for narcotics and to lie about pain. One could imagine what it would be like in the hospital if cigarettes were only available by prescription and administered by nurses.

These social and policy factors aggravate the problem of trust introduced by the subjectivity of pain. A fairly straightforward moral value, compassionate response to pain, can become confounded beyond the best moral judgment by background social and economic problems. Since nurses are in a good position to discuss these issues with clients, further research from nurses on the complex psychological, sociological, and clinical problems here would be helpful.

O.A.'s case introduces a further issue. It is increasingly the practice to respect a patient's struggle near death as meaningful and terminal insights as valuable. Narcotics can be used to maintain a variety of levels of consciousness and pain from acute awareness through bad dreams to virtual oblivion. What level should be sought? This is a difficult and complex question on which health professionals would gladly have guidance from clients and which deserves further study. Although we cannot be certain, O.A. appears to have little potential for alertness that would justify keeping her at an uncomfortable level of consciousness.

Values and Responsibilities

Although many discussions about treating dying patients emphasize client choice and the right to die with dignity, the key concepts of this chapter are values and responsibilities. Value questions underly such decisions as terminating therapy and administering pain medication. Value questions are also involved in identifying who should be responsible for decisions near death.

What constitutes a compassionate response to suffering experienced while dying? According to one perspective, living well involves a struggle against death: Since it is worthwhile to live as long as possible, clinicians demonstrate care by committing tremendous resources to therapy as long as rescue seems faintly possible. According to another perspective, a long life is independent from living well: It is better to have convivial company and relief from pain than a long struggle against the inevitable. Although individuals prefer different perspectives, individual choices are represented collectively by institutions and available services. Can we develop health care resources so that both choices are readily available?

Most people view the issue of who should make decisions as resting on involvement, interest, and expression of individual identity. Although this is appropriate, another way to answer questions about decision-making power is to ask what values are represented by decision makers. In this chapter, I argue that nurses should be involved actively in decisions surrounding dying partly because they have a right and obligation to avoid hands-on responsibility for what they perceive as cruel acts. More importantly, however, nurses as professionals represent commitment to the value of compassionate care of suffering clients. Nurses should be involved in decisions about dying so that this value is voiced in decision processes.[47]

[47]For additional arguments favoring more active nursing participation in decisions about dying patients, see Catherine P. Murphy, "Nurses and Nontreatment Decisions," in *Dilemmas of Dying*, eds. Cynthia B. Wong and Judith P. Swazey (Boston: G. K. Hall & Co., 1981); Inge B. Corless, "Physicians and Nurses: Roles and Responsibilities in Caring for the Critically Ill Patient," *Law, Medicine & Health Care* (April 1982), 72–76; and Robert J. Levine, "Do Not Resuscitate Decisions and Their Implementation," in Wong and Swazey, *Dilemmas of Dying*, p. 29.

Because I see decision makers as representing values, I am troubled by those who foster hospice care mainly because it is cheaper than intensive care unit medicine. Hospices created primarily to help reduce the national health care budget are not likely to express compassion effectively. Compassionate care requires a budget adequate to provide staff for it, and this means that those who appreciate its value need to be heard when resources are allocated to care of the dying.

Responsibility issues arise for the dying and those who work with them. To become involved in the sequence of actions, causes, and omissions near death is to risk liability responsibility (see p. 137) for the results of one's participation. But the trajectory of death is uncertain in its duration and visibility: Who is dying? Who is salvageable? At the extremes, clinicians risk neglect or cruel heroism. This uncertainty limits the value of consequentialist approaches to decisions about death and encourages clearly intended devotion to one's clients. A certain formalism protects participants from too burdensome guilt feelings: Instituting care should be discernible from discontinuing it, and discontinuing therapy should be distinguishable from bringing death about. Such distinctions keep our compassion from resolving all suffering in the oblivion of death.

Apparently, where nurses normally have an active role in decisions about dying, that is, in deciding whether to refer ECF clients with pneumonia to acute care, little research has been done. The invisibility of these nursing decisions contrasts sharply with the extensive literature on DNR orders, final responsibility for which is generally held to rest with physicians. This instance is one among many where important issues are regrettably silent because they are nursing, not medical, decisions. When I argue that nurses play a central role in health care, I base this claim on the view that they represent the central and most significant value of health care—a compassionate response to suffering. Because this value is central, I believe nurses have a central moral responsibility for the conduct of health care. Patient advocacy is another important source of this responsibility, and the moral significance of advocacy also rests on the vulnerability of those who are ill and suffering. The central moral responsibility of nurses for the conduct of care needs at least to be expressed through open and active reliance on nurses' professional insights in decisions about dying patients.

Summary

Hospital nurses witness and provide compassionate care for many forms of suffering. How to respond to human suffering is a historically important ethical problem. Since providing a humane response to suffering is a morally central function of health care, nurses have a central role in relation to the ethical goals of health care.

Compassionate care of dying patients requires sensitive attention. Such care may require decisions about when to terminate therapy. Deciding when to discontinue therapy involves considering the effectiveness of therapy, the client's wishes, the amount of suffering involved, and the availability of resources. On rare occasions, active euthanasia may be morally acceptable. Allowing patients to die by withholding cardiopulmonary resuscitation (CPR) is common in hospitals. Orders not to resuscitate should be openly discussed and documented.

Physical pain is a common source of suffering. The ethics of using medication for pain relief is complicated by health hazards, legal restrictions, and social problems such as drug abuse. Nurses have an important responsibility to assess patients' needs for pain medication accurately and to use pain medication with justice and respect for persons.

FURTHER READINGS

General Works

AIKEN, LINDA H., AND MARTITA M. MARX, "Hospices: Perspectives on the Public Policy Debate," *American Psychologist,* 37 (1982), 1272–79.

ARIES, PHILIPPE, *Western Attitudes toward Death.* Baltimore: Johns Hopkins University Press, 1974.

BALDWIN, ANN, "The Nurse as Survivor of Right-to-Die Situations." Unpublished manuscript, University of California, San Francisco.

BAYLES, MICHAEL D., AND DALLAS M. HIGH, EDS., *Medical Treatment of the Dying: Moral Issues.* Cambridge, Mass.: Schenkman Publishing Co., Inc., 1981.

BEAUCHAMP, TOM L., AND SEYMOUR PERLIN, EDS., *Ethical Issues in Death and Dying.* Englewood Cliffs, N.J.: Prentice-Hall, Inc. 1978.

CASSELL, ERIC J., "Dying in a Technological Society," in *Death inside Out,* eds. Peter Steinfels and Robert M. Veatch, pp. 43–48. New York: Harper & Row, Publishers, Inc., 1975.

CASSEM, NED H., "Controversies Surrounding the Hopelessly Ill Patient," *Linacre Quarterly,* 42 (1975), 89–98.

DAVIS, ANNE J., "Ethics Rounds with Intensive Care Nurses," *Nursing Clinics of North America,* 14, 1 (March 1979), 45–55.

DUFF, RAYMOND S., "Guidelines for Deciding Care of Critically Ill or Dying Patients," *Pediatrics,* 64 (1979), 17–23.

EARLE, A., *The Nurse as Caregiver for the Terminal Patient and His Family.* New York: Columbia University Press, 1976.

EPSTEIN, CHARLOTTE, *Nursing the Dying Patient.* Reston, Va.: Reston Publishing Company, Inc., 1975.

GLASER, BARNEY G., AND ANSELM L. STRAUSS, *Time for Dying.* Chicago: Aldine Publishing Co., 1968.

GOROVITZ, SAMUEL, "Dealing with Dying," in *Medical Treatment of the Dying: Moral Issues,* eds. Michael D. Bayles and Dallas M. High. Cambridge, Mass.: Schenkman Publishing Co., Inc., 1981.

JACKSON, CHARLES O., "Death Shall Have No Dominion: The Passing of the World of the Dead in America," *Omega,* 8, 3 (1977) 195–203.

KALISH, RICHARD A., "Death and Dying in a Social Context," in *Handbook of Aging and the Social Sciences,* eds. Robert H. Binstock and Ethel Shanas, pp. 483–507. New York: Van Nostrand Reinhold Company, 1976.

KASS, LEON R., "Death as an Event: A Commentary on Robert Morison," *Science,* 173 (1971), 698–702. Reprinted in *Readings on Ethical and Social Issues in Biomedicine,* ed. Richard W. Wertz (Englewood Cliffs, N.J.: Prentice-Hall, Inc., 1973), pp. 109–13; and *Ethical Issues in Death and Dying,* ed. Robert F. Weir (New York: Columbia University Press, 1977), pp. 70–81.

LADD, JOHN, ED., *Ethical Issues Relating to Life and Death.* New York: Oxford University Press, 1979.

MAXWELL, MARY B., "Nurse Practitioner Chemotherapy Clinic," *Cancer Nursing* (June 1979), 211–18.

MORISON, ROBERT S., "Death: Process or Event?" *Science,* 173 (1971), 694–98. Reprinted in *Readings on Ethical and Social Issues in Biomedicine,* ed. Richard W.

Wertz (Englewood Cliffs, N.J.: Prentice-Hall, Inc., 1973), pp. 105–9; *Death inside Out: The Hastings Center Report,* eds. Peter Steinfels and Robert M. Veatch (New York: Harper & Row, Publishers, Inc., 1975), pp. 63–70; and *Ethical Issues in Death and Dying,* ed. Robert F. Weir (New York: Columbia University Press, 1977), pp. 57–69.

NAGEL, THOMAS, "Death," *Nous,* 4, 1 (1970), 73–80.

SONTAG, SUSAN, *Illness as Metaphor.* New York: Farrar, Straus, & Giroux, Inc., 1978.

STEINFELS, PETER, AND ROBERT M. VEATCH, EDS., *Death inside Out: The Hastings Center Report.* New York: Harper & Row, Publishers, Inc., 1975.

VEATCH, ROBERT M., *Death, Dying and the Biological Revolution: Our Last Quest for Responsibility.* New Haven, Conn.: Yale University Press, 1976.

WEIR, ROBERT F., ED., *Ethical Issues in Death and Dying.* New York: Columbia University Press, 1977.

Psychological Aspects

BECKER, ERNEST, *The Denial of Death.* New York: The Free Press, 1973.

BROWN, ESTHER LUCILE, *Newer Dimensions of Patient Care,* Appendix 2, Part 1, "Nurse's Perceptions of Things and People as Sources of Comfort during Hospitalization," pp. 126–42. New York: Russell Sage Foundation, 1961.

CASSEM, NED H., "Stress on the Nurse and Therapist in the Intensive Care Unit and the Coronary Care Unit," *Heart and Lung,* 4, 2 (1975), 252–59.

———, AND THOMAS P. HACKETT, "Sources of Tension for the CCU Nurse," *American Journal of Nursing,* 72 (1972), 1426–30.

GEIZHALS, JUDITH SUSAN, "Attitudes toward Death and Dying: A Study of Occupational Therapists and Nurses," *Journal of Thanatology,* 3 (1975), 243–69.

GERMAIN, CAROL P., "Nursing the Dying: Implications of Kübler-Ross' Staging Theory," *Annals of the American Academy of Political and Social Science,* 447 (January 1980), 46–58.

LEE, ROBERT E., AND PATRICIA A. BALL, "Some Thoughts on the Psychology of the Coronary Care Unit Patient," *American Journal of Nursing,* 75 (September 1975), 1498–1501.

LEVINE, CAROLE WEINSTEIN, "Nursing Grand Rounds: The Dying Patient: Can You Help When You Care Too Much?" *Nursing '77,* 7, 3 (1977), 40–43.

MAXWELL, MARY, "Confessions of a Cancer Nurse: Toward Better Pain Management in a Nurse Practitioner Clinic," *Oregon Nurse,* 44, 2 (June 1979), 1–4.

PATTISON, E. MANSELL, ED., *The Experience of Dying.* Englewood Cliffs, N.J.: Prentice-Hall, Inc., 1977.

PRILOOK, MARION E., "What Can You Give for Grief? Care," *Patient Care,* 13, 6 (1979), 100.

QUINT, JEANNE C., "Awareness of Death and the Nurse's Composure," *Nursing Research,* 15 (1966), 49–55.

SHNEIDMAN, EDWIN S., "Some Aspects of Psychotherapy with Dying Persons," in *Psychosocial Care of the Dying Patient,* ed. Charles A. Garfield, pp. 201–18. New York: McGraw-Hill Book Company, 1978.

SONSTEGARD, LOIS, ET AL., "The Grieving Nurse," *American Journal of Nursing,* 76 (1976), 1490–92.

STRAUSS, ANSELM, "Family and Staff during Last Weeks and Days of Terminal Illness," *Annals of the New York Academy of Science,* 164 (1969), 687–95.

Death Decisions

AROSKAR, MILA A., JOSEPHINE FLAHERTY, AND JAMES M. SMITH, "The Nurse and Orders Not to Resuscitate," *Hastings Center Report,* 7, 4 (1977), 27–28.

BANDMAN, ELSIE L., AND BERTRAM BANDMAN, "The Nurse's Role in Protecting the Patient's Right to Live or Die," *Advances in Nursing Science,* 1, 3 (April 1979), 21–35.

BASSON, MARC D., ET AL., "Under What Circumstances Should Euthanasia Be Performed?" in *Ethics, Humanism, and Medicine,* ed. Marc D. Basson, pp. 37–56. New York: Alan R. Liss, Inc., 1980.

BEAUCHAMP, JOYCE M., "Euthanasia and the Nurse Practitioner," *Nursing Forum,* 14, 1 (1975), 56–73.

BEHNKE, JOHN A., AND SISSELA BOK, EDS., *The Dilemma of Euthanasia.* Garden City, N.Y.: Doubleday & Co., Inc., Anchor Press, 1975.

BENOLIEL, JEANNE QUINT, ET AL., "Helping the Patient to Die," in *Critical Incidents in Nursing,* eds. Loretta Sue Bermosk and Raymond J. Corsini, pp. 54–65. Philadelphia: W.B. Saunders Company, 1973.

BOK, SISSELA, "Personal Directions for Care at the End of Life," *The New England Journal of Medicine,* 295 (1976), 367–69.

BRANSON, ROY, ET AL., "The Quinlan Decision: Five Commentaries," *Hastings Center Report,* 6, 1 (1976), 8–19.

CAPRON, ALEXANDER, "Death and the Law: A Decade of Change." *Soundings,* 95 (Fall 1980), 290–320.

CAWLEY, MICHELE ANNE, "Euthanasia: Should It Be a Choice?" *American Journal of Nursing,* 77 (1977), 859–61.

CRANE, DIANA, "Decisions to Treat Critically Ill Patients: A Comparison of Social Versus Medical Considerations," *Milbank Memorial Fund Quarterly,* 53 (Winter 1975), 1–33.

————, *The Sanctity of Social Life: Physicians' Treatment of Critically Ill Patients.* New York: Russell Sage Foundation, 1975.

CUSHING, MAUREEN, "'No Code' Orders: Current Developments and the Nursing Director's Role," *Journal of Nursing Administration* (April 1981), 22–29.

DAVITZ, LOIS JEAN, *Interpersonal Processes in Nursing: Case Histories,* "A Matter of Responsibility," pp. 127–31. New York: Springer Publishing Co., Inc., 1970.

DOWNING, A.B., ED., *Euthanasia and the Right to Die.* New York: Humanities Press, Inc., 1970.

DUFF, RAYMOND S., "Patients, Families, and Health Professionals: Deciding the Use of Heroic Life-Sustaining Measures," *Journal of the Medical Society of New Jersey,* 75, 1 (January 1978), 43–47.

EUTHANASIA EDUCATIONAL COUNCIL, "A Living Will," Appendix 1, in *The Dilemmas of Euthanasia,* eds. John A. Behnke and Sissela Bok, pp. 153–56. New York: Doubleday & Co., Inc., Anchor Press, 1975.

FROMER, M., "The Suicidal Client: Philosophical Bases for Nursing Intervention," *Nursing Law and Ethics,* 2 (January 1981), 1–3+.

FURLOW, THOMAS W., JR., "Euthanasia and the Tyranny of Technology," in *Beneficent Euthanasia,* ed. Marvin Kohl, pp. 169–79. Buffalo: Prometheus Books, 1975.

FURUKAWA, EDWARD F., ET AL., "The Doctor Lets the Patient Die," in *Critical Incidents in Nursing,* eds. Loretta Sue Bermosk and Raymond J. Corsini, pp. 127–33. Philadelphia: W.B. Saunders Company, 1973.

GLASER, ROBERT J., "A Time to Live and a Time to Die: The Implications of Negative Euthanasia," in *The Dilemmas of Euthanasia,* ed. John A. Behnke and Sissela Bok, pp. 133–50. New York: Doubleday & Co., Inc., Anchor Press, 1975.

GLOVER, JONATHAN, *Causing Death and Saving Lives.* New York: Penguin Books, 1977.

HAUG, MARIE, "Aging and the Right to Terminate Medical Treatment," *Journal of Gerontology,* 33, 4 (1978), 586–91.

HISCOE, SUSAN, "The Awesome Decision," *American Journal of Nursing,* 73, 2 (1973), 291–93.

HORAN, DENNIS J., AND DAVID MALL, EDS., *Death, Dying, and Euthanasia.* Washington, D.C.: University Publications of America, Inc., 1977.

HULL, RICHARD T., "Codes or No Codes?" *Kansas Nurse*, 55, 10 (November 1980), 8–12.

HUSHEN, SUSAN C., "Dilemmas in Practice: Questioning TPN as the Answer," *American Journal of Nursing*, 82 (1982), 852, 854.

In the Matter of Karen Quinlan: The Complete Legal Briefs, Court Proceedings, and Decision in the Superior Court of New Jersey. Arlington, Va.: University Publications of America, Inc., 1975.

JACKSON, D.L., AND S. YOUNGNER, "Patient Autonomy and 'Death with Dignity': Some Clinical Caveats," *The New England Journal of Medicine*, 301 (1979), 404–8.

KOHL, MARVIN, ED., *Beneficent Euthanasia*. Buffalo: Prometheus Books, 1975.

LEFF, ELLEN, "Dilemmas in Practice: Keeping a Promise," *American Journal of Nursing*, 82 (1982), 1136, 1138.

LEWIS, FRANCES MARCUS, "Experienced Personal Control and Quality of Life in Late-Stage Cancer Patients," *Nursing Research*, 31, 2 (March/April 1982), 113–19.

MCCORMICK, R.A., "To Save or Let Die: The Dilemmas of Modern Medicine," *Journal of the American Medical Association*, 229 (1974), 172–76.

MCINTYRE, KEVIN M., "Cardiopulmonary Resuscitation and the Ultimate Coronary Care Unit," *Journal of the American Medical Association*, 244 (1980), 510–12.

MEAD, MARGARET, "The Right to Die," *Nursing Outlook*, 16, 10 (1968), 20–21.

MOSER, DOROTHY, AND JEAN MARIE COX, EDS., "Perspectives: Resolving an Ethical Dilemma," *Nursing '80*, 10, 5 (May 1980), 39–43.

National Conference on Cardiopulmonary Resuscitation (CPR) and Emergency Cardiac Care (ECC), "Standards and Guidelines for Cardiopulmonary Resuscitation (CPR) and Emergency Cardiac Care (ECC)," *Journal of the American Medical Association*, 244 (1980), 453–509.

PRATO, SUE ANN, "Ethical Decisions in Daily Practice," *Supervisor Nurse*, 12, 7 (July 1981), 18–20.

SCHOWALTER, JOHN E., JULIAN B. FERHOLT, AND NANCY M. MANN, "The Adolescent Patient's Decision to Die," *Pediatrics*, 51, 1 (1973), 97–103.

SEIDEN, R.H., "Suicide: Preventable Death," *Public Affairs Report*, 15 (1974), 1–6.

STORLIE, FRANCIS J., ET AL., "Nursing Grand Rounds: Caring for a Patient Who Wants to Die: Should You Let Her?" *Nursing '80*, 10, 2 (February 1980), 50–55.

SWYTER, JAI, "When Is Life Without Value? A Study of Life-and-Death Decisions on a Hemodialysis Unit," *Omega*, 9 (1978–79), 369–80.

Pain and Suffering

BAKAN, DAVID, *Disease, Pain and Sacrifice: Toward a Psychology of Suffering*. Chicago: University of Chicago Press, 1968.

DAVITZ, LOIS L., AND JOEL R. DAVITZ, WITH CHARLENE FISCHI RUBIN, *Nurses' Responses to Patients' Suffering*. New York: Springer Publishing Co., Inc., 1980.

ENGEL, GEORGE L., "'Psychogenic' Pain and the Pain-Prone Patient," *American Journal of Medicine* (June 1959), 899–918.

HACKETT, THOMAS P., "The Pain Patient: Evaluation and Treatment," in *Massachusetts General Hospital Handbook of General Hospital Psychiatry*, eds. Thomas P. Hackett and Ned M. Cassem, pp. 41–63. St. Louis: The C.V. Mosby Company, 1978.

LIPP, MARTIN R., *Respectful Treatment: The Human Side of Medical Care*, Chap. 6, "Pain and Addiction," pp. 74–85. New York: Harper & Row Publishers, Inc., 1977.

MCCAFFREY, MARGO, "A Question of Ethics: Sedating the Dying," *Nursing Life* (November/December 1981), 41–43.

———, "When Your Patient's Still in Pain, Don't Just *Do* Something: Sit There," *Nursing*, 11, 6 (June 1981), 58–61.

PATENAUDE, ANDREA FARKAS, AND JOEL M. RAPPEPORT, "Surviving Bone Marrow Transplantation: The Patient in the Other Bed," *Annals of Internal Medicine,* 97 (1982), 915–18.

TWYCROSS, R.G., "The Use of Narcotic Analgesis in Terminal Illness," *Journal of Medical Ethics,* 3 (1977), 10–17.

CHAPTER 16

Technology
and Humanism:
The Newborn
Intensive Care Unit

The growth of bioethics as a field is often attributed to advances in medical technology, and difficult questions are often seen as arising from our growing ability to keep people alive. For instance, respirators and kidney dialysis can sustain life for long periods but can pose difficult questions about the quality of life. It is important to recognize, however, that many of these issues are not new ones. Many decisions that take place in technologically advanced units have ample historical precedents. Active euthanasia and abortion, for instance, were discussed in ancient times.[1] Another important set of debates surrounds the treatment of infants with birth defects or difficult deliveries. Infanticide has been practiced in many cultures, and vigils over premature infants are an inevitable part of human experience.

Although many bioethics issues are ancient, new technology creates situations that challenge one's ability to make ethical judgments and provide humane treatment. The more technologically oriented units—coronary, neurological, pediatric, newborn, and adult intensive care—are common sources of nursing ethics questions. An entire nursing ethics text could be organized according to hospital units and reflect the particular issues of each one. However, in this text we will confine our attention to one: the newborn intensive care unit (NICU). First, it is as good an instance as any of the problems posed by new technology. Second, it poses these problems in an acute form. NICU decisions have a tremendous impact on infants and families over the long term; the patient is unable to express views and has no personality or history on which to base decisions; the ability of infants to experience what is being done with them is a matter for speculation; and NICU interventions are often experimental and uncertain in their long-term effects. It is thus virtually impossible to develop a secure model for making decisions in NICUs or to obtain

---

[1]David Michael Feldman, *Birth Control in Jewish Law: Marital Relations, Contraception, and Abortion as Set Forth in the Classic Texts of Jewish Law* (New York: New York University Press, 1968); John T. Noonan, Jr., *The Morality of Abortion: Legal and Historical Perspectives* (Cambridge, Mass.: Harvard University Press, 1970); *Encyclopedia of Bioethics*, 1978 ed., s.v., "Euthanasia and Sustaining Life: Historical Perspectives," by Gerald J. Gruman.

any widespread agreement on how aggressively to treat newborns with health problems.

Newborn intensive care units treat critically ill infants with birth defects, low birth weights, genetic disorders, and conditions due to prematurity. NICUs are equipped with isolettes, respiratory and heart monitors, alarms, special lights, ventilators, and lots of plastic tubing. The isolettes are small and arranged so that many patients are within easy reach. Work goes on constantly; the lights are on day and night. Nurses on the unit combine simple care and comfort, such as changing diapers and holding, handling, and feeding babies, with supportive care for families, highly skilled care for infants needing constant management, and complex monitoring and assessment of infants and machines.

Although the work requires skill and is challenging, the NICU is a common source of stress for nurses.[2] Long hours of intense work with, and emotional investment in, infants who are sometimes very sick and whose future is completely uncertain can be very draining. Nurses wonder whether they are doing good for these patients in the long run. While puncturing the heel of a baby who knows nothing about the future and less about the purpose of the blood sample, it is easy for a nurse to ask, "Why am I doing this?" "What am I doing here?"

Infants Too Sick to Treat

A classic bioethics question arises in the NICU: Are there any infants so seriously ill, premature, or defective that they should not be treated, but instead should be allowed to die? Although some react in horror to the thought of allowing a vulnerable and helpless infant to die, most have given a cautious and definite "yes" to this question.[3] Treatment should be withheld from those infants (1) who will surely die during treatment, (2) whose only mental life will be to produce seizures, (3) who will have only a vegetative existence, or (4) who have multiple and grotesque anomalies. To treat all infants is to fall into the grip of the *technological imperative*. Our power to keep infants alive on respirators and with tube feedings is much greater than our power to correct defects and prevent suffering. One NICU openly reported statistics on the number of infants allowed to die so that "earlier death and relief from suffering would occur."[4]

Many infants are not easily categorized. They are not sick enough to be allowed to die, but they are too sick to be sure they will be normal. Are there any principles on which to think about these borderline cases? Most writers state conditions based on the infant's potential to attain the basic elements of worthwhile human life. This is sometimes put in terms of an infant's capacity for "personhood" or to be "human." Considerations include the potential for loving relations with other humans, the likelihood of survival to adulthood, the possibilities for developing a concept of self, the expectation of freedom from intractable pain, and

[2]Susan Blackburn, "The Neonatal ICU: A High-Risk Environment," *American Journal of Nursing*, 82 (1982), 1708–12.

[3]Albert R. Jonsen and Michael J. Garland, eds., *Ethics of Newborn Intensive Care* (Berkeley, Calif.: University of California, 1976).

[4]Raymond S. Duff and A.G.M. Campbell, "Moral and Ethical Dilemmas in the Special Care Nursery," *The New England Journal of Medicine*, 292 (1973), 75–78.

the intentions and capacities of parents. But one often cannot predict whether these criteria will be met. These criteria are of little help in evaluating the most common problem in NICU infants—prematurity with low birth weight, respiratory distress syndrome, and possible neurological damage. In some units physicians react to this uncertainty by treating all such infants and seeing what happens. Consequently, nurses frequently provide prolonged care for infants who eventually die in the NICU.[5]

Down's Syndrome: The Benchmark Case

In 1963 a baby born with Down's syndrome at Johns Hopkins Hospital was allowed to die, and a number of people disturbed by the case publicized it widely. However, the case is not typical of NICU ethics problems. There was a definite diagnosis with a well-studied prognosis, and the parents were very clear about their position. Often parents struggle to decide what to do. For all its difficulties, the case is a relatively simple one:

> CASE EXAMPLE. A baby boy was born to a couple in their mid-thirties. At birth he was diagnosed clinically as having Down's syndrome complicated by duodenal atresia.
>
> Down's syndrome occurs in about one out of every 700 live births. Raised at home, Down's syndrome children will usually achieve an IQ showing mild (IQ 50–69) to moderate (IQ 35–49) mental retardation. Their tested social competence will often range from low normal to close to normal. Down's syndrome children raised in institutions generally fare significantly worse with regard to these measures.
>
> Down's syndrome children are usually readily identifiable shortly after birth by many clinical signs, including slack muscle tone, a characteristic facial gestalt, and creases in the palm. Down's syndrome is usually attributable to an extra or unusual configuration of the twenty-first chromosome. A confirming cytogenetic study can be done, but it takes days or weeks to perform.
>
> The mental retardation of Down's syndrome is incurable, and other health problems are often associated with Down's. The most frequent serious medical complication is congenital heart disease, occurring in about 12 percent of Down's syndrome children. Frequent infection; seizure disorders; and blood, joint, and eye abnormalities are also common. Most of these conditions are treatable. If a Down's syndrome child lives five years, he or she is only 6 percent less likely than a normal child to live to forty years of age.
>
> Duodenal atresia, in which the gut is closed off at the duodenum, is an uncommon complication of Down's syndrome. Without surgery, a child cannot pass or digest food. Since feeding by mouth will kill the child, the child can only be nourished intravenously. Duodenal atresia can be corrected by a simple surgical procedure with a high probability of success.

[5]In the late 1970s, about 200,000 infants received intensive care each year. Of these, about 75,000 had problems related to prematurity. Twenty-five thousand of these died each year of respiratory problems. About 3,000 Down's syndrome babies were born per year. Albert R. Jonsen, "Justice and the Defective Newborn," in *Justice and Health Care*, ed. E. Shelp (Boston: D. Reidel, 1981), p. 98.

The baby's mother, a nurse, had experience working with Down's syndrome children. She believed it would be unfair to her other two children to raise them with a Down's syndrome child. Therefore, she refused to give consent to the operation. Her husband concurred, deferring to her greater experience with mentally retarded children. The hospital staff acquiesced in this decision after discussion with the parents. The baby was placed in a side room and died over a period of two weeks of dehydration and starvation.[6]

This case has become a benchmark in NICU decisions. Most commentators, including some participants, agree that the case was mishandled. A minority of commentators think, on humanitarian grounds, that the infant should have been dispatched more efficiently. However, the majority judge that he definitely should have been kept alive. In the absence of a clear definition of "personhood" this case provides an intuitive limit: Infants whose expected quality of life is no worse than this one should be treated.

"It's Not a Nursing Issue"

The decision in the Down's syndrome case was about whether or not to perform surgery. Since surgery is the province of physicians, some clinicians conclude that the decision was therefore not a nursing issue. But many features of this case also make it a nursing issue. The considerations relevant to surgery are broad and include the overall health and welfare of the infant, the welfare of the family as a whole, the views of the parents, the goals of therapy, and basic human values. Since these are areas of nursing knowledge and reflection, decision making would benefit from the active participation of nurses in it.

Some NICUs experience staff conflicts and stress because they do not allow nurses to participate actively in decisions with regard to newborns. At morning rounds on such units, attendings, residents, and fellows move from bed to bed and discuss cases. Nurses listen in the background and go about their work. Occasionally they are asked for information. The medical director of the unit is rarely present; he or she is out reporting research results or raising funds. Such units invite awkward moments; for instance, a nurse may have to stand by while a pediatrician gives a glowing report to parents about a baby the nurse perceives as a "bad" baby. Sometimes referring pediatricians unfamiliar with birth defects are so upset by them that they are unable to make decisions. Sometimes nurses go out to transport an infant to the NICU only to discover that the infant ought to have been allowed to die. The infant may have been "dumped" on the unit because no one was willing to take the responsibility for stopping treatment.[7] When attending physicians fail to take responsibility for decisions in some units, there is no one to step in and ensure that difficult questions are faced and decisions made. Care may be escalated be-

---

[6]Based on a well-filmed reenactment, "Who Should Survive?" (Joseph P. Kennedy, Jr., Foundation, 1971); Richard A. McCormick, "To Save or Let Die: The Dilemma of Modern Medicine," *Journal of the American Medical Association,* 229 (1974), 172–76; James S. Gustafson, "Mongolism, Parental Desires, and the Right to Life," *Perspectives in Biology and Medicine,* (1973), 529–57; and an unpublished case prepared by Carol Beresford, M.D., University of California San Francisco, 1980.

[7]NICU nurses ask, however, where dying babies should be managed. Is the neonatal hospice just around the corner?

cause there is no one to call a halt, or it may be reduced without adequate evaluation. Along with emotional and ethical stress, nurse–physician conflicts are a common source of stress for nurses in the NICU. An angry nurse describes an incident:

> CASE EXAMPLE. A very jaundiced baby . . . was admitted from another hospital. Notes from the referring hospital showed the nurses had noticed the baby was jaundiced at two days and told the doctor about it every day. He ignored them. The parents kept asking us if there would be brain damage and if it would have been better if their doctor had transferred the baby earlier. It made me mad that the nurses' careful observations were disregarded and that in addition we had to keep quiet about it because there could be a lawsuit if the parents knew all the facts.[8]

In other units, no infant is discussed unless the nurse attending the infant is present and actively participating. The medical director of the unit and the social worker also participate in such meetings. The director acts less as a decision maker and more as a coordinator of the decision process. Conducted well, staff meetings on decisions in the NICU make it possible to share responsibility for difficult decisions and, it is to be hoped, produce decisions ethically more sound than those made by individuals without consultation. In team-oriented NICUs nurses may actively plan follow-up studies of infants, develop criteria for treatment in terms of quality of life outcomes, and assess new technology.

This is not to say that all NICU decisions should be made by nurses. But it is to say that nurses should have more than "input" into decisions, although that input is more than nurses now have in many units. Nurses should contribute their clinical and ethical judgments to a consensual decision process. On some issues—such as nursing values, assessment of the infant's condition, and the attitude of the family—they may have special knowledge and expertise. On other issues, such as basic human values, they may have as much as others, and no more, to contribute. NICU decisions are like those about terminating therapy in adults: Even if nurses had no special knowledge, they would have a responsibility and right to express views on therapy because of their intimate involvement in performing procedures. Where one is performing work that feels cruel, or where one looks at an infant and says, "If this were my infant, I would not want it treated," it is crucial to participate in the overall care plan, so that one can discover good reasons for supporting it, participate in changing it, or give good reasons for refusing to participate in it.

The Role of the Parents

In contrast to ancient times, parents today cannot exercise absolute power over their children. Once born, infants exist on their own as citizens and persons entitled to respect. Their welfare, not just that of the family, becomes a central focus of decision making, and parents need not be consulted on every infant. Where it is clear that an infant deserves treatment, as in cases of mild prematurity, or where the infant clearly cannot be treated, as in Trisomy-18, the staff can make decisions

---

[8]Sharol P. Jacobsen, "Stressful Situations for Neonatal Intensive Care Nurses," *MCN: The American Journal of Maternal Child Nursing*, 3 (1978), 146.

on clear medical indications. Where decisions are more doubtful, the family's views are extremely significant but still not conclusive. There may be good reasons to support the life of a child over the family's objections, or to refuse to treat an infant the family wants treated. This view is based mainly on the extension of the notion of equality of respect to children: Youth and dependency on parents are not generally seen as good reasons to treat children differently from adults with regard to life support.

The staff observes premature infants closely during the first hours after birth. If the baby is very premature and in need of increasing amounts of oxygen,

> . . . the family is told that the outcome is highly questionable, and asked if life-sustaining care should be continued. The following is a composite quote about this situation from one ward:
>
> "The response can be everything from the father who says 'Where are the autopsy papers?' to the one who says, 'I don't care if he's blind and retarded, save him'. . . In most instances, the family will say, 'Withdraw support.' If we can't read the family, or if the family says they want the baby to survive, we will go great guns."[9]

It is important to consult the family about borderline infants, partly because they will be the most important factor in the infant's future welfare, and partly because the infant's impact on the family gives them a significant interest in their child's treatment. Although parents are very stressed during such crises, they have often thought about possible defects and are able to address the issue. Parents' participation in decisions and the time they spend with the infant will affect their feelings about the infant, and staff can learn much about the parents' ability to care for their child by consulting them.

Potential conflicts of interest between the child and the family raise problems of moral judgment for NICU staff. A severely handicapped child requires great labor and sacrifice from its family. At the same time, a handicapped child usually has the best chance for maximal development at home. The staff feels torn between winning the family over on behalf of the infant and defending the family from a potentially burdensome baby. In these cases, a frank presentation of the issues to the family is important. If they are to engage in a difficult lifelong enterprise, parents are entitled to consider what they are getting into.

Some families cannot handle such decisions or information, and sometimes staff cannot resolve issues. Where there are significant conflicts of views or interests, turning to a court is a morally acceptable recourse. A court can hear broad questions, take a more distant perspective than those involved, and command the obedience of participants. Consultation with a hospital ethics committee may also be a suitable means of resolving differences of opinion.

The Graduates of NICUs

It is not difficult to defend treating the Down's syndrome infant. He met all of the minimum conditions for a worthwhile life except parental support (p. 245): He

[9]Carolyn Wiener et al., "Trajectories, Biographies and the Evolving Medical Technology Scene: Labor and Delivery and the Intensive Care Nursery," *Sociology of Health & Illness*, 13 (1979), 269. Reprinted with permission of Routledge & Kegan Paul, Ltd.

could reasonably be expected to live to adulthood; be able to communicate, love, and be loved; possess a sense of identity; and live without intractable pain. Moreover, it would be difficult to defend stricter criteria for therapy: Perfectionism about individual capacities makes people judgmental about each other and fails to respect the importance of interdependence in ordinarily worthwhile lives. It is distressing to think that he might live in an institution, but where institutions are inadequate we should think in terms of modifying them to meet conditions of humanity, rather than modifying our conception of what is human to suit our institutions.

Although we may be clearly able to say that infants with prospects better than Down's syndrome should be treated, decisions with regard to other conditions are less clear. For instance, prematurity is not comparable to Down's syndrome. A premature infant may be healthy at birth; the only question is whether the infant can survive, grow, and develop normally. This is a question of probabilities to which no definite figure can be given. All we can say is that lower weight at birth and shorter gestation periods decrease the probability of intact survival.

Rather than attempt finer distinctions in a rapidly changing realm of practice, it would be more useful to step back and reflect on the context in which these decisions are made—the NICU itself. What are the overall social gains and losses of NICUs? What controls their development, and how do new techniques shape decision processes in units? What values should control the development of NICUs? These questions so far do not have definite answers, and they require both empirical and philosophical research. Many people in health care support NICUs, and some are even enthusiastic. However, I give them much more qualified support and want to present some considerations favoring a cautious policy with regard to highly technological life support, of which NICUs are an important instance.

NICUs are one example of technological approaches to birth. Fetal monitors and cesarean sections are also increasingly used.[10] The NICU has also grown alongside similar hospital units, such as adult intensive care units and burn units. The arguments for these new units and techniques are generally based on the claim that outcomes improve as a result of their use and that we are progressing toward even better outcomes in the future. But, contrary to common belief, these highly technological modes of practice expanded *without* evidence that they produce better overall patient outcomes. Efforts to find out whether ICUs actually improve outcomes were made *after* they developed, and for the most part, the results of the evaluations are equivocal.[11] Moreover, most studies employ global outcome mea-

[10]See, for example, Ian M. Kelso et al., "An Assessment of Continuous Fetal Heart Rate Monitoring in Labor: A Randomized Trial," *American Journal of Obstetrics and Gynecology,* 131 (1978), 526–32; and Ronald L. Williams and Peter M. Chen, "Identifying the Sources of the Recent Decline in Perinatal Mortality Rates in California," *The New England Journal of Medicine,* 306 (1982), 207–14.

[11]Results are not yet in on NICUs. One study shows overall U.S. NICUs are resulting in a lower *proportion* but a larger *number* of handicapped children (p. 38 in Peter Budetti et. al., "The Costs and Effectiveness of Neonatal Intensive Care," in *The Implications of Cost-Effectiveness Analysis of Medical Technology,* Washington, D.C.: Office of Technology Assessment, 1980). Compare analogous findings in the development of other critical care units. See, for example, Howard Waitzkin, "A Marxian Interpretation of the Growth and Development of Coronary Care Technology," *American Journal of Public Health,* 69 (1979), 1260–68. The development of adult ICUs without studies to show their outcomes is reviewed in Louise B. Russell, *Technology in Hospitals: Medical Advances and Their Diffusion* (Washington, D.C.: The Brookings Institution, 1979). Fetal monitoring has also grown in spite of studies showing neither good nor harm from it. See Kelso, above, and Albert D. Haverkamp, "The Evaluation of Continuous Fetal Heart Rate Monitoring in High-Risk Pregnancy," *American Journal of Obstetrics and Gynecology,* 125 (1976), 310–20; and Albert D. Haverkamp, "A Controlled Trial of the

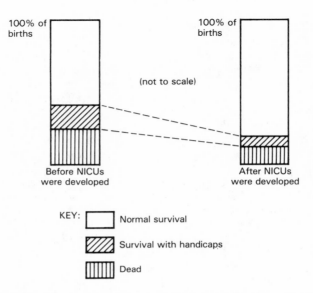

Figure 16.1. The Case for Newborn Intensive Care Units

sures such as morbidity and mortality rather than more subtle considerations of quality and meaningfulness of life.

The argument for NICUs is presented visually in Figure 16.1. At birth, children fall roughly into three categories: normal, handicapped, and dead or dying. The theory claims that NICUs increase the number of normal children and decrease the dying and the handicapped. Reducing the number of dead children is not the most important measure; it is most important to reduce the number of handicapped children, because they suffer the most. But no one knows whether NICUs reduce the number of handicapped children.

This means that *overall* outcomes of NICUs are not known to be better than outcomes before their use. I assume that since we do not know that they reduce the number of handicaps, NICUs do not reduce their number very much; otherwise, the reduction would be obvious.[12] Can we justify extensive investment in NICUs in order to reduce the number of handicapped children slightly? Perhaps we can, but the overall reduction, assuming that there is one, is the result of the difference between the number of normal children who would otherwise have been handicapped *minus* the number of handicapped children who would otherwise have died at birth: Our cure rate must be balanced by the handicaps that we cause through NICUs.[13] But our moral responsibility is greater for the handicaps that we *cause*

Differential Effects of Intrapartum Fetal Monitoring," *American Journal of Obstetrics and Gynecology,* 134 (1979), 399–408. The efficacy of therapies is a necessarily controversial subject. My position is consistent with the fact that critical care therapies have good outcomes for some conditions. A unit may improve some conditions and *as a whole* have little impact on morbidity and mortality.

[12]Budetti et al. report an overall impact of NICUs in the U.S. as resulting in 15,075 fewer deaths, 1,356 fewer moderately abnormal infants, 16,043 more normal infants, and 349 more severely abnormal infants ("Costs and Effectiveness," p. 39).

[13]I do not consider cost issues here. They are also equivocal and much more complicated. For a discussion of the costs of care, see Chapter 17 (pp. 267–70).

through NICU treatment than the handicaps we *permit* by omitting to use NICUs. My admittedly controversial suggestion is that if we assume approximate numerical equality between NICU-prevented handicaps and NICU-induced handicaps, we are marginally morally worse off by creating NICUs.[14]

Moreover, investment in NICUs should be balanced against investment in other modes that could accomplish the same ends as well. Many countries with less investment in NICUs appear to have lower rates of infant mortality than the U.S.[15] It is thus plausible that we can improve infant survival rates by means other than NICUs, such as better maternal nutrition and prenatal care.[16] Controlling such factors as exposure to substances that cause birth defects could also be of crucial importance.

The numerical argument could be met by being more selective about treating infants in the NICU. Although good statistics are not available, my observations indicate that some NICUs would decide to treat a premature infant with poor prospects of intact survival rather than allow an opportunity to rescue the infant to slip by. By allowing such infants to die, NICUs could cause fewer handicaps, but allowing high-risk infants to die would mean slower progress toward learning how to treat them. Infants for whom poor outcomes are expected are treated partly in the hope that future infants will be benefited, and thus much therapy in NICUs falls under the heading of therapeutic research (p. 109). It is done not only for the sake of infants, but also out of confidence in medical progress and for the sake of future infants.

Medical Progress

Proponents of NICU technology point out that medical knowledge is constantly changing and progressing.[17] They claim that we have not yet seen the outcomes of the latest NICU techniques, and we will eventually have even better ones. The argument for continuing to develop NICUs thus rests on confidence in future results.

But what are the next steps in NICU technology? One important development is treating increasingly smaller and more premature infants. Infants weighing less than 500 grams are occasionally saved, but the majority of them die in treatment. Care of these infants involves much more time and equipment than of infants with

---

[14]Compare arguments on allowing to die versus killing in Chapter 15 (pp. 231–33) and the discussion of lying versus failing to disclose in Chapter 12 (p. 173).

[15]Among countries with relatively complete birth statistics, the United States ranks about seventeenth in infant mortality rates. See, Ann Ashworth, "International Differences in Infant Mortality and the Impact of Malnutrition: A Review," *Human Nutrition: Clinical Nutrition,* 36C (1982), 7–23.

[16]Bernard Guyer, Lee Anne Wallach, and Sharon L. Rosen, "Birth-Weight-Standardized Neonatal Mortality Rates and the Prevention of Low Birth Weight: How Does Massachusetts Compare with Sweden?" *The New England Journal of Medicine* 306 (1982), 1230–33.

[17]NICU outcomes are improving rapidly as measured by the rate of normal survivals. For instance, Budetti reports that for infants born at less than 1,000 grams, 1.7 percent survived without deficit in 1960, but 36.9 percent survived without defects in 1978. Nevertheless, in 1960, 6.3 percent survived with abnormalities, and in 1978, 13 percent survived with abnormalities ("Cost and Effectiveness," p. 38).

birth weights greater than 1,000 grams. Neonatal heart surgery is becoming increasingly sophisticated. Fetal surgery is a related development; for instance, in a sophisticated operation a ureter can be delicately cleared during gestation to prevent kidney damage.[18] In some ways, these technological achievements are awesome, and they are extremely valuable in particular cases. But they require tremendous investments of highly skilled personnel and costly equipment for treating fewer and fewer cases.

This conception of technological progress does not necessarily arise from a deep commitment to save human lives. If we had such a commitment, we would do many other things to preserve life, such as eliminate the 1,100 known carcinogens from the workplace,[19] reduce the stockpile of nuclear weapons, and build safer automobiles. We need to look both at how many lives we save and how we save them; how we treat each other in saving lives; and how we see the meaning of the processes by which we foster life. We thus should not make too much of counting lives. Just as in the care of the dying, the quality of life is significant, not just its amount.

We could imagine turning technology in the opposite direction and moving toward much simpler modes of life. If we found such modes of life meaningful, it is by no means clear that we would be worse off, even if such changes shortened life expectancies. It is conceivable that life under different technological priorities would be *incomparable* to life with present technologies. We cannot say, for example, whether Navajos led better or worse lives before the arrival of the Europeans than San Franciscans now do. The quality of a way of life cannot be measured *simply* by longevity, infant mortality rate, or even the per capita quantity of automobiles, radios, telephones, and the like. In choosing a simpler life-style, a mother who gives birth at home and refuses a fetal monitor cannot be shown wrong by presently available statistics.[20] The nurse's question, "What am I doing here?" thus expresses a legitimate concern. Given the availability of NICU technology, we have an obligation to use it to save babies, but we can reasonably doubt whether our investment in the enterprise is wise.

Why do people place so much faith in technologies with uncertain effects and speculative futures? Answering this question is beyond the scope of this book, but a better understanding of the ideological functions of medicine helps explain the sense of moral distress that some nurses feel in the NICU. In addition to caring for the sick, medicine serves an *ideological* function in our culture; it expresses a set of beliefs which, regardless of their truth or falsity, help to maintain our social order. Advanced industrial countries like the United States are committed to continuing development of new technology. Medicine supports this commitment by using new

---

[18]Michael R. Harrison, Mitchell S. Golbus, and Roy A. Filly, "Management of the Fetus with a Correctable Congenital Defect," *Journal of the American Medical Association*, 246 (1981), 774–77.

[19]Thomas R. Donahue, "Technology: Using It Wisely," *American Federationist* (September 1979), p. 1.

[20]Research does not show any significant difference between home and hospital births for low-risk mothers with experienced attendants. See Lewis E. Mehl and Gail H. Peterson, "Home Birth versus Hospital Birth: Comparisons of Outcomes of Matched Populations" (paper presented at the annual meeting of The American Public Health Association, Miami, Fla., October 20, 1976); Lewis E. Mehl, "The Outcome of Home Delivery Research in the United States," in *The Place of Birth*, eds. S. Kitzinger and J.A. Davis (New York: Oxford University Press, 1978); and G. David Adamson and D.J. Gare, "Home or Hospital Births?" *Journal of the American Medical Association*, 243 (1980), 1732–36.

technology to cure the ills that society causes. In short, medicine says to us: "Technology will save us from the ills of technology."

To give up faith in technological progress in medicine would require us to be even less hopeful about less well intended and less beneficial new technological developments. Medicine hastens to find a way to cure cancer with radioactive materials, when about 50,000 nuclear weapons threaten many more lives than cancer.[21] The petrochemical industry produces both carcinogenic by-products and pharmaceuticals that treat cancer.

As an ideology, medicine has many uses. (1) It defines health problems in biological terms, and thus encourages technological rather than social solutions. (2) It defines illness as an individual problem, thus limiting our ability to approach health as a collective problem and supporting victim-blaming explanations of disease. (3) It serves a social control function. Nurses and physicians write excuses from work and school and allocate Workers' Compensation Benefits. Problems of daily life may be given psychiatric interpretations and receive medical responses. (4) Medicine provides explanations of disease that support race, gender, and social class stratification.[22] (5) Medical ideology maintains the dominance and high status of physicians through esoteric and expensive forms of practice.[23]

These themes are displayed in NICUs: Upset mothers who refuse treatment for their infants may be labeled as mentally ill; the NICU concentrates intensive care on a few individuals; neonatologists, NICU directors, and suppliers of equipment are well paid; NICUs have received much more development than prenatal nutrition; follow-up of NICU "graduates" is limited; record keeping needed for demographic studies to identify causes of birth defects meets opposition from physicians; and so on.

I am not saying that modern medicine is bad, only that it is not under the control of humane values. It has had major successes, such as the treatment of polio, syphilis, and TB, and we should make a serious attempt to sort out the valuable practices from the unsound. But this is not easy to do, partly because appropriate information is very hard to obtain: For instance, a former state health department official described the process of obtaining statistics needed to assess health risks and publicize the dangers of widely used products as "like being hit by a Mack truck." Information is also hard to obtain because hospitals integrate many specific treatments into a mode of practice for which it is hard to sort out effects. The ideological aspects of medicine indicate that medical progress may not be as much an established fact as a faith or ideology, and that the supposed facts supporting belief in medical progress either beg the question or are limited by being seen through the spectacles of established medical practice.

[21]Bernard Lown et al., "The Nuclear Arms Race and the Physician," *The New England Journal of Medicine,* 304 (1981), 726–28. Some people believe that nuclear war, which could easily cause 60 to 140 million immediate deaths in the U.S. alone, is possible in the next 20 years. In the next 20 years, about 7.5 million U.S. cancer deaths are likely. Which poses the more serious health problem?

[22]*Encyclopedia of Bioethics,* 1978 ed., s.v. "Racism and Medicine," by James H. Jones; and Barbara Ehrenreich and Deidre English, *Complaints and Disorders: The Sexual Politics of Sickness* (Old Westbury, N.Y.: The Feminist Press, 1974).

[23]Howard Waitzkin, "A Marxist View of Medical Care," *Annals of Internal Medicine,* 89 (1978), 264–78.

Nursing and Technology

This discussion is important to nursing and nursing ethics because nursing is in a very interesting, promising, and difficult position with regard to medical technology. On one hand, nurses represent "nontechnology" in health care—the moral and humane residue of ancient practice. In health care

> . . . there is a large body of what might be termed "nontechnology." . . . It consists of what is sometimes called "supportive therapy." . . . It is what is meant by the phrases "caring for" and "standing by." It is indispensable. . . . It also involves lots of nursing, lots of involvement with nonmedical professionals in and out of the hospital.[24]

On the other hand, nursing grew up in conjunction with hospitals, which embody health care technology, and nursing practice is largely shaped by and committed to the same technology as medical practice. The solution to this conflict is not for nurses to divorce themselves from technology. Instead, it would be better to develop "appropriate technology." Instead of trying to squeeze humanism into current techniques, the problem for nurses is to use humane ideals in shaping technological development.

For example, the high level of NICU technology often blinds people to the most elementary features of emotional life. Staff members have little opportunity to express their feelings or use them in making clinical judgments. Medical language displays this poverty of human feelings: "Thus, at rounds one hears that the patient has a stable cardiac rhythm, not how well the child is doing."[25] A pediatric resident, asked what to do if a baby is inhaling air when nursing, suggested a nasogastric tube; burping the baby never occurred to him. Architecture, for example, could take into better account the emotional needs of clients, staff, and families.[26] The room provided for parents to visit the NICU is often a tiny afterthought in the hall. As things stand now, those who work in hospitals are surrounded and overwhelmed by technological development which is out of the control of humane principles. In this setting, moral uncertainty about the goals of practice comes to consciousness primarily through distress at difficult decision points.

"Nontechnological" Skills

For the professional, the so-called "nontechnological" aspects of clinical practice require clarity, theoretical analysis, and skilled application. So the humane elements of health care can also be considered a "technology." To make these values more concrete, it is important to develop specific characterizations of what

[24]Lewis Thomas, "The Technology of Medicine," in *The Lives of a Cell: Notes of a Biology Watcher* (New York: Viking Penguin Inc., 1974), pp. 36–37.

[25]Joel E. Frader, "Difficulties in Providing Intensive Care," *Pediatrics,* 64 (1970), 10–16.

[26]See, for example, Roslyn Lindheim, "An Architect's Perspective," in *Humanizing Health Care,* eds. Jan Howard and Anselm Strauss (New York: John Wiley & Sons, Inc., 1975), 293–303. Lindheim refers to architecture as "frozen ideology."

people generally mean by *humane* health care. Common criteria include seeing the client as having inherent worth and as an irreplaceable whole, sharing in decisions with clients, maintaining equality of status with clients, and displaying empathy and good feelings.[27] One problem for the "scientist" of humanism is to translate these criteria, or more appropriate ones, to the NICU. Unfortunately, these criteria apply more readily to parents than infants. What would be criteria of humane care for infants?

Skills in relationship to *feelings* would be a subject for study under a humane approach to health care. For example, some health professionals were surprised to learn that cancer patients who show negative feelings seem to do better than more controlled patients.[28] Feelings are informative; if we interpret them rightly we can learn things about our environment that are invisible to the "objective" eye. For example, how does it feel to work in the NICU? What are the causes of good and bad feelings there? Feelings also express and direct us to moral judgments and guide us in managing the care of patients. For instance, the feeling that one is being cruel to infants should not be ignored.

The feelings of a woman visiting her dying mother in the hospital constitute a damning moral assessment of the hospital setting.

> When I walk into the room, there is no oxygen, no air. No contrast. No real light. There is no place to exercise. There is no touching; no beauty. I feel I'm made tighter and smaller. No good smells. No hot and cold. No physical stimulation to keep your senses alive. No quiet; no beautiful sounds. Dinner comes in sealed plastic cups with numbers, tags, and ingredients. My mother's body is controlled from without, from desks in another room. I stopped breathing. It was a hostile environment.

As suggested in Chapter 15, nursing appears to be directed to more immediate and experiential goals than medicine: A compassionate response to suffering is more closely identified with nursing than with medicine. Nurses also more often express an interest in disease prevention and health maintenance than physicians. Nurses are less wedded to the physiological theories and diagnostic modes of medical practice. And nursing has a more global and unified science approach to health care. For these reasons, I believe nurses are in a better position than physicians to make use of these "nontechnological" skills and to more clearly direct technological development in the hospital toward humane goals. Some physicians also reject the traditional clinical model of detached concern and are developing more humane ways to practice medicine. Physicians can speed this project by listening to, learning from, and allying with nurses.

Summary

Advances in health care technology make it difficult for clinicians to apply humane conceptions of patients' health and welfare. Newborn intensive care units

[27]Jan Howard, "Humanizing and Dehumanizing of Health Care: A Conceptual View," in Howard and Strauss, *Humanizing Health Care*, pp. 57–102.

[28]Leonard R. Derogatis, Martin D. Abeloff, and Nick Melisaratos, "Psychological Coping Mechanisms and Survival Time in Metastatic Breast Cancer," *Journal of the American Medical Association*, 242 (1979), 1504–08.

(NICUs) exemplify modern technological advances in health care and are an important source of bioethics disputes. NICUs treat premature infants and those with birth defects. Some infants are born with such serious problems that they should be allowed to die. Others should be treated, even though they will suffer from mental retardation and other health problems, as in the case of a Down's syndrome infant who needs surgery. NICU nurses, with a significant "hands-on" role in caring for infants, have a responsibility to take an active part in making decisions with regard to providing and withholding treatment in the NICU. Parents also have an important but not decisive role in these decisions.

Nurses experience moral uncertainty working in NICUs for three reasons. (1) The uncertain future of newborns makes many decisions difficult. (2) Some units do not permit nurses to participate actively in decisions. (3) Legitimate moral questions can be raised about the wisdom of highly technological approaches to birth and perinatal care. Humane and compassionate goals should direct development of health care technology and hospital architecture, rather than ethically less certain goals such as efficiency and small differences in morbidity and mortality rates. Since nurses have important skills in humane aspects of patient care, they should play an important role in directing the future development of health technology.

FURTHER READINGS

Birth Defects

ADAMSON, G. DAVID, AND DOUGLAS J. GARE,   "Home or Hospital Births?" *Journal of the American Medical Association,* 243 (1980), 1732–36.

BEEBE, JOYCE E., AND HENRY O. THOMPSON,   "A Paradigm of Ethics for the Maternal Child Nurse," *MCN: American Journal of Maternal Child Nursing,* 4 (May/June 1979), 141.

BEHLMER, GEORGE K.,   "Deadly Motherhood: Infanticide and Medical Opinion in Mid-Victorian England," *Journal of the History of Medicine,* 34 (1979), 403–27.

CAMPBELL, A.G.M.,   "Which Infants Should Not Receive Intensive Care?" *Archives of Disease in Childhood,* 57 (1982), 569–71.

CHINN, PEGGY L.,   "Issues in Lowering Infant Mortality: A Call for Ethical Action," *Advances in Nursing Science,* 1, 3 (April 1979), 63–78.

DE LEON SIANTZ, MARY LOU,   "Human Values in Determining the Fate of Persons with Mental Retardation," *Nursing Clinics of North America,* 14, 1 (March 1979), 57–67.

DUFF, RAYMOND S.,   "Counseling Families and Deciding Care of Severely Defective Children: A Way of Coping with 'Medical Vietnam,'" *Pediatrics,* 67 (1981), 315–20.

ELLIS, T.S., III,   "Letting Defective Babies Die: Who Decides?" *American Journal of Law & Medicine,* 7 (1982) 393–424.

Encyclopedia of Bioethics, 1978 ed., s.v. "Children and Biomedicine," by Norman C. Fost.

FLETCHER, JOHN,   "Abortion, Euthanasia, and Care of Defective Newborns," *The New England Journal of Medicine,* 292 (1975), 75–80.

————,   "Attitudes towards Defective Newborns," *Hastings Center Studies,* 2, 1 (January 1974), 21–32.

FOST, NORMAN,   "Counseling Families Who Have a Child with a Severe Congenital Anomaly," *Pediatrics,* 67 (1981), 321–24.

FRADER, JOEL E.,   "Difficulties in Providing Intensive Care," *Pediatrics,* 64 (1979), 10–16.

———— AND CHARLES L. BOSK,   "Parent Talk at Intensive Care Unit Rounds," *Social Science and Medicine,* 15E (1981), 267–74.

Gustafson, James M., "Mongolism, Parental Desires, and the Right to Life," *Perspectives in Biology and Medicine* (Summer 1973), 529–57.

Haire, Doris, "The Cultural Warping of Childbirth," in *The Cultural Crisis of Modern Medicine,* ed. John Ehrenreich, pp. 185–200. New York: Monthly Review Press, 1978.

Hauerwas, Stanley, "The Demands and Limits of Care—Ethical Reflections on the Moral Dilemma of Neonatal Intensive Care," *American Journal of the Medical Sciences,* 269 (1975), 222–36.

Heymann, Philip B., and Sara Holtz, "The Severely Defective Newborn: The Dilemma and the Decision Process," *Public Policy,* 23 (1975), 381–417.

Horan, Dennis J., "Infanticide: When Doctor's Orders Read 'Murder'" *R.N.* (January 1982), 75.

Jonsen, Albert R., et al., "Critical Issues in Newborn Intensive Care: Conference Report and Policy Proposal," *Pediatrics,* 55 (1975) 756–68.

Kass, Leon R., "'Making Babies' Revisited," *Public Interest* (Winter 1979), 32–60.

Knapp, Ronald J., and Larry G. Peppers, "Doctor-Patient Relationships in Fetal/Infant Death Encounters," *Journal of Medical Education,* 54 (October 1979), 775–80.

Korsch, Barbara M., et al., "Experiences with Children and Their Families during Extended Hemodialysis and Kidney Transplantation," *Pediatric Clinics of North America,* 18, 2 (May 1971), 625–37.

Langham, Paul, "Parental Consent: Its Justification and Limitations," *Clinical Research,* 27 (December 1979), 349–58.

Lee, K.S., et al., "Neonatal Mortality: An Analysis of the Recent Improvement in the United States," *American Journal of Public Health,* 70 (1980), 15–21.

McCarthy, J.T., et al., "Who Pays the Bill for Neonatal Intensive Care?" *Journal of Pediatrics,* 95 (1979), 755–61.

McCormick, Richard A., "To Save or Let Die: The Dilemma of Modern Medicine," *Journal of the American Medical Association,* 229 (1974), 172–76.

Mnookin, Robert H., "Children's Rights: Legal and Ethical Dilemmas," *Pharos,* 41, 2 (April 1978), 2–7.

Nelson, Katherine, "The First Twenty-four Hours," *Neonatal Network* (October 1982), 24–9.

Normand, I., "Dilemmas in Neonatal Care," *Midwives Chronicle,* 91 (October 1978), 285–8.

Phibbs, Ciaran S., Ronald L. Williams, and Rodrick H. Phibbs, "Newborn Risk Factors and Costs of Neonatal Intensive Care," *Pediatrics,* 68 (1981), 313–21.

Pomerance, J.J., et al., "Cost of Living for Infants Weighing 1000 Grams or Less at Birth," *Pediatrics,* 61 (1978), 908–10.

Robertson, John A., "Involuntary Euthanasia of Defective Newborns: A Legal Analysis," *Stanford Law Review,* 27 (1975), 246–61.

Shaw, Anthony M., and Iris A. Shaw, "Dilemmas of 'Informed Consent' in Children," *The New England Journal of Medicine,* 289 (1973), 885–90.

Smith, D.H., "Letting Some Babies Die," *Hastings Center Studies,* 2, 2 (May 1974), 37–46.

Stinson, Robert, and Peggy Stinson, *The Long Dying of Baby Andrew.* Boston: Little, Brown & Company, 1979.

Thompson, Theodore, and John W. Reynolds, "The Result of Intensive Care Therapy for Neonates: I. Overall Neonatal Mortality Rates. II. Neonatal Mortality Rates and Long-Term Prognosis for Low Birth Rate Neonates," *Journal of Perinatal Medicine,* 5, 2 (1977), 57–99.

Philosophy of Technology

Barrett, William, *The Illusion of Technique: A Search for Meaning in a Technological Civilization.* Garden City, N.Y.: Doubleday & Co., Inc., Anchor Press, 1978.

BERMAN, MORRIS, *The Reenchantment of the World.* Ithaca, N.Y.: Cornell University Press, 1981.

CARLSON, RICK J., "Holism and Reductionism as Perspectives in Medicine and Patient Care," *Western Journal of Medicine,* 6 (1979), 466–70.

Encyclopedia of Bioethics, 1978 ed., s.v. "Philosophy of Technology," by Carl Mitcham and Jim Grote.

HABERMAS, JÜRGEN, *Toward a Rational Society: Student Protest, Science and Politics,* Chap. 6, "Technology and Science as Ideology," pp. 81–122. Boston: Beacon Press, 1971.

HOCHSCHILD, ARLIE RUSSELL, "Emotion Work, Feeling Rules, and Social Structure," *American Journal of Sociology,* 85, 3 (1979), 551–75.

MUMFORD, LEWIS, *Technics and Civilization.* New York: Harcourt Brace & Jovanovich, Inc., 1934.

ROUCEK, JOSEPH, "A History of the Concept of Ideology," *Journal of the History of Ideas,* 5 (1944), 479–88.

Humanistic Health Care

BARNETT, KATHRYN, "A Theoretical Construct of the Concepts of Touch as They Relate to Nursing," *Nursing Research,* 21 (1972), 102–10.

CARPER, B., "The Ethics of Caring," *Advances in Nursing Science,* 1, 3 (April 1979), 11–19.

CRAWSHAW, RALPH, "A Lesson from Chinese Medicine: The Humanitarian Imperative," *Journal of the American Medical Association,* 240 (1978), 2257–59.

EHRENREICH, JOHN, ED., *The Cultural Crisis of Modern Medicine.* New York: Monthly Review Press, 1978.

GOULD, GRACE THERESA, ED., "Symposium on Compassion and Communication in Nursing," *Nursing Clinics of North America,* 4, 4 (1969), 651–729.

KRIEGER, DOLORES, "Therapeutic Touch: The Imprimatur of Nursing," *American Journal of Nursing,* 75 (1975), 784–87.

MARTIN, MORGAN, "Native American Medicine: Thoughts for Post-traditional Healers," *Journal of the American Medical Association,* 245 (1981), 141–43.

PATERSON, JOSEPHINE G., AND LORETTA T. ZDERAD, *Humanistic Nursing.* New York: John Wiley & Sons, Inc., 1976.

PURTILO, RUTH B., "Loneliness, the Need for Solitude, and Compliance," in *Communication and Compliance in a Hospital Setting,* eds. David J. Withersty, James M. Stevenson, and Roger H. Waldman, pp. 91–115. Springfield, Ill.: Charles C Thomas, Publisher, 1980.

"High Tech" Health Care

BERLINER, HOWARD S., "Emerging Ideologies in Medicine," *Review of Radical Political Economics,* 9 (1977), 116–23.

BLUMHAGEN, DAN W., "The Doctor's White Coat: The Image of the Physician in Modern America," *Annals of Internal Medicine,* 91 (1979), 111–16.

CARLSON, RICK J., *The End of Medicine,* Chap. 2, "The Impact of Medicine," pp. 6–29. New York: John Wiley & Sons, Inc., 1975.

CASSELL, ERIC J., "Dying in a Technological Society," in *Death Inside Out,* eds. Peter Steinfels and Robert M. Veatch, pp. 43–48. New York: Harper & Row, Publishers, Inc., 1975.

CHALMERS, THOMAS C., "The Impact of Controlled Trials on the Practice of Medicine," *The Mt. Sinai Journal of Medicine,* 41, 6 (1974), 753–59.

CONNORS, DENISE DONNELL, "Sickness unto Death: Medicine as Mythic, Necrophilic and Iatrogenic," *Advances in Nursing Science,* 2 (1980), 39–51.

Downs, Florence S., "Technological Advance and the Nurse-Family Relationship," *Nursing Digest* (1975), 22–24.

Dubos, René, *Mirage of Health—Utopias, Progress, and Biological Change.* Garden City, N.Y.: Doubleday & Co., Inc., Anchor Press, 1959.

Epstein, Samuel S., *The Politics of Cancer.* Garden City, N.Y.: Doubleday & Co., Inc., Anchor Press, 1979.

Fagerhaugh, Shizuko, et al., "The Impact of Technology on Patients, Providers, and Care Patterns," *Nursing Outlook,* 28, 11 (November 1980), 666–72.

Harding, Sandra, "Value-Laden Technologies and the Politics of Nursing," in *Nursing: Images and Ideals: Opening Dialogue with the Humanities,* eds. Stuart F. Spicker and Sally Gadow, pp. 49–75. New York: Springer Publishing Co., Inc., 1980.

Hiatt, Howard H., "Lessons of the Coronary-Bypass Debate," *The New England Journal of Medicine,* 297 (1977), 1462–64.

Kass, Leon R., "Regarding the End of Medicine and the Pursuit of Health," *Public Interest,* 40 (1975), 11–42.

Navarro, Vicente, "Work, Ideology, and Science: The Case of Medicine," *Social Science and Medicine,* 14C (1980), 191–205.

Vreeland, R., and G.L. Ellis, "Stresses on the Nurse in an Intensive-Care Unit," *Journal of the American Medical Association,* 208 (1969), 332–34.

Wright, Robert D., "The Immorality of Excellence in Health Care," *Virginia Quarterly Review* (April 1974), 175–86.

Zola, Irving Kenneth, "Medicine as an Institution of Social Control," in *The Cultural Crisis of Modern Medicine,* ed. John Ehrenreich, pp. 80–100. New York: Monthly Review Press, 1978.

CHAPTER 17

Social
and Political
Responsibilities
of Nurses

At home after an eight- or twelve-hour hospital shift, one feels morally justified in setting aside thoughts of broader social concerns. One has already paid one's dues to health and humanity with the day's work. Yet many nurses return home with a nagging sense that they have left much undone for the health of their clients and the public. Clients' health is entwined with their lives as a whole, and since their health is a basic value, it invites nurses' full devotion. So nurses seldom view their clients simply in terms of what they have done for them during a shift.

The sense of work undone is felt most concretely when patients are discharged from the hospital. What will happen to the old woman returning to a tiny apartment and a solitary life? What will happen to a battered child who has no better place to return to than the home of his abusive parents? How long will it be before "Old George" is found lying in the street again? Why are the only available nursing home placements fifty miles out of town? It is hard to admit, but nurses must, that "We just patch them up and send them back out." One clinician described the problem vividly:

> You know, sometimes I feel like this. There I am standing by the shore of a swiftly flowing river and I hear the cry of a drowning man. So I jump into the river, put my arms toward him, pull him to shore and apply artificial respiration. Just when he begins to breathe, there is another cry for help. So I jump into the river, reach him, pull him to shore, apply artificial respiration, and then just as he begins to breathe, there is another cry for help. So back in the river again, reaching, pulling, applying, breathing and then another yell. Again and again, without end, goes the sequence. You know, I am so busy jumping in, pulling them to shore, applying artificial respiration, that I have *no* time to see who the hell is upstream pushing them all in.[1]

---

[1]From Irving K. Zola, "Helping—Does it Matter? The Problems and Prospects of Mutual Aid Groups," address to the United Ostomy Association, 1970, quoted in John B. McKinlay, "A Case for Refocusing Upstream: The Political Economy of Illness," in *Patients, Physicians, and Illness,* 3rd ed., ed. E. Gartley Jaco (New York: The Free Press, 1979), p. 9.

Nurses tend to be acutely aware of the limitations of "downstream" acute modes of care because they have been broadly educated in health maintenance skills and concepts which go well beyond the limits of hospital care. Martha Rogers, for example, argues that nursing, as a humanistic science, should view human beings in their social and natural context. Nursing interventions should therefore emphasize health promotion and prevention of illness more than tertiary care.[2]

This broad perspective is awakened by several aspects of nurses' roles:

Patient care: Sickness raises problems for clients' overall welfare. Phone calls may be needed to relatives or the landlord, or referrals to a dentist or lawyer. Disparate factors in patients' lives affect their health, such as jobs, housing, finances, transportation, families, and community.

Clients' effects on others: One's client may carry a contagious disease or threaten harm to others. To what extent are nurses responsible for looking out for the family and friends of clients?[3]

Possible patients: There are millions of people out there who are not now clients. It would be ideal if these possible patients never needed to be actual patients. A concern for *public health* is a sensible way to fulfill one's responsibility as a nurse, since prevention is better than therapy.

Public welfare: Many nonhealth factors affect public health: working conditions, speed limits, and so on. Many public issues also have a major health impact even though health is not central to them. Racism, for example, has important health consequences.

Health: The concept and value of health undergird nursing practice. Nurses study philosophy, sociology, and anthropology in order to assume responsibility for the conceptual foundations of practice.

Nursing practice: Hospital working conditions, standards of admission to the profession, legislative support of nursing, nursing education, wages and fringe benefits, and so on are all concerns for which nurses have a responsibility.

Professional nursing associations generally recognize these sources of social and political responsibility. The last three points of the ANA Code for Nurses, for example, address working conditions of nurses, public education about health issues, and cooperative work for public health and welfare on a national scale.

There is a tension in this concern and a limit to it. Health is so inextricably linked with all aspects of peoples' lives that a concern for it tempts one to take responsibility for *everything*. The World Health Organization went overboard in this direction in its famous definition of health:

---

[2]Martha Rogers, *An Introduction to the Theoretical Basis of Nursing Practice* (Philadelphia: F.A. Davis Co., 1970), pp. 122–23.

[3]Patients with infectious diseases can be dangerous to others. See Henry S. Perkins and Albert R. Jonsen, "Conflicting Duties to Patients: The Case of a Sexually Active Hepatitis B Carrier," *Annals of Internal Medicine,* 94 (1981), 524–30. A classic dilemma involves a psychiatrist whose patient confided that he might murder his girl friend. Should the psychiatrist have warned her? A California court ruled yes after the patient murdered her. See Tarasoff v. Regents of University of California, 551 P.2d 223 (Ca. 1976).

Health is a state of complete physical, mental and social well-being and not merely the absence of disease or infirmity.[4]

But nurses cannot claim a professional level of competence in everything. A good nurse is not necessarily a good politician, physical education instructor, highway engineer, dietitian, building safety inspector, or anything else. But the limitations of individual nurses are compensated for partly by the ability of the nursing profession as a whole to take collective responsibility for some of these problems. It can fulfill some of its social and political responsibilities through public health nursing, home care, nursing law, health administration, lobbying, nursing research, occupational health nursing, and so on.

A brief text on ethics cannot do justice to the broad social and political issues facing nursing, nor can one philosopher have competence in them all. So this chapter will sample some of these issues: the right to health and health care, the costs of care, and racism in nursing.

The Right to Health and Health Care

For two decades, much attention was devoted to the right to health care. Then suddenly, concern about the high costs of care rose to public attention and talk of rights diminished. It seemed futile to claim a right to something we cannot realize. But it is all the more important to speak of rights when there are conflicts over the use of limited resources. The language of rights can still be used to defend access to health care of those in need, even when some health care services must be limited. To say that we have a right to health care is to say that health care is a basic good that should be distributed justly. To appreciate the reasons for saying that we have a right to health care, we thus need to discuss justice.

Two Concepts of Justice

People differ about what it means to distribute health care justly (see p. 133). For instance, sociologists who interviewed health care providers in European countries with socialized health care systems found a consensus that health care should express and support *equality* and be distributed according to *need*.[5] In the United States, in contrast, we are sharply divided about the meanings of justice in health care. One American view follows principles that might be roughly labeled *market justice:* Personal liberty, self-reliance, free enterprise, and economic efficiency should guide our decisions. The other view follows principles closer to those identi-

[4]From the preamble to the constitution of the World Health Organization, adopted by the International Health Conference, New York City, June 19–July 22, 1946. Reprinted in *Contemporary Issues in Bioethics*, 2nd ed., eds. Tom L. Beauchamp and LeRoy Walters (Belmont, Calif.: Wadsworth Publishing Co., Inc., 1982), p. 48.

[5]Ruth Purtilo, *Justice, Liberty, Compassion—"Humane" Health Care and Rehabilitation in the U.S.: Some Lessons from Sweden* (New York: World Rehabilitation Fund, Inc., 1981); and Charles Lockhart, "Values and Policy Conceptions of Health Policy Elites in the United States, the United Kingdom, and the Federal Republic of Germany," *Journal of Health Politics, Policy, and Law*, 6 (1981), 98–119.

fied in studies of Europeans. We can call these principles *public health justice:* distribution of health care according to need, collective approaches to public health problems, equal access to services, and humane and compassionate care.[6] This dividedness on the issue of justice in health care makes it hard to manage health services in a rational way. When we look at health care from the standpoint of *providers* of health care, we often express market concepts of justice. And when we look at the same services from the point of view of *consumers,* we express public health justice principles. But providers and consumers are part of the same system, and one system cannot be guided by two conflicting principles of justice.

In Chapter 10, we defended the principles of *need* and *equal respect* in distributing health care. The Swedish writer Alva Myrdal explains the concept of equal respect in health care.

> Equality means that where nature has created great and fundamental differences in abilities, these must *not* be allowed to determine the individual's chances in life, but rather that society should "restore the balance." These differences, in the form of physical or intellectual handicaps, can never be eliminated, but they can be reduced in a generous social climate, and one can work against their leading to social discrimination. Disadvantages inflicted by nature should not be accepted as something we can do nothing about.[7]

The concept of need in health care means two different things. Need has an *instrumental* meaning when we talk of therapies which restore and maintain health. In this sense of *need,* a need is a necessary means to an end. But need also has an evaluative and *humane* meaning. People who are sick or disabled can suffer a great deal. They are sometimes *needy.* Humane health care may not be able to cure their ills, but it can provide compassion, care, and comfort. Solace is the least a society can offer to us when we are, it is hoped temporarily, among the worst off. If we support principles of public health justice, we will also support a right to both the humane and instrumental functions of health care. Since we have conflicting conceptions of justice and there is pressure to withdraw resources from health and use them for other purposes, it is important to defend a right to health care in terms of principles of public health justice.

The right to health care is not an *established legal right* to health care. Health care is not written in the Constitution as a basic right, and those who lack access to care cannot legally enforce a claim to it. By a right to health care most people mean a *fundamental* or *basic* right that should, for reasons of justice, be recognized by law. When we ask Is our society adequately governed and can we feel justified in giving it allegiance? we need some sort of checklist of conditions that we agree society must meet. This checklist should not be too long, lest we endorse controversial values, nor too short, lest we overlook some of the basic conditions of a just society. The United States Declaration of Independence asserts rights to life, liberty, and the pursuit of happiness. It can be argued that the right to *health* is a fundamental right like these. For instance, the President's Commission on the Health Needs of the Nation claimed in 1952 that "access to the means for the

---

[6]Dan E. Beauchamp, "Public Health as Social Justice," *Inquiry,* 13 (1976), 3–14, uses the labels *market justice* and *public health ethic.*

[7]Alva Myrdal Report (1971) quoted in Purtilo, *Justice, Liberty, Compassion,* p. 17.

attainment and preservation of health is a basic human right."[8] A right to health *care* can be defended on the grounds that we have a right to health.

The Right to Health

Those who would like to see health on this list do so because almost *everything,* as noted in the introduction to this chapter, affects health and is affected by it. They would like to see a concern for health reflected in all our public policy decisions. They believe health should weigh heavily in decisions about growing and processing food, organization of manufacture, use of chemicals and radioactive materials, urban planning, water supplies, automobile design, and so on.

We already display some concern about these things, but proponents of a right to health want more attention given to them. They believe that we are doing an *injustice* if health is not given *priority* in production, commerce, transportation, and so on. The government should not be able to say, when resources are short, that our first priority is to protect commerce, that is, market justice, and not health.

Proponents of a right to health are legitimately concerned about the clarity of our social commitment to health. For instance, in the nineteenth century, the federal government's right to establish quarantine laws during yellow fever epidemics was litigated in the courts. Quarantine required that ships loaded with goods stand out from port for long periods of time. This was good for public health but bad for business. Courts repeatedly decided that the federal government's role was limited to protecting commerce, not health.[9] Similarly, in 1981 the government was able to dismantle many health programs because it could argue that people have no legal right to them.

Those who don't think health is a fundamental right are usually uncomfortable with the vagueness of the concept of health. *Physical* health defines too narrowly what we mean, but the phrase "physical, mental, and social well-being" is too broad. And how much health are we talking about? Are we trying to create some superspecies with eternal life? Or should people just be able to drag themselves to work every day for twenty years and then perish? Opponents are also worried that society is limited in its ability to protect health; for instance, thunderstorms, droughts, genes, volcanos, and so on powerfully affect health. Proponents of a right to health respond that the concept of health is no more vague, and no less a candidate for the list, than life, liberty, and the pursuit of happiness. Society is equally limited in its ability to guarantee these. Proponents are only saying that society should make health a top priority in basic social decisions.

Opponents of a right to health also argue that it is a controversial value. They point out that if people genuinely valued health, they would behave differently: Many people neglect and abuse their health. Proponents reply that when people become ill, they realize the importance of health and really want it, even if they

---

[8]Quoted in the President's Commission for the Study of Ethical Problems in Medicine and Biomedical and Behavioral Research, *Securing Access to Health Care: A Report on the Ethical Implications of Differences in the Availability of Health Services, Vol. I: Report* (Washington, D.C.: U.S. Government Printing Office, 1983), p. 4.

[9]Carleton B. Chapman and John M. Talmadge, "The Evolution of the Right to Health Concept in the United States," *The Pharos of Alpha Omega Alpha,* 14 (1971), 30–51.

abuse it. Although health may not be first in most people's minds, they *need* it to enjoy other pursuits. Proponents also claim that the observed tendency to neglect health does not arise as much from the desires of individuals as from social arrangements that fail to support the desire for health.[10] Most urban areas, for example, make automobile travel relatively convenient but lack pleasant places to exercise. Highly specialized organization of labor places people in repetitive factory work or sedentary desk jobs that leave little time or motivation for compensatory exercise. One could ask how healthy nursing work is and observe the difficulties nurses face in maintaining good health.

The Right to Health Care

Health *care* is a much more specific and concrete concept than health and lacks the splendid breadth and vagueness that health shares with life, liberty, and happiness. Along with adequate shelter, a clean water supply, and similar measures alluded to above, health care is a significant and limited factor in maintaining good health. Insofar as health care is instrumental in restoring and maintaining health, preventing illness, and providing functional substitutes for health such as eyeglasses and artificial limbs, proponents of a right to health would also want to support a right to health care.

But these curative or *instrumental* aspects of health care are only a limited part of the activities of health care institutions. The most prevalent diseases in the U.S. are either incurable or self-limiting. Health care is somewhat effective in reducing the overall impact of these chronic and limited diseases, but if we were to limit health care only to activities improving health, we would limit it very much indeed. Health care also expresses justice by meeting needs in a humane and evaluative sense of the term (p. 264). It provides a wide range of services oriented to the care, comfort, and protection of the sick. People need these functions of health care whether they restore health or not. Proponents of a right to health care would thus also support a right to these aspects of it. As has been argued in earlier chapters, these functions of health care are more closely associated with nursing than medicine. In 1983, a Presidential commission concluded that "society has an ethical obligation to ensure equitable access to health care for all," on the basis of both the instrumental and humane functions of health care.[11]

Realizing the Right to Humane Health Care

Some proponents of a right to humane health care argue that it cannot be realized in a free market system. Only some form of socialized health care can

---

[10]For example, most alcoholics would prefer to drink an alcohol substitute that would taste like alcohol and get them drunk, but would not destroy livers and neurons. People do not normally drink *in order* to destroy their health but *in spite of* destroying their health. The link between the value of getting high and the disvalue of liver disease is a result of the dual nature of alcohol. We cannot do much about this except restrict the use of alcohol. But many links between disease and other values are entirely subject to *social arrangements*. For example, gasoline need not have lead in it, textile factories can be well ventilated, and so on.

[11]President's Commission for the Study of Ethical Problems in Medicine and Biomedical and Behavioral Research, *Securing Access to Health Care*, p. 4.

express the principles of public health justice. For example, in 1979 California Representative Ron Dellums proposed a bill in Congress to create a national health care delivery system. The bill contains provisions that address neighborhood and workplace health problems. It provides for democratic control of the health care system by clients, the public at large, and health providers.[12]

Some health professionals worry that recognizing a right to health care will force them to treat patients whom they hate or force them to live in undesirable places.[13] However, this need not be the case. Socialized systems can work much like market systems: They can create jobs and offer salaries for them. No one has to take a particular job; rather, one chooses or competes for it. The difference is that decisions about where to allocate jobs are made by patients and providers according to needs, instead of being subject to the forces of the market system. Such a system need not be expensive either, as decisions can be made to limit salaries and services.[14]

Similar conflicts over public-health and market justice, humane and instrumental functions, costs and services, and so on, arise in business, public welfare, government, and law. It may not be possible to create a health care delivery system conforming to public health justice while other social institutions conform to market justice. Recognizing a right to health care may thus require that we realize a more humanistic perspective in society at large.

The High Cost of Care

In the late 1970s, a growing consciousness arose that health care costs too much. People wondered whether we should set an age limit on eligibility for highly technological care, such as dialysis or heart transplants. Training programs were introduced to sensitize physicians to the costs of diagnostic tests and therapies. This cost consciousness reflects a virtue emphasized in early nursing ethics texts—the virtue of *economy* or *frugality*. Historically, nurses were expected to protect the hospital budget from waste, whether by careless use of supplies or excessive ordering by physicians.[15] However, few who discuss the problem of costs analyze what it means to say that health care costs are *high* or that health care *costs too much*. Usually large dollar figures are mentioned, and analysis moves immediately to cutting these figures. Sometimes the problem is expressed in terms of the increasing

[12]U.S., Congress, The Health Service Act, HR 2969, *Congressional Record* 25, 3, 96th Cong., 1st sess. (March 19, 1979).

[13]Robert M. Sade, "Medical Care as a Right: A Refutation," *The New England Journal of Medicine,* 285 (1971), 1288–92; and Mark Siegler, "A Physician's Perspective on a Right to Health Care," *Journal of The American Medical Association,* 244 (1980), 1591–96.

[14]The American Nurses' Association in 1977 favored a national health insurance program as one element of a policy to realize "the belief that health care is a basic right of all people." American Nurses' Association, "A National Policy of Health Care: Principles and Positions" (Kansas City, Mo.: American Nurses' Association, 1977).

[15]The duty or virtue of economy was discussed by Isabel Hampton Robb, *Nursing Ethics: For Hospital and Private Use* (Cleveland: J.B. Savage, 1900). She associated it with principles of "practical household economy," a "branch of woman's work" (p. 42). Charlotte A. Aikens included a chapter on "Ethics and Economy" in *Studies in Ethics for Nurses* (Philadelphia: W.B. Saunders Company, 1916), pp. 80–96.

percent of the Gross National Product devoted to health care, in which case our discussion must be about what it means to spend *too much* of the GNP on health care.

When discussing the problem of high costs, it is important not to be overawed by large dollar figures. For instance, in 1980 the federal government spent approximately $1 billion on hemodialysis and kidney transplant. But in 1980, dollar figures for all major programs were large. Here are some concrete comparisons:

The cleanup and repair bill for the Three Mile Island nuclear reactor incident is estimated at about $1 billion.

One billion dollars is the approximate price of two B-1 bombers or one Trident submarine equipped with nuclear missiles.

One billion dollars spent in 1975 for defense supported about 75,000 jobs, but supported about 140,000 jobs in health care.

Pacific Telephone budgeted $3 billion in 1981 to change from mechanical to electronic switching.

Americans spent $2.6 billion to go to the movies in 1980. They spent $21.6 billion on TVs, radios, records, and musical instruments; $6.4 billion on books; $4.5 billion on flowers, seeds, and potted plants; and about $7 billion on toys.

U.S. corporations spent $44 billion in 1980 to buy other corporations.

Cigarette and pharmaceutical advertising each cost their manufacturers more than $1 billion in 1980.[16]

Moreover, dollar amounts and percent of GNP are poor measures of *costs*. When somebody spends money, that is, incurs dollar costs, somebody else *makes* money, that is, receives dollar benefits. We cannot tell from giving a dollar amount whether we are better or worse off as a people by the exchanges. We need to know more concrete information about these exchanges. Who is paying? Who is getting? For what? A significant reduction in health care expenditures would mean a significant reduction in health care incomes, and incomes benefit people. The University of California, San Francisco, makes this point in the introduction to its general catalog:

UCSF is one of the largest employers in San Francisco and attracts many millions of dollars to the city and state each year. As a result, UCSF is one of the city and state's most important economic resources.[17]

Nurses and physicians sometimes complain about paying taxes for health care and express resentment toward Medicare and Medicaid clients whose health care is paid for by public funds, as though such clients received money from the government, when actually the money goes to doctors and nurses themselves. In concrete terms, the claim that health care costs too much has three very different meanings, each of which calls for a different remedy.

[16]I found these estimates here and there. Readers can supply their own figures from the daily newspaper.

[17]University of California, San Francisco, "General Catalogue 1980–1981," *UCSF*, 20, 6 (July 1980), 5.

WE CAN'T AFFORD IT.   The claim that health care costs too much can mean that we are allocating too much of our labor and capital to health care, we need these resources in other areas, and we should divert our energies from health care into other activities. This is a global claim and hard to assess even in a limited case. For example, during 1977 and 1978, the state of Oregon's syphilis screening program for newlyweds cost an astonishingly large amount—$1,290,000—per case discovered. The money for tests came from fees paid by newlyweds.[18] What would happen to this money if it were not spent on VD tests? Perhaps it would be spent on wine and flowers to celebrate weddings. We can then ask two questions. Was this too much to pay in forsaken wine and roses for this case? And would it have benefited society more if the money had gone to vintners and florists rather than to clinicians, lab technicians, and state bureaucrats? We need to express expenditures in concrete alternatives like wine and roses before we even begin to consider what we can afford.

The only significant increase in the federal budget for fiscal year 1982 was for military purposes.[19] As I see it, this shift in expenditures indicates a shift in national priorities toward military development at the expense of investment in health care. I am wholly antagonistic to this trend. I would feel a much stronger sense of conflict about what health care we can afford, if it were shown that we had to make a choice, for instance, between neonatal intensive care units and prenatal care. I would also be more concerned by what we can afford if *concrete* resources for health care were scarce; however, unemployment rates are high and many licensed RNs are not working in health care. I do not know to what extent health care exhausts natural resources, and this consideration is relevant to what we can afford, but dollar amounts give no indication of what we can afford in labor and resources.

HEALTH CARE IS NOT WORTH IT.   The claim that health care costs too much might mean that we are getting too little from our investment in it. To consumers and health professionals interested in quality health services, this is the most humane interpretation of the claim that health care costs too much. Remedying this problem involves discontinuing services of negligible value. We do not have to think in terms of sending the needy away, because no one needs ineffective health care. Everyone has favorite targets for reducing health care costs. Some of mine are drugs prescribed for nonindicated conditions, drugs not taken anyway, intensive care unit services for obviously dying patients, redundant diagnostic tests, diagnostic tests not relevant to therapy, excessive ordering of nursing observations and vital signs, and expensive therapies of unestablished value. These recommendations need not be taken too seriously; careful evaluation is required to eliminate useless and unwanted therapies. In order to identify ineffective therapies, we need to have a clearer humanistic perspective on the goals of health care, a task that I argued in Chapter 16 is a special responsibility of nurses (pp. 255–56).

WE'RE BEING OVERCHARGED.   This claim says that health care services may well have value, but somebody is making too much money from them. Indeed, health care has been charged with excessive profits and income (see pp. 103–7).

---

[18]They found one case in a year. David B. Polonoff and Michael J. Garland, "Oregon's Premarital Blood Test: An Unsuccessful Attempt at Repeal," *Hastings Center Report*, 9, 6 (1979), 5–6.

[19]". . . by again taking a hard line on social spending, Mr. Reagan will be able to provide bargaining room and be able to protect much of his five-year, $1,600 billion program for military increase" (*New York Times*, November 20, 1982, pp. 1, 10).

The solution to this problem is not to cut patient care services but to find ways to limit profiteering in health care. Limiting access to health services is entirely irrelevant to this problem.

Efforts were being made to cut back health care expenditures in the early 1980s. Hospital administrators began talking about setting upper age limits on care, and ability to pay became a more attractive factor in accepting patients. But my analysis of costs suggests that cost-limiting measures can first be taken which better respect the right to health: limiting extraneous therapies, cutting income at the top, and not diverting resources to less worthwhile enterprises than health.

Limits on health expenditures present challenges and opportunities for nursing. On one hand, nurses only began in the late 1970s to make much progress toward better salaries and respect for their work; tighter budgets and layoffs threaten these advances. The need for real charity, that is, unpaid work, raises once again the danger of exploiting nurses' conscientious devotion to health needs. On the other hand, nurses increasingly offer many health services more cheaply than physicians and so may be able to find new opportunities for work.[20] Moreover, nurses can clearly defend the humane aspects of health care and resist abuse of clients as health services become more limited.

Corporate and profit-making institutions are increasing their influence in health care. They argue that competitive institutions will make health care more efficient and improve services in spite of contracting resources.[21] Although many support this view, I do not believe that institutions operating on market conceptions of justice can make health care more humane. Large health care corporations may offer services cheaply, but in the long run, savings will not be returned to the consumer and will be used instead for corporate growth and profit. I would hold that we have to replace market justice in health care with a socialized system that allocates resources on humane terms rather than on commercial terms,[22] and that nurses should support socialized modes of health delivery in order to protect a humane conception of the right to health care.

Racism in Nursing

It is surely no news to anyone that the U.S. is a race-stratified society. Nor should it be news that the health care system reflects this stratification. Table 17.1 illustrates that overall U.S. health employment figures show a lower percentage of minorities (blacks, Hispanics, Asians, Native Americans) in higher income job categories. This stratification can be seen more vividly when one looks at specific job categories. Table 17.2 indicates the race and sex makeup of representative job

[20]Claire M. Fagin, "Nursing as an Alternative to High-Cost Care," *American Journal of Nursing,* 82 (1982), 56–60.

[21]The leading version of the market approach in 1981 was introduced by Alain C. Enthoven. See "Health Care Cost Control through Incentives and Competition: Consumer-Choice Health Plan," *Socioeconomic Issues of Health* (Center for Health Services Research and Development, American Medical Association, 1979); and Alain C. Enthoven, "The Competition Strategy: Status and Prospects," *The New England Journal of Medicine,* 304 (1981), 109–12.

[22]Richard Titmuss describes the allocation of blood through the nonmarket system of donation in the British National Health Service. See *The Gift Relationship: From Human Blood to Social Policy* (New York: Random House, Inc., 1972).

Table 17.1. Minority and Women Workers in U.S. Health Occupations, 1981

Job Category	Percentage of Minority	Percentage of Women
RNs	12.3	96.8
LPNs & LVNs	19.9	97.8
Physicians	14.5	13.7
Administrators	6.8	49.8
Dietitians	23.8	93.7
Aides, orderlies, attendants	29.0	86.6

NOTE: About 17 percent of the U.S. population are minorities. About 75 percent of all health workers are women and about 30 percent are nonwhite.
SOURCE: U.S. Bureau of the Census, *Statistical Abstract of the United States: 1982–83*, 103rd ed. (Washington, D.C.: U.S. Government Printing Office, 1982), pp. 32, 109.

classifications at a large university health sciences center in 1980. Racial imbalances are strongest at the extreme ends of the salary scale.

Nursing has not escaped racism. Nonwhite graduates of nursing schools pass RN licensure examinations less often than white graduates. In California, for example, 80 percent to 90 percent of all whites pass, while 55 percent of Hispanics, 40

Table 17.2. Minority and Women Workers in a Large Urban Health Sciences Center in the U.S., 1980

Selected Job Categories, in Descending Order of Average Monthly Income	Percentage of Minority	Percentage of Women
Full Professor	7	9
Administrative Nurse* (Grades I–V) (RNs)	10	97
Clinical Nurse* (Grades I–V) (RNs)	17	96
Clinical Laboratory Technician†	48	84
Hospital Laboratory Technician II†	41	62
Respiratory Therapist I	38	31
Administrative Assistant	31	92
Senior Vocational Nurse (LVNs)	73	92
Senior Hospital Assistant	79	74
Secretary II	25	94
Senior Custodian	95	40
Senior Linen Service Worker	100	73
Food Service Worker	90	37

NOTE: In 1980, the proportion of minorities in the city in which this health sciences center is located was about 55 percent. Minority admissions to the hospital averaged about 31 percent.
SOURCE: Figures are from the university's affirmative action records. The table is compiled from selected representative titles. For example, the full-professor category combines the two most populous full-professor titles; Secretary II was chosen in preference to Secretary I or III because it is by far the most populous secretarial category.
*Administrative and clinical nurse grades overlap in average salary.
†Average monthly salaries in these titles overlap salaries in nursing grades.

percent of blacks, 25 percent of Asians, and about 14 percent of Filipinos pass the state examinations.[23]

One result of this phenomenon is that those who do not pass the state boards but wish to continue working in nursing must take jobs as LVNs or aides. The two-class system that divides RNs and LVNs thus supports race stratification in nursing. Table 17.1 shows that about 12 percent of RNs, and about 25 percent of LVNs, aides, orderlies and attendants are minority people.

In about 1980, hospitals in California and other states began exploiting this stratification. There was a shortage of nurses in California and elsewhere. In order to fill positions, hospitals recruited nurses from abroad—from England, Ireland, Wales, and Scotland, but more often from the Philippines. Since fair employment recruitment procedures do not apply abroad, hospitals can bypass them, and nurses coming to the U.S. on temporary visas are tied to the hospitals that recruit them almost as indentured servants.[24]

These conditions impose ethical dilemmas on foreign-trained nurses, as shown by this case:

> CASE EXAMPLE.   I am an immigrant nurse living but one year in this country. I have not been able to get a work permit as a registered nurse because I did not pass the examinations of this new country although I sat for them twice. My family is in a difficult financial situation, and I must send money to them. The owner of a small private hospital, whom I met socially, asked me to work in his hospital under the title of nurse aide on condition that I carry the responsibility of the senior nurse on night duty. I know that I could do this work competently and safely as I had a good training and many years of experience in similar hospital nursing. However, it is clear that I am being cheated of the proper salary, and also asked to break the law by doing work of a nurse while carrying another title. In addition, accepting these conditions will contribute to the exploitation of nurses. I have decided to take the job, but am very uncomfortable about it.[25]

Foreign nursing school graduates have an especially difficult time with the California licensure exams. For example, only 7 percent of Filipinos pass.[26] Since standard educational testing in the U.S. has a history of racial bias, there is reason to believe that the tests are discriminatory.[27] The point of a licensure exam should not be to limit professions to privileged classes of people, but to make sure that only qualified nurses become licensed.

[23]California Department of Consumer Affairs.

[24]Information supplied by Pat Franks, Institute for Health Policy Studies, University of California, San Francisco, September, 1981.

[25]From Barbara L. Tate, ed., *The Nurse's Dilemma: Ethical Considerations in Nursing Practice* (Geneva: Florence Nightingale International Foundation, International Council of Nurses, 1977), pp. 69–70. In the case cited, "this country" does not necessarily refer to the U.S., as cases in *The Nurse's Dilemma* are not identified by nationality.

[26]California Department of Consumer Affairs.

[27]Stephen Jay Gould, "Racist Arguments and IQ," and Peggy R. Sanday, "On the Causes of IQ Differences between Groups and Implications for Social Policy," in *Race and IQ*, ed. Ashley Montagu (New York: Oxford University Press, 1975).

It would be fairer to revise the examinations and make them more equitable for nonwhite and foreign nurses. Another important step is for nursing associations and unions to help foreign nurses become familiar with U.S. practices and examination skills. In addition to showing humanity to easily exploited newcomers, this encourages their loyalty to nursing. A historical precedent for recognizing the problem of racism in nursing was set by the ANA in the 1950s when it encouraged direct membership in the national organization for black nurses who were excluded from state chapters.[28] The moral and political problem for nurses is to continue to break down racial stratification in nursing and keep hospitals from exploiting differences among nurses, while at the same time, keeping judgments of excellence in practice in the hands of nurses rather than those who have traditionally exploited them.

Unresolved Issues of Justice

There are many social and political issues on which nurses could provide more leadership by virtue of their familiarity with health problems, their access to clients, and their position in health care institutions. Examples include public payment for abortion, treatment of the aged, prevention of nuclear war, treatment of the disabled and mentally ill, occupational health hazards, disaster planning, financing and organizing health care services, smoking and alcoholism, long-term institutional care, sexism and employment, and improved nutrition. There are so many issues that nurses must set priorities on time and energy for addressing such concerns.

Criticisms of the cost controversy presented in this chapter were inspired by a belief that it is important to resist concepts of scarcity that result in unnecessary limitations on patient care. In spite of these criticisms, scarcity of time, energy, and human resources is always a real concern. What should nurses do when, wisely or unwisely, clinical resources are so limited that practitioners must choose whom they can serve and limit available services? In clinical settings, scarcity presents so many faces and affects so many decision points, it is difficult to be certain how cost concerns do and should affect patient care. Allocating resources for patient care is seldom a life-and-death issue. Instead, such decisions involve complex considerations such as the choice of a procedure from several uncertain ones, the number of nurses available per patient, the complexity of required nursing tasks, the severity indices, the placing of patients in types of institutions, the admitting of patients to special care units, the bumping of patients to the wards, and the acceptance of ambulances at the emergency department. The effects of such factors on client welfare involve tendencies and probabilities. It is thus sometimes hard to tell whether clinicians are being consistent and equally respectful in selecting clients for therapy when services are scarce.

When need is established as the main criterion for justly distributing scarce resources and resources continue to be scarce, other considerations must affect treatment priorities. Clinicians appeal to a wide variety of considerations. The likelihood of successful therapy, the projected quality of life, the impact of care on

[28]Lucie Young Kelly, *Dimensions of Professional Nursing*, 4th ed. (New York: Macmillan, Inc., 1981), p. 542.

other patients, and the wishes of client and family are often given great weight. Other criteria may affect clinical practice strongly even though they are not especially relevant to clients' needs, such as fear of malpractice, personal feelings about individual clients, research protocols, the motivation to conquer disease, and the technological imperative. Still other considerations sometimes used by clinicians could be argued to be morally questionable, such as past or prospective social worth, blameworthiness of clients for their health, age, and ability to pay.

The soundness of the *need* criterion in equitably allocating services also requires assessment. Proponents of humane health care tend to emphasize allocating health resources by both need *and* prevention. But prevention measures do *not* express health care needs; they are the antithesis of need in that they prevent needs from occurring. Preventive services are primarily directed to the healthy—those not in need. This disparity invites exploration and may even present a dilemma. Perhaps a more utilitarian concept of justice in health care should be developed which better expresses overall public welfare. Or perhaps prevention can be seen as expressing a collective need. Nurses who study the clinical aspects of scarcity, need, and public health can contribute to the philosophical debate over priorities in health care delivery.

Summary

Since health is not an isolated quality of clients' lives, nurses' professional concern for their clients' health leads them to take responsibility for a wide range of issues affecting the health and welfare of clients and the public.

One of these issues is the right to health care. Our health care system displays conflicts between two concepts of justice—*market* justice and *public health* justice. The concept of public health justice supports the claim that we have a right to *health*. A right to the *instrumental* functions of health care is justified by supporting the right to health. A right to the *humane* functions of health care is also supported by principles of justice.

Another issue of concern to nurses is the high cost of care. We may mean by *high costs* that we can't *afford* health care, that it is not *worth* it, or that we are being *overcharged* for it. What we should do to remedy the high costs of care depends on which of these meanings most concerns us.

A third issue of concern to nurses is race stratification in nursing. Barriers to entry are important in maintaining quality of care and the bargaining power of the profession. But these have traditionally had discriminatory consequences. Employers may exploit race conflict in nursing in order to maintain control over the nursing profession. Thus, ways need to be found to eliminate race stratification without eliminating nursing influence on the conduct of care.

There are many additional public issues on which nurses can have important input because of their skills and acquaintance with health aspects of these problems. Although individual nurses may not be able to do very much, the profession acting collectively has the ability, and recognizes the responsibility, to address them. One important task is to find a just balance between devoting health care resources to acute needs and using resources to prevent such needs from arising.

FURTHER READINGS

Health and Public Policy

DAVIS, ANNE J., "Nursing's Influence on Health Policy for the Eighties," in *Nursing's Influence on Health Policy for the Eighties,* ed. American Academy of Nursing, pp. 3–12. Kansas City, Mo.: American Nurses' Association, 1979.

DEJONG, GERBEN, "A Political Economy Critique of the American Welfare State," *Journal of Sociology and Social Welfare,* 5 (1978), 1–45.

FLAHERTY, DIANE, ET AL., EDS., *Review of Radical Political Economics,* special issue on "The Political Economy of Health," 9, 1 (Spring 1977).

GEORGE, VIC, AND PAUL WILDING, *Ideology and Social Welfare.* London: Routledge & Kegan Paul, 1976.

JONSEN, ALBERT R., AND ANDREW L. JAMETON, "Social and Political Responsibilities of Physicians," *Journal of Medicine and Philosophy,* 2 (1977), 376–400.

KELMAN, SANDER, "Toward the Political Economy of Medical Care," *Inquiry,* 8, 3 (September 1971), 30.

KLEIN, RUDOLF, "Reflections on the American Health Care Condition," *Journal of Health Politics, Policy and Law,* 6, 2 (Summer 1981), 188–204.

LOMASKY, LOREN E., "Medical Progress and National Health Care," *Philosophy & Public Affairs,* 10 (1981), 65–88.

MECHANIC, DAVID, "Some Dilemmas in Health Care Policy," *Milbank Memorial Fund Quarterly,* 59 (1981), 1–15.

TELFER, E., "Justice, Welfare and Health Care," *Journal of Medical Ethics,* 2 (1976), 107–11.

VEATCH, ROBERT, AND ROY BRANSON. *Ethics and Health Policy.* Cambridge, Mass : Ballinger Publishing Co., 1976.

WILLIAMS, FRANK C., AND CAROLYN A. WILLIAMS, "Ethical Issues in Health Care Policy," in *Current Perspectives in Nursing: Social Issues and Trends,* eds. Michael H. Miller and Beverly C. Flynn, pp. 3–13. St. Louis: C.V. Mosby Company, 1977.

Health Rights

ARRAS, JOHN, AND ANDREW JAMETON, "Medical Individualism and the Right to Health Care," in *Intervention and Reflection: Basic Issues in Medical Ethics,* ed. Ronald Munson, pp. 462–73. Belmont, Calif.: Wadsworth Publishing Co., Inc., 1979.

DANIELS, NORMAN, "Health-Care Needs and Distributive Justice," *Philosophy & Public Affairs,* 10 (1981), 146–79.

FRIED, CHARLES, "Equality and Rights in Medical Care," *Hastings Center Report,* 6 (February 1976), 29–37.

———, "Rights and Health Care—Beyond Equity and Efficiency," *The New England Journal of Medicine,* 293 (1975), 241–45.

GUTMANN, AMY, "For and against Equal Access to Health Care," *Milbank Memorial Fund Quarterly,* 59 (1981), 542–60.

KING, MAURICE, "Personal Health Care: The Quest for a Human Right," in *Human Rights in Health, Ciba Foundation Symposium 23* (new series), pp. 227–43. Amsterdam: Elsevier, 1974.

MCCULLOUGH, LAURENCE B., "The Right to Health Care," *Ethics in Science & Medicine,* 6 (1979), 1–9.

SPARER, EDWARD V., "The Legal Right to Health Care: Public Policy and Equal Access," *Hastings Center Report,* 6, 5 (October 1976), 39–47.

WILLARD, L. DUANE, "Needs and Medicine," *The Journal of Medicine and Philosophy,* 7, (1982), 259–74.

Costs and Scarce Resources

"The Ailing Health Care System—Medical Staff Conference, University of California, San Francisco," *Western Journal of Medicine*, 128 (June 1978), 512–26.

BROWN, LAWRENCE D., "Competition and Health Cost Containment: Cautions and Conjectures," *Milbank Memorial Fund Quarterly*, 59 (1981), 145–89.

CULLEN, D.J., "Results and Costs of Intensive Care," *Anesthesiology*, 47 (1977), 203–16.

Encyclopedia of Bioethics, 1978 ed., s.v. "Rationing of Medical Treatment," by James F. Childress.

ENTHOVEN, ALAIN C. "The Competition Strategy: Status and Prospects," *The New England Journal of Medicine*, 304 (1981), 109–12.

HIATT, HOWARD H., "Protecting the Medical Commons: Who is Responsible?" *The New England Journal of Medicine*, 293 (1975), 235–41.

VLADECK, BRUCE C., "The Market vs. Regulation: The Case for Regulation," *Milbank Memorial Fund Quarterly*, 59 (1981), 209–23.

WEINER, STEPHEN M., "On Public Values and Private Regulation: Some Reflections on Cost Containment Strategies," *Milbank Memorial Fund Quarterly*, 59 (1981), 269–96.

WIENER, CAROLYN, ET AL., "What Price Chronic Illness?" *Society* (January/February 1982), 22–30.

Health and Social Problems

BERMAN, DANIEL M., *Death on the Job: Occupational Health and Safety Struggles in the United States*. New York: Monthly Review Press, 1978.

BUTLER, LEWIS, ET AL., *Low Income and Illness: An Analysis of National Health Policy and the Poor*. Health Policy Program Discussion Paper, San Francisco, University of California School of Medicine, February 1980.

BUTLER, ROBERT N., *Why Survive? Being Old in America*. New York: Harper & Row Publishers, Inc., 1975.

DOWD, JAMES J., *Stratification among the Aged*. Monterey, Calif.: Brooks/Cole Publishing Co., 1980.

EISDORFER, CARL, "Care of the Aged: The Barriers of Tradition," *Annals of Internal Medicine*, 94 (1981), 256–60.

FORMAN, PAT, "Scandal at Gauley Bridge," *Health/PAC Bulletin*, no. 79 (November/December 1977), 9–16.

JOHNSON, DOUGLAS, "Abuse of the Elderly," *Nurse Practitioner* (January/February 1981), 29.

KAPLAN, JEROME, "In Search of Policies for Care of the Aged," in *Ethics of Health Care: Papers on the Conference on Health Care and Changing Values, November 27–29, 1973*, ed. Laurence R. Tancredi, pp. 281–303. Washington, D.C.: National Academy of Science, 1974.

LORION, RAYMOND P., "Patient and Therapist Variables in the Treatment of Low-Income Patients," *Psychological Bulletin*, 81 (1974), 344–54.

ORWELL, GEORGE, "How the Poor Die," in *Shooting an Elephant and Other Essays*, pp. 19–31. New York: Harcourt Brace Jovanovich, Inc., 1950.

SLOAN, PATRICIA E., "Commitment to Equality: A View of Early Black Nursing Schools," in *Historical Studies in Nursing*, ed. M. Louise Fitzpatrick, pp. 68–85. New York: Teachers College Press, 1978.

Patient Selection for Scarce Resources

BASSON, M.D., "Choosing among Candidates for Scarce Medical Resources," *Journal of Medicine and Philosophy*, 4 (1979), 313.

BEECHER, HENRY K., "Scarce Resources and Medical Advancement," in *Experimentation with Human Subjects,* ed. Paul A. Freund, pp. 66–104. New York: George Braziller, Inc., 1970.

CHILDRESS, JAMES F., "Who Shall Live When Not All Can Live?" *Soundings,* 3 (1970), 339–55.

GOROVITZ, SAMUEL, "Ethics and the Allocation of Medical Resources," *Medical Research Engineering,* 5 (1966), 5.

RESCHER, NICHOLAS, "The Allocation of Exotic Medical Lifesaving Therapy," *Ethics,* 79 (1969), 173–86.

CHAPTER 18

Making
Hard Choices

Case discussions in this text have an open structure. Rarely have definite conclusions been drawn as to the right choice. Instead, relevant principles and values were discussed, clinical details were highlighted, worst options were ruled out, and questions were opened. This approach is consistent with the limited power of ethical inquiry.[1] Only on the easy cases can definite answers be given. To resolve the hard cases, one has to supplement ethical considerations with political, social, and historical interpretations of events and personal commitments. In the end, one has to make a personal judgment appropriate to the problem at hand. Ethical theory and reflection end in choice.

This chapter discusses two common sources of hard choices. What should nurses do who find they are working with someone who is incompetent or abusing patients? And, should nurses participate in such collective job actions as strikes?

Dealing with Medical Incompetence

There is an old joke that beds are dangerous because so many people die in them. From that point of view, hospital beds are particularly dangerous. In 1964, a study showed that 20 percent of patients on the wards of a teaching hospital suffered iatrogenic harm.[2] *Iatrogenic* illness is that caused by medical, nursing, or other health care interventions. In a more recent study reported in 1981, the combined medical, nursing, and other health care error rate was 36 percent. Nine percent of these errors were life threatening, and 2 percent killed patients (or .7 percent of all

---

[1]Ethics could be taken to mean "everything we need to consider in order to make a decision," but then the subject of ethics would have no boundaries.

[2]Elihu M. Schimmel, "The Hazards of Hospitalization," *Annals of Internal Medicine*, 60 (1964), 100–110.

patients admitted). This is a *conservative* estimate; if there was any doubt about the medical source of an untoward event, it was not counted. The authors attributed the 150 percent increase in errors since 1964 to increasingly complex medical technology.[3] A recent study of surgical errors with adverse outcomes found fewer errors but worse consequences. It found a 1 percent error rate, an overall mortality rate of 55 percent, average excess hospital costs of $40,000 per client, and forty days average excess hospitalization.[4] Another recent study found nearly a threefold increase in mortality among hospital patients who acquired nosocomial urinary-tract infections.[5]

These studies do not show that clients should stay out of the hospital; clients may have been even worse off at home. Instead, the studies show that coping with errors is an everyday part of hospital work. What should nurses do when they detect mistakes in their own or others' work? What is the responsibility and moral liability of nurses for the wrongdoing of others with whom they work? Physicians, nurses, other health care staff, and clients all make mistakes. Mistakes are normal and accepted phenomena of daily life; we do not regard all of them as being culpable or blameworthy. Sorting out blameworthy from acceptable errors is an important problem, but we will only touch on it in passing here (see also p. 82). Where errors are culpable, the ANA "Code for Nurses" gives a straightforward though partial answer to the question of professional responsibility. It states unequivocally:

> Point 3: The nurse acts to safeguard the client and the public when health care and safety are affected by incompetent, unethical, or illegal practice of any person. (ANA, 1976)[6]

It is unprofessional, therefore, to cooperate in acts which in the nurse's judgment unethically impose risks on patients. But this is merely the beginning of the inquiry. Is it morally wrong to fail to respond in accordance with Point 3 of the code? What practical recourse does a nurse have when culpably incompetent practice occurs? To consider the issue, let us look at an extreme case, not the excusable mistakes of a competent clinician, but the chronic mistakes of an incompetent one. The following incident took place in the late 1970s in a medium-sized private teaching hospital.

> CASE EXAMPLE. Dr. Hyde performed four surgeries at Mt. Citadel Hospital during a four-month period. All four were for slowly growing cancers in debilitated elderly patients. All four patients died slow, painful deaths in the Intensive Care Unit. There was a consensus among ICU nurses and residents that Dr. Hyde performed the surgeries for marginal indications; that he performed them badly, and that he atrociously mismanaged their follow-up

[3]Knight Steel et al., "Iatrogenic Illness on a General Medical Service at a University Hospital," *The New England Journal of Medicine,* 304 (1981), 638–42.

[4]Nathan P. Couch et al., "The High Cost of Low-Frequency Events: The Anatomy and Economics of Surgical Mishaps," *The New England Journal of Medicine,* 304 (1981), 634–37.

[5]Richard Platt et al., "Mortality Associated with Nosocomial Urinary-Tract Infection," *The New England Journal of Medicine,* 307 (1982), 637–42.

[6]The AMA code has a similar provision. "A physician should deal honestly with patients and colleagues, and strive to expose those physicians deficient in character or competence, or who engage in fraud or deception" (AMA, 1980).

care in the unit. Said Nurse Robin, "He wrote orders that were just ridiculous."

The ICU nurses did their best to see that each of Dr. Hyde's patients got the best care possible under the circumstances. They carried out the instructions of residents as quickly as possible and delayed filling Dr. Hyde's less competent instructions.

Nurses did not complain through hospital channels. In their opinion, the head nurse and the medical director were weak and would not help. The residents concurred in this judgment and complained through very indirect channels. Staff were not yet sure whose side the new Director of Nursing was on. Moreover, seeing her would require going over the head nurse's head.

They hesitated to use any "outside" channels, not because they feared losing their jobs, but because they feared a possible libel suit. When they looked at the case records, they could not find any obvious defects in them. Only the patients were in bad shape.

They did not discuss their concerns with Dr. Hyde because they hated him. Everybody hated him. Besides, they were sure that he knew he was incompetent, and his air of theatrical insincerity discouraged frank discussion.

They did not discuss it with any of the clients' families. Only Mr. Apple had family actively involved in his care. His sister suspected that Dr. Hyde was not managing the case well. The nurses stood by when she asked Dr. Hyde how Mr. Apple was doing. "He's doing fine," said Dr. Hyde.

The sister asked Ms. Robin privately, "Why is he still in a coma?" "What could I say?" commented Ms. Robin months later, "The patient has rotted for a month. It is too late to say, 'Somebody blew it.' I am just a nurse. All I know is that his patients don't do well. At this point, confidence in the doctor was about all the health care we had to offer."

The nursing staff hoped that Mr. Apple's sister would ask if a second opinion was needed. When they induced her to ask this, the nurses said, "YES!" The sister consulted the Director of Surgery at the hospital, an excellent surgeon whom the nurses regarded as beyond reproach. But he whitewashed the case in his report to the sister and in his notes in the record. No problems were mentioned about the indications for surgery, surgery itself, or postsurgical management. Nurse Robin said, "I felt physically ill."

The staff nurses created rituals to ease their tension. When Dr. Hyde's four patients filled half the ICU beds and Mr. Apple's sister came to visit, the staff lined up all four patients in exactly the same position with their respirator hoses in exactly parallel alignment. They labeled this part of the ICU "The Dr. Hyde Memorial Isolation Room." When the last patient died, Ms. Robin cowled herself in a sheet like a nun "to escort Mr. Apple to his Heavenly Rest."

Before Dr. Hyde got to a fifth patient, a quiet, informal agreement was reached between him and the Chief of Surgery: He was not to perform any surgeries at Mt. Citadel without first consulting with the Chief, and all surgery had to be performed with another surgeon.

A month after Mr. Apple died, Ms. Robin ran into his sister on the street. She asked again what the nurses thought of Dr. Hyde. Ms. Robin still could not bring herself to say anything critical. That she never talked openly with his sister remains for her one of the most painful doubts about her own actions. Ms. Robin asks, "What do you do when you know what you have no right to know?"[7]

Cases like these are extremely painful and complex. There are three questions that we should ask about it. First, what was Ms. Robin's role-responsibility to say something to her client or do something about the problem? Second, what courses of action were available to her? And third, did she really have a choice?

There are many things she rightly considered in ascertaining her obligation; some of the most immediate are the following:

WAS SHE SURE THE DOCTOR WAS INCOMPETENT?   Absolute certainty that there is a problem is not required. Clinicians always work under conditions of uncertainty. The unit might have had a false picture of Dr. Hyde, but since his orders appeared "ridiculous" to everyone, surely there was evidence adequate to raise the issue.

WAS THIS AN ISSUE OF PROTECTING THE PATIENT?   The ANA Code is clear that protection is owed to the patient, but in this case the primary harm had already been done. Although it was too late to protect Mr. Apple from surgery, further harm to him might have been prevented by discussing the issue with his sister. After he was dead, or nearly dead, protecting him was no longer the issue; instead, the issue became one of protecting future patients.

WOULD THE PATIENT OR THE FAMILY LOSE FAITH IN HEALTH CARE?   We don't know what would have happened. The sister might have doubted Ms. Robin instead of Dr. Hyde, but her confidence in him was already weak. Moreover, health care should not be an article of faith. Admitting errors to clients can help them better understand what is happening when unexpected side effects occur. In addition, patients may appreciate the trust shown them by frankness.

DOES THE PATIENT WANT TO KNOW?   If the patient asks, then there is good reason to think the patient wants to know. In this case, Mr. Apple's sister, who can be regarded as an ethically legitimate proxy for him, asked. If clients do not ask, matters are less clear. Some hold that clients' views should prevail, and so we should not challenge those who choose incompetent clinicians. Clients know more about their needs than we do as observers, and so they may be obtaining rewards from seemingly bad practice that we overlook.

This position will not do, however. It is the responsibility of a profession to make judgments about its practitioners. Dr. Hyde may have had a prepossessing bedside manner, but the client was also entitled to a professional judgment of his surgical competence. Assessing basic competencies of practitioners is not like trying to judge acupuncturists or faith healers, who claim a different *kind* of competence. Ms. Robin is a nurse; Dr. Hyde is a physician. Although they are not members of the same profession, their professions overlap, and so she had the expertise needed to make judgments about his competence.

WOULD DISCLOSURE EXPOSE MS. ROBIN TO PERSONAL RISKS?   Every health professional who thinks of whistle blowing rightly worries about retaliation. Ms. Robin might have been seen as a troublemaker and thereby have lost the confidence and cooperation of other nurses and physicians. Moreover, patients are

---

[7]I chose a nurse–doctor problem because such problems are so often discussed by nurses. I am unsure whether coping with the incompetence of nurses is mentioned less often because it is an easier or a more difficult problem for nurses.

natural hostages for retaliation. A physician may react to a request for a second opinion by dropping the patient or creating difficulties with a subsequent patient. Nurses who blow the whistle are sometimes fired—never for blowing the whistle, but for some unrelated infraction of the rules. Would this have happened in this case? We just don't know.

ARE THERE ANY CONFLICTING OBLIGATIONS? Hospital workers owe some loyalty to each other, as indicated in Chapter 9. But in this case, Ms. Robin owed Dr. Hyde no *personal* loyalty; indeed, she hated him, and the *professional* loyalty she owed him is explicitly limited by the ANA "Code for Nurses." She had a much stronger relationship with Mr. Apple's sister and felt some loyalty to the comatose Mr. Apple. Discussing the matter with the client's sister might also have helped to break down the professional–patient barrier we have identified as an obstacle to ethical decision making (see Chapter 14).

WERE HER MOTIVES PURE? Was Ms. Robin displacing on Dr. Hyde her justifiable hostility toward physicians in general or her own guilt feelings about the inadequacies of Mt. Citadel Intensive Care? Did her decision not to disclose arise mainly from her desire to avoid trouble and protect herself? This kind of self-knowledge is acquired only through time and by looking at one's other choices. Do I admit my *own* errors? Am I complaining about everything?

There is the beginning here of a case for disclosure. Mr, Apple's sister asked for information; Ms. Robin had information on which she was pretty sure. Protecting the client was at issue. Countervailing considerations were present, but they were not as strong in this case as in many others.

Cooperation in Wrongdoing

Hospitals present a chiaroscuro-like pattern of beneficial and harmful practices. From one point of view, to labor in the hospital is to labor in the pits. Like Eugene O'Neill's Hairy Ape (the coal stoker at the ship's furnaces below deck),[8] nurses, respiratory therapists, and residents stoke the furnaces of suffering under an unceasing fluorescent glare, along clattering halls coated not in soot, but painted pale green, white, or pink. Attendings, like wealthy passengers on the catwalk above, stop briefly to marvel at the spectacle and depart to their private dining room. From another point of view, this picture is outrageously distorted. Health care is noble and beautiful. The health care team heals the sick and succors the dying. Intimate contact with human suffering elevates us. Medical techniques, although not perfected, are glowing marvels compared to dark remedies of the past. Health professionals express the most powerful tradition of humane ideals of any occupation.

Since urgent good and gruesome evil cohabit in the hospitals, nurses work in ambiguity and contradiction. Since they do both good and bad things to patients, nurses ask themselves whether the enterprise as a whole justifies continuing cooperation with the things that are in their judgment reprehensible. Since nurses are "hands on" in many procedures, the fact that someone else generally makes the decision to undertake a risky procedure does not relieve their feelings of complicity in wrongdoing.

[8]Eugene O'Neill, *Anna Christie; The Emperor Jones; The Hairy Ape* (New York: Random House, Inc., 1973).

Nurses feel guilt and real moral distress when they perform procedures that they feel are morally wrong and can find no way to avoid. Incompetent practice and "medically justified" pain (p. 223) are common causes of nurses' distress. Typical instances are:

1. An oncology nurse is assigned to perform a painful test on a child. The child is dying, and the nurse believes that the test is irrelevant to the child's welfare.
2. A nurse assists a medical resident who inserts a catheter into a deep vein. The resident has failed to insert it eight times and is now trying for the ninth time. The nurse believes that a more skilled physician should have taken over this painful task after the second or third try.
3. In the newborn intensive care unit, a nurse cares for a severely damaged infant who she feels in her heart cannot survive. She punctures his heel each day to take blood samples.
4. The nurse is tending a patient who is about to have surgery and has signed the consent forms for it. Yet the nurse can tell from the patient's conversation that the patient has no comprehension of the seriousness of the choice.
5. A surgeon fails to wash his hands before examining a patient in the ICU and ignores the nurse's reminder.[9]

These cases are more than failures to realize an ideal: They involve what nurses judge to be morally wrong. Nurses can thus be very critical of the hospitals in which they work. "I wonder if we should even work here. It seems like an immoral place to work," said one Coronary Care Unit nurse just before she quit her job. Francis J. Storlie reports similar remarks: "Politics, or catering to the doctors— that's what counts around here." "There is an overriding feeling of doing McDonald's nursing."[10] Staff nurses rarely undertake what they regard as questionable procedures on their own initiative or as team leaders. They usually find themselves involved in bad practice through cooperation with others. General considerations to keep in mind in setting limits on cooperation are these:

What is the seriousness of the harm involved? The more serious the danger posed to this patient or to future patients, the stronger the call to action. The practitioner causing the harm may be competent, incompetent, well meaning, or uncaring— these considerations are not as relevant as the amount of harm.

Does this happen often? The more chronic a problem is in one's institution, the more reason one has to address it. A case which is an instance of a more general problem gains in importance, since, whether noncooperation succeeds or not in a particular case, it can make a vivid statement about the more general problem.

[9]For case studies related to hospital infections, see Katherine Hill Chavigny and Ann Helm, "Ethical Dilemmas and the Practice of Infection Control," *Law, Medicine & Health Care* (September 1982), 168–70, 174. For rates of hand washing, see Richard K. Albert and Francis Condie, "Hand-Washing Patterns in Medical Intensive-Care Units," *The New England Journal of Medicine*, 304 (1981), 1465–66. In relation to patient contacts, nurses wash their hands about twice as often as physicians. But since nurses have the bulk of contact with patients, most unwashed contacts are with nurses. Respiratory therapists are *tops* at hand washing.

[10]Frances J. Storlie, "Burnout: The Elaboration of a Concept," *American Journal of Nursing*, 79 (1979), 2108.

Are there ways to prevent the harm or future occurrences of it? Refusing to participate in the care of a patient or speaking to the head nurse or supervisor may prevent an incident or lead to changes in the future. Even if there is no recourse, some acts are so wrong that one should not cooperate in them, whatever the consequences.

What is the nurse's role in causing the harm? One's liability increases as one becomes more closely involved in causing the harm. A nurse is morally and legally liable for administering a harmful medication, although the act is done on the instructions of a physician.[11] The nurse who cares for a patient after a questionable surgery is in a morally safer position than the nurse who prepares the patient for surgery.[12]

What is the nurse's attitude with regard to the harm? A nurse who wholeheartedly supports a questionable procedure is more actively responsible for it than a nurse who acts reluctantly.[13]

In brief, nurses are in general *accountable* for harmful practices in which they are involved, even though they do not themselves initiate them. As the profession becomes more autonomous, the responsibility of nurses for health practices increases. Thus, if health care continues to have problems, nurses will become responsible for them not merely as accomplices, but also as principal agents.

How to Proceed with Complaints

What should one do about the mistakes of other nurses and physicians? What should one do first? The ANA "Code for Nurses" is specific about what steps to take. First,

> . . . concern should be expressed to the person carrying out the questionable practice and attention called to the possible detrimental effects upon the client's welfare.

The next step, if needed, is "the responsible administrative person." Then,

> if indicated, the practice should then be reported to the appropriate authority within the institution, agency, or larger system.

---

[11]Helen Creighton, *Law Every Nurse Should Know*, 4th ed. (Philadelphia: W.B. Saunders Company, 1981), pp. 111, 117.

[12]In this and the next point, I reflect a distinction made in some Catholic ethics texts between *formal* and *material* cooperation. To cooperate in evil *formally* is either to choose or to desire the evil act itself, or to cooperate knowingly in actions that are a means to that evil act. To cooperate *materially* is to be involved neither as a means nor to wish for the evil outcome. I *formally* cooperate when I loan my sister my car when she asks me if she can use it to rob a bank. If she comes to me after the robbery and asks me to hide her, and this is the first I have heard of it, hiding her would only be *material* cooperation. Formal cooperation is morally more culpable than material cooperation. See Joseph B. McAllister, *Ethics: With Special Application to the Medical and Nursing Professions*, 2nd ed. (Philadelphia: W.B. Saunders Company, 1955), pp. 97–98.

[13]One cannot find permanent refuge in mental reservations, except under the most repressive conditions. Chronic reluctance eventually becomes bad faith and as morally problematic as wholehearted cooperation in evil.

The "Code" states that health care institutions should have

. . . an established mechanism for the reporting and handling of incompetent, unethical, or illegal practice within the employment setting so that such reporting can go through official channels and be done without fear of reprisal.

The "Code" also says that

local units of the professional association should be prepared to provide assistance . . .

Finally, if problems persist,

the problem should be reported to other appropriate authorities such as the practice committees of the appropriate professional organizations or the legally constituted bodies concerned with licensing of specific categories of health workers or professional practitioners.[14]

One of the problems is that there are *many* ways one can proceed. And there are more ways than the ANA mentions. One can speak to the client or the client's family. One can go the the courts, the newspapers, or one's union.

Virtually all hospitals have established a mechanism for filing *incident reports*. Nurses and other staff are expected to file these reports on every untoward incident—a bad drug reaction, a fall or spill, a drunken practitioner—whether or not such incidents are blameworthy. Hospitals like to have these as a documentary basis should any legal action occur, and they also use them to assess and modify procedures. Although staff and head nurses sometimes discuss them, they are primarily designed as administrative instruments.[15]

Coping with bad *medical* practice can be an extremely delicate matter. Not only are nurses relatively powerless in relation to physicians in these matters, but also physicians regard the problem of bad medical practice as one of extreme delicacy. Most procedures are complex and mined with legal pitfalls.[16]

In California, the Board of Medical Quality Assurance oversees licensure and discipline of physicians. It has a procedure by which *anyone* can make a complaint simply by filing a form. The Board will always respond with an investigation. The Civil Code

. . . provides nearly absolute immunity for persons who communicate ". . . information . . . to any hospital, hospital medical staff, professional society, medical or dental school, professional licensing board or division, committee or panel of such licensing board, peer review committee, or underwriting committee . . . when such communication is intended to aid in the evaluation of the qualifications, fitness,

[14]All five quotes are from Point 3.2 of the American Nurses' Association "Code for Nurses" (1976).

[15]Physicians regularly practice the ritual of the Morbidity and Mortality Conference. In this conference, physicians confess their errors and discuss them openly and critically. This is a way of improving practice and displaying frankness, humility, and competence. See Charles L. Bosk, "Occupational Rituals in Patient Management," *The New England Journal of Medicine*, 303 (1980), 71–76. To the best of my knowledge, nurses have no similar protected, regular setting in which to discuss mistakes openly.

[16]William E. Mitchell, Jr., "How to Deal with Poor Medical Care," *Journal of the American Medical Association*, 236 (1976), 2875–77.

character, or insurability of a practitioner of the healing arts and does not represent as true any matter not reasonably believed to be true."[17]

In spite of these options, and in spite of written assurances of protection, many nurses view whistle blowing as a hazardous and ineffective venture.

"I don't know why I bother to fill this out," she complained. "I've worked in this unit for more than seven years, and in that time I've filed exactly three reports about medical practice. Nothing is ever done. . . . You document what you observed, and you darn well better have proof. You know it doesn't matter when a doctor is complaining about a nurse. No one asks for proof of what he says, but if I complain about a physician's practice, I'm just not taken seriously. . . . Nothing is ever done."[18]

Are nurses right in this judgment? In spite of these problems, 80 percent of respondents to an *R.N.* survey reported that they had been able to take effective action in response to medical errors.[19] Using procedures more widely and actively may also strengthen them. The only way to find out whether they work is to use these mechanisms, and where they fail, to create new ones.

Conscientious Objection

The forms of recourse above follow established channels. Another form of recourse is simply to refuse to cooperate with a procedure even if ordered to do it. The model for refusal is noncooperation with the law, where it is called *conscientious objection* or *civil disobedience*. Refusals to cooperate in employment situations are similar to civil disobedience where noncooperation violates the employer's policies or one's conditions of employment and where protest is based on issues of conscience.

Civil disobedience in order to make a public point about a moral issue has been prominent in the birth control movement. Emma Goldman, Van Kleek Allison, Margaret Sanger, and Ethel Byrne all violated laws in the early part of the century in order to marshal support for the legalization of contraception. While she was in jail, Margaret Sanger tried to distribute birth control information among other prisoners.[20]

The issue of conscientious objection has arisen recently in connection with abortion. Although abortions are legal, some nurses object to them strongly on grounds of conscience. Nurses who object should not be required to cooperate with them, not because they might provide bad care, but because they should not be required to cooperate in what they regard as wrong. Thelma Schorr, for example, argues:

[17]California Medical Association and Board of Medical Quality Assurance, "Physician Responsibility . . . . A Joint Statement," January, 1980. This pamphlet quotes from California Civil Code, sec. 43.8.

[18]Storlie, "Burnout," p. 2110.

[19]Linda Stanley, "Dangerous Doctors: What to Do When the M.D. Is Wrong," *R.N.*, 42, 3 (March 1979), 25.

[20]*Encyclopedia of Bioethics*, 1978 ed., s.v. "Civil Disobedience in Health Services," by Edward H. Madden and Peter H. Hare.

There are many nurses who see an abortion as an unconscionable act, and certainly they should never be placed in the position of having to nurse patients who have chosen to have their pregnancies terminated. Just as a patient's freedom to choose must be respected, so must a nurse's. But it is also that nurse's responsibility to protect both the patient's freedom and her own by refusing to work in a situation which she finds morally offensive.[21]

Institutions should make arrangements to make conscientious noncooperation possible. For example, the International Labour Conference recommended:

Nursing personnel should be able to claim exemption from performing specific duties, without being penalized, where performances would conflict with their religious, moral, or ethical convictions and where they inform their supervisor in good time of their objection so as to allow the necessary alternative arrangements to be made to ensure that essential nursing care of patients is not affected.[22]

Analogously, bad nursing and medical practice can also be seen as issues of conscience or integrity; if not of private conscience, then at least of professional conscience.[23] It is not at all unusual for nurses to refuse to carry out questionable orders by physicians. Physicians perform the procedure in question themselves without much conflict. A nurse may refuse to work on a unit until a mishandled case is resolved. This may galvanize the nurses and physicians who remain into holding the meetings needed to get the problem resolved promptly.

If one felt strongly about an issue, one could go further. A nurse could say "Anyone who comes near this patient does so at his or her peril," and physically prevent procedures from being done. In 1974, the Feminist Women's Health Center in Los Angeles stole the equipment from a substandard abortion clinic in order to prevent its operation.[24] In another case, aides at a nursing home sued their employers because supervisors were ordering aides to engage in abusive procedures, such as disciplining patients with cold showers.

Nurses and physicians have found highly varied ways with which to cope with conflicts between their standards of practice and the rules under which their work is conducted. For example, when it was the law in California that newborn babies' eyes must be washed with silver nitrate as a prophylactic against gonorrhea, this was regarded by clinicians as unnecessary in many cases. When parents refused to consent to the procedure, newborn units varied in their reactions. One unit insisted on performing the procedure because it was required by law. If they had to, they signed and filed the consent forms themselves. In another unit, they simply forgot about it. In another, they would do it and not tell the parents. In another, they documented doing the procedure and didn't do it. In another, they made up a very light wash of silver nitrate and washed it out very quickly. This variety of reactions

[21]Thelma Schorr, "Issues of Conscience," *American Journal of Nursing,* 72 (1972), 61.

[22]International Labour Conference, "Text of the Recommendation Concerning Employment and Conditions of Work and Life of Nursing Personnel, Submitted by the Drafting Committee," *Provisional Record,* 36th sess., Geneva, 1977, p. 21B/5.

[23]For an excellent analysis of integrity in nursing, see Christine Mitchell, "Integrity in Interprofessional Relationships," in *Responsibility in Health Care,* ed. George J. Agich (Dordrecht, Holland: D. Reidel Publishing Company, 1982).

[24]Madden and Hare, "Civil Disobedience," p. 160.

indicates the depth and difficulty of finding ways to proceed when one is morally distressed and facing institutional constraints.

Is There Really a Choice?

Many of the practices that we regret in institutions appear to us as constraints—like natural laws that limit our actions. There are many things we just can't do—for example, make a hospital committee listen to an unwelcome complaint. In some conceivable sense of *can*, perhaps, one can make it listen, but to do so would require nearly impossible quantities of energy and involve great personal risks or violations of principles. Indeed, there are really two very different kinds of limits on our ability to choose: There are limits of physical and psychological possibility, and limits of conventions and ethics.

An important viewpoint on human possibility is that of Jean Paul Sartre.[25] He believed that we are completely free to choose, no matter what circumstances we are in. He emphasized that what ethics says one can and cannot do does not exhaust the possibilities open to one. Ethics, for example, says that we *should* not force a committee to listen to us by waving a gun at its members, but we still *can* force it to do so.

Sartre believed that most of us find this freedom awesome and frightening. It makes us responsible for everything that goes on around us. So we try to escape this freedom. We pretend to ourselves that we are forced to do things when we are not. When a nurse, for example, tells a patient "You must do this because the doctor ordered it," both the nurse and patient pretend that they must act because of the doctor's order, but in fact either one could make another choice.

We may try to use ethics to escape this freedom. A nurse who asks a bioethicist "What should I do?" may be told that ethics does not provide a definite answer. Instead of rejoicing that ethics leaves room for choice, the nurse regrets that no rule or principle forces a definite course of action. Although Sartre saw this regret as natural, he offered no comfort for it. He believed that there is no significant morality except that of honest choice and personal responsibility.

This is one of the deeper meanings of *accountability*.[26] Nurses who work in hospitals are accountable for their choices because they choose to work in them and make choices in that setting when they could be making other choices. Many nurses leave nursing precisely because they morally reject hospital working conditions, and thus burnout can be a moral statement.[27] Since the good that nurses do in hospitals must also be credited to their account, it is a legitimate choice to stay in the

[25]For a brief account of Sartre's views, see "Existentialism Is a Humanism," in *Existentialism from Dostoevsky to Sartre,* ed. Walter Kaufmann (Cleveland: The World Publishing Company, 1956), pp. 287–311.

[26]Sally Gadow, "Existential Advocacy: Philosophical Foundation of Nursing," in *Nursing: Images and Ideals: Opening Dialogue with the Humanities,* eds. Stuart Spicker and Sally Gadow (New York: Springer Publishing Co., Inc., 1980).

[27]Ann M. McElroy, "Burnout—A Review of the Literature with Application to Cancer Nursing," *Cancer Nursing* (June 1982), 211–17; Frances J. Storlie, "Burnout: The Elaboration of a Concept," *American Journal of Nursing,* 79 (1979), 2108–11; and Ayala Pines and Christina Maslach, "Characteristics of Staff Burnout in Mental Health Settings," *Hospital & Community Psychiatry,* 29 (1978), 233–37.

hospital, to accomplish as much as one can there, and to struggle for change. What Sartre wants to emphasize is that such courses of action represent *choices,* not necessities. In remaining in the hospital setting, nurses thereby become responsible for complicity in wrongs done there.

Another point of view emphasizes the limits on individuals set by ethical claims of institutions. Immanuel Kant gives expression to this position:

> Many affairs which are conducted in the interest of the community require a certain mechanism through which some members of the community must passively conduct themselves with artificial unanimity, so that the government may direct them to public ends, or at least prevent them from destroying those ends.[28]

The government is not the only institution that demands "artificial unanimity." Any large, complex enterprise requires the smooth cooperation of many persons to accomplish its ends. If the hospital were to become the site of daily discussions on the aims, goals, and morality of health care, there would be little time left for work. It is difficult for us to reconcile our conception of ourselves as autonomous agents with the need of major productive endeavors for orderly cooperation.

A basic choice is forced on those who work in hospitals by the existence of prevalent and systematic problems in health care. If one fails to resist exploitation, incompetence, and corrupt practices, one becomes responsible for them. If one resists them, one enters into conflict with conventional conceptions of behavior for employees and thereby risks reprisals. One has to choose between complicity and self-sacrifice, or enter the uncomfortable middle ground of irony. Ethics does not give a clear answer as to which one must choose. Instead, one is free to move in the direction of the kind of world one personally desires to create.

Reviewing the Case

These brief reflections do not produce, even in retrospect, a definite course of action for Nurse Robin to have pursued in regard to Dr. Hyde. Yet they help to clarify the moral problems created by the case and underline the considerations relevant to making a decision.

To review the case in terms of the discussion; on one hand, the harm Dr. Hyde was doing was serious and recurrent. But on the other hand, Ms. Robin was for the most part indirectly involved in it. Her main direct involvement was to carry out Dr. Hyde's instructions for Mr. Apple's postoperative care. On one hand, it is a standard professional responsibility for nurses to protect patients from harm due to incompetence. But on the other, Ms. Robin also had less well defined responsibilities to future patients. And on one hand, the simpler and less dramatic remedies prescribed by the ANA code looked unpromising. But on the other, she could have taken less standard measures if professional conscience demanded it. Ms. Robin might have chosen to circumvent the head nurse and go directly to the new Director of Nursing, refuse to work on the unit until the problem was solved, speak privately with Mr. Apple's sister, or inform the Medical Director of the unit that she intended to speak with the family unless something were done about Dr. Hyde.

[28]Immanuel Kant, "What Is Enlightenment," in *Foundations of the Metaphysics of Morals and What Is Enlightenment,* trans. Lewis White Beck (Indianapolis: The Bobbs-Merrill Co., Inc., 1959), p. 87.

These more forceful steps were shrouded by their uncertain impact and personal risk. It is understandable that she did not consider undertaking any of them to be a light matter. The liability Ms. Robin incurred should be placed in the context of collective responsibility. She did less than she might have in a context where others habitually did less than they could and where institutional lacunae made remedies difficult. The unavailability of simple remedies was the result of collective actions and omissions attributable to the hospital and the health professions.

Speaking to Mr. Apple's sister would have had an uncertain impact on Dr. Hyde's future practice, but there was still something clearly to be gained from approaching her. Nurse Robin might have given the family a clearer opportunity to seek legal redress for malpractice, an action which appears on its face justified. The least strong reason for not answering the sister's questions was probably the most powerful cause for withholding information: There is sometimes a deep gulf between professionals and lay persons that resembles the tension between separate cultures. More reasonable considerations for not answering the sister's questions may have included tacit acceptance of responsibility as a hospital employee not to foster suits against it, rejection of malpractice as a sound mode of professional discipline, or general distaste for retribution.

Doubt about what direction to move in is best resolved by considering what sort of health care delivery system Ms. Robin would like to see created in the long run. Would she like to see the separation between professionals and patients fostered, or would she like to see patients have more information about and control over their care? Whatever the actual consequences of her action might have been, speaking to the sister could have performed a symbolic function toward this end. If she aspired to a more open health care system, then speaking to Mr. Apple's sister was certainly justified.

The only question remains whether it would have been heroic to do so or not (see pp. 214–16). The personal risks Ms. Robin might have exposed herself to by other choices are inestimable, since none of these roads were taken. We can only judge that her actual course of action was not heroic. Although Ms. Robin later regretted her inaction, she and other staff apparently did something about the problem that was partially successful. Dr. Hyde's practices were brought to the attention of the Chief of Surgery, and although he was not willing to act for the record, he restricted Dr. Hyde's activities at Mt. Citadel Hospital.

The case is a good example of a class of cases common in the study of ethics in health care. It is sufficiently complex that sorting out the ethical considerations is itself an interesting and thought-provoking task, and coming to a judgment requires appeal to at least three different kinds of considerations. (1) Relatively concrete events in the case play a crucial role in giving direction to final judgments about the case. For example, that Mr. Apple's sister asked more than once for information rules out a host of considerations about the nurse's responsibility to manage information for patients and their families. (2) What might be called "political" considerations—the nurse's long-run hopes for the structure of health care delivery—provide specific commitments needed to resolve uncertainty about consequences and ethical principles. (3) General philosophical considerations help us to identify the ethical issues and to appreciate their generality, but general philosophical questions do not have to be resolved in order to make a decision with regard to the case. For example, the question of balancing self-interest against the interest of others, although relevant to understanding the case, does not have to be answered to make a judgment. Indeed, the more specific responsibilities of professionals for patients provide much clearer direction, and even these falter before the realities of the working world.

Philosophical principles do not so much provide a resolution to problems like these as they help us to appreciate the significance of a resolution. Cases of this kind are valuable to the study of ethics partly because they help us to understand philosophical principles more concretely and to indicate what issues philosophers should address. The appropriate role of philosophy in such cases is not *application* of ethical theory to cases, as suggested by the common ascription of the rubric "applied ethics" to the study of ethics in health care.[29] Instead, such cases provide important information and direction for the continuing growth and development of philosophical theory.

Strikes and Other Collective Actions

Individual nurses depend on institutional support in order to do their jobs well (pp. 82–83). When hospitals deliver poor health care and exploit patients and staff, they threaten the competence of individual nurses. Individual competence is thus a collective problem. Similarly, our concept of individual responsibility makes us individually responsible for cooperation in the acts of those around us. The converse of this is that those who work with us are responsible for their cooperation in our individual actions. If an incompetent practitioner works among us, we all become responsible for that practitioner's actions. Thus, individual responsibility quickly becomes group or collective responsibility.

Since individual competence and responsibility are closely related to collective responsibility, it is justifiable to consider collective actions in order to cope with hospital problems. Such actions reflect loyalty (pp. 118–19) among professionals and workers and are more powerful than individual actions. Hospitals, corporations, nonprofit health care institutions, pharmaceutical corporations, and the like are forms of collective organizations which manage work and production. They have no more legitimacy than our acceptance of them creates. They are no more legitimate or important than unions, professional organizations, or other ways of allocating work and rewards that we might devise. The study of ethics need not focus merely on the conduct of individuals in institutions. It can also look at the structure of institutions from a moral point of view. The ethicist asks, Should professional associations and unions exercise power to improve health care? The answer is of course yes, and much can be done.

Stratification and complex division of labor are prominent features of health care institutions. Specialties, professions, and occupations abound, and each group vies for status against others. Unions and professional organizations compete with each other to represent nurses, workers, and professionals. Meanwhile, corporate organizations increase their legal, financial, and administrative hold on the conduct of health care delivery through ever-growing corporate organization. Because of these obstacles, hospital employees can seldom organize widespread collective power around improving health care.

From the point of view of ethics, one hopes that employee organizations in

---

[29]See also, Art Caplan, "Can Applied Ethics Be Effective Health Care and Should It Strive to Be?" *Ethics*, 93, 2 (January 1983), 311–19.

health care will be able to develop enough power to prevent increased exploitation of workers, professionals, and clients by growing financial interests and fiscal crises in health care. And one hopes that employee organizations can exercise power in the congruent defense of *both* the self-interest of employees and the quality of patient care.

Professional organizations have traditionally fostered nursing education, research, and communication and supported the identity and status of their members. They have also protected the power of their members by restricting entry into the professions. Important from the point of view of ethics, professional organizations uphold ideals of good patient care, autonomy, and collegiality among practitioners. They have increased their activities in defense of practitioners by bargaining on their behalf and leading such job actions as strikes.

But they have defects. In giving support to status-seeking (pp. 32–33) and to professional identity, professional organizations have not cooperated strongly with other professions and occupations. The American Nurses' Association has not well represented the interests of LVNs and LPNs, for example, and the American Medical Association has done little to empower nurses. Indeed, it has tended to dominate nursing and other employee organizations.[30]

Historically, unions have more clearly recognized the need for broad unity to protect the welfare of workers, especially workers not protected by licensure and entry requirements. They have also been traditionally less embarrassed about using power overtly: slowdowns, strikes, negotiations, grievance procedures, arbitration, picket lines, and cooperation with other unions during conflicts. However, unions also have defects. In the United States, unions have tended to focus largely on wages, benefits, and job security for workers. Like some hospitals, large unions may become bureaucratic and their leadership alienated from workers. Few major U.S. unions have clearly tackled the problems of autonomy and democracy in the workplace or the ideals and meaning of work.[31] They seldom have codes of ethics. There is no reason in principle why professional organizations cannot cooperate more actively with other professional groups and unions. Nor is there any reason in principle that unions cannot articulate ideals of work more clearly and emphasize quality-of-care issues among their bargaining considerations.[32] Indeed, professions and unions each sometimes do both sorts of things.

Both physicians and nurses, in their historical mix of cooperation and conflict, play an important role in upholding standards of care. On one hand, it is important for nurses to weaken the power of physicians over nurses and their practice. On the other, it would be damaging for nurses to weaken the ability of physicians to uphold professional standards against the growing power of corporations in health care. Although many observations in this text are critical of physi-

[30]Committee on Nursing, "Medicine and Nursing in the 1970s: A Position Statement," *Journal of the American Medical Association*, 213 (1970), 1881–83; Beatrice J. Kalisch and Philip A. Kalisch, "An Analysis of the Sources of Physician-Nurse Conflict," and Mariann C. Lovell, "Daddy's Little Girl: The Lethal Effect of Paternalism in Nursing," in *Socialization, Sexism, and Stereotyping: Women's Issues in Nursing*, ed. Janet Muff (St. Louis: The C.V. Mosby Company, 1982); and Chapter 3, pp. 42–46.

[31]See for example Richard Sennett and Jonathon Cobb, *The Hidden Injuries of Class* (New York: Random House, Inc., 1972).

[32]Lily M. Hoffman, "Housestaff Activism: The Emergence of Patient-Care Demands," *Journal of Health Politics, Policy and Law*, 7 (1982), 421–39.

cians, and although I believe nurses have a central position of moral leadership in health care, I believe that nurses and physicians with similar ideals of health care practice can work most effectively together to reform health care.[33] Similarly, it may be necessary for LVNs and RNs to organize along separate lines to do different kinds of work. But it would be damaging to the interests of both to cross each other's picket lines. Needed, then, are organizations which represent the bulk of health care workers and which combine representing the interests of workers with raising the quality of care.

What about the welfare of patients during strikes? Is it ethical for a nurse to go on strike? Isn't a strike a matter of refusing to do work, and aren't patients vulnerable hostages who might be hurt or neglected in a strike? A strike could hurt patients, and that would violate the professional ethics of nursing. But it is not necessary that strikes do so. Much health care can be delayed. Indeed, some clients may even be better off during a strike.[34] During any strike, a union should plan to provide emergency and needed care for patients who might be harmed. Where supervisors and scabs continue to work, they can care for these needs, but those on strike should generally accept a responsibility to provide necessary health care.[35]

Moreover, patients and their organizations sometimes support strikes, especially those that are over quality-of-care issues. Exchanging support with patients' organizations can expand the unity of interest and welfare possible through collective organization. Patients are often members of unions and professional organizations themselves, just as nurses are sometimes patients.

Ethics and the Future of Nursing Practice

Bioethics came of age in a period of conflict and crisis in health care. Basic problems in the organization of health care delivery created many questions among practitioners about the ethics of their work. Moral uncertainties, distress, and dilemmas testified to the depth of reactions of nurses and other health professionals to this crisis. These moral problems call for two very different but closely related responses. On one hand, they call for better philosophical and intellectual analysis. They call for clearer consciousness of the problems, clearer statements of conflicting principles, and thorough efforts to analyze them reflectively. In this work, philosophers can be most helpful.

On the other hand, this approach is limited. Distinctions can only become so subtle before they become laughable. A choice in a dilemma may be painful, but it can be resolved for the moment by the toss of a coin as soundly as by a too nicely drawn distinction. Instead, we need to inquire why we are caught in these dilemmas at all. Why is there a conflict between loyalty to other professionals and to clients?

[33]Carol J. Peterson, "The New Nurse and the New Physician," *Annals of Internal Medicine*, 96 (1982), 374–75; and David Mechanic and Linda H. Aiken, "A Cooperative Agenda for Medicine and Nursing," *The New England Journal of Medicine*, 307 (1982), 747–50.

[34]Reduced death rates from decreased numbers of elective operations during a physicians' strike were noted by James J. James, "Impacts of the Medical Malpractice Slowdown in Los Angeles County: January 1976," *American Journal of Public Health*, 69 (1979), 437–43.

[35]James L. Muyskens, "Nurses' Collective Responsibility and the Strike Weapon," *Journal of Medicine and Philosophy*, 7 (1982), 101–12.

Why do lifesaving methods reduce the quality of life? Why do we do so little about prevention? Where does the doctor/nurse game (pp. 44–45) come from? What values are represented by standard health care techniques? We need to be conscious of the conditions which create ethical dilemmas and struggle to change them. The solution to moral problems is not limited to finding a new intellectual analysis; it includes improved modes of life and work. In this realm of nursing ethics, philosophers must follow the lead of nurses and the nursing profession.

Articulating moral principles and solutions to moral problems requires some care. If we use our ideas about ethics to set hard-edged and unrealistic ideals or if we use them to articulate principles meaninglessly distant from life, we only invite disillusionment. Such exercises may be valuable as exhortation or analysis, but they do not express what we think we *really* should do.[36] On the other hand, if we were so complacent in our ethical thinking as to endorse the world as it is, we would fail again at ethics. We know that the world is not as it should be.

The world will change; nursing practice and health care organizations will change; present dilemmas will pass and others come to the fore. Nurses are gaining in power and influence, and nursing is increasingly accepted as a profession. But this is taking place at a time when professions in health care are under attack from many directions. It is hard to guess what will result from this struggle. What we choose to say through our moral principles and solutions to problems is important to the struggle of nurses for power and recognition. The study of ethics should strengthen nurses, rather than limit or discourage them. At the same time, by supporting one direction more than another, ethics can make a goal more readily attainable by directing and focusing our energies toward it. Ethics should express what we hope for in what we sense is possible.

Nursing has been an important humanizing force in health care. Compassion for ill and dying patients, protection of vulnerable clients, health education, and skillful treatment of the sick are all basic human goods that express our idealism about the ability of human beings to care for each other. There are many forces that threaten our ability to express humane ideals in the world—economic inequality, scarce resources, burgeoning military weaponry, sexism, racism, and so on. By carrying on a tradition of humane ideals, nurses can be friends to both humanity and themselves. Ethics supports the power of nursing in its expression of this tradition.

Summary

Ethics is limited in its ability to tell us what to do, and so we still have to make hard choices. Hospital work is a source of hard choices for nurses. When nurses participate in procedures they believe to be wrong, they face the ethical problem of complicity in wrongdoing. Issues of complicity arise when nurses cooperate with incompetent medical practitioners. In such cases, possible harm to patients and the professional obligation to protect patients must be balanced against limited remedies available and possible retaliation against nurses. Despite institutional constraints, nurses have a variety of realistic alternatives and are responsible for the choices they make. To decide what to do, nurses can supplement ethical considerations with political and personal aspirations.

[36]Susan James, "The Duty to Relieve Suffering," *Ethics*, 93 (1982), 4–21.

Chronic difficulties in patient care may be approached collectively, for instance, by unions and professional organizations. Strikes can be morally acceptable ways of improving patient care, protecting working conditions of nurses, and maintaining adequate pay and benefits. But those on strike should take responsibility for providing care for patients in serious need. Collective actions should be directed toward both improving patient care and increasing cooperation among all those who provide health care. Nursing represents a tradition of humane ideals. The study of ethics supports the power of nurses to uphold this tradition.

FURTHER READINGS

Making Mistakes

GOROVITZ, SAMUEL, AND ALASDAIR MACINTYRE, "Toward a Theory of Medical Fallibility," *Journal of Medicine and Philosophy*, 1 (1976), 51–71.
HERBERT, V., "Medical, Legal and Ethical Considerations in the Use of Drugs Having Undesirable Side Effects," *American Journal of Clinical Nutrition*, 28 (1975), 555–60.
HOFLING, CHARLES K., ET AL., "An Experimental Study in Nurse-Physician Relationships," *Journal of Nervous and Mental Disease*, 143 (1966), 171–80.
KIRSCH, JONATHAN, "A Death at Kaiser Hospital," *California* (November 1982), 78–81, 164–75.
MCCULLOUGH, LAURENCE B., AND CHARLES E. CHRISTIANSON, "Ethical Dimensions of Diagnosis: A Case Study and Analysis," *Metamedicine*, 2 (1981), 121–35.

Complicity

FAGOTHEY, AUSTIN, *Right and Reason: Ethics in Theory and Practice*, pp. 280–84. St. Louis: The C.V. Mosby Company, 1963.
HILL, THOMAS E.,JR., "Symbolic Protest and Calculated Silence," *Philosophy and Public Affairs*, 9 (1979), 83–102.
LADD, JOHN, "The Ethics of Participation," in *Nomos XVI: Participation in Politics*, eds. J. Roland Pennock and John Chapman, pp. 98–125. New York: Lieber-Atherton, Inc., 1975.
MURPHY, JEFFRIE G., ED. *Civil Disobedience and Violence*. Belmont, Calif.: Wadsworth Publishing Co., Inc., 1971.
SAGAN, LEONARD A., AND ALBERT JONSEN, "Medical Ethics and Torture," *The New England Journal of Medicine*, 294 (1976), 1427–30.
THOREAU, HENRY D., "Civil Disobedience," in *Civil Disobedience: Theory and Practice*, ed. Hugo Adam Bedau, pp. 27–48. New York: The Bobbs-Merrill Co., Inc., 1969.

Handling Mistakes

ANDERSON, ROBERT M., ET AL., *Divided Loyalties: Whistle-Blowing at BART*. West Lafayette, Ind.: Purdue University, 1980.
BERMOSK, LORETTA SUE, AND RAYMOND J. CORSINI, EDS., *Critical Incidents in Nursing* (see especially Esther Blanc et al., "The Nurse Is a Drug Addict"; George J. Breen et al., "Toppling the Tyrant"; Maureen Brown et al., "A Difference of Opinion"; Sharon Gedan et al., "Questioning the Dose"; and Roberta F. Hirsch et al., "When No One Answers"). Philadelphia: W.B. Saunders Company, 1973.
BLAKE, BONNIE LOU KESSRO, "Quality Assurance: An Ethical Responsibility," *Supervisor Nurse*, 2, 2 (February 1981), 32.

CHAYET, NEIL L., AND THOMAS M. REARDON, "Trouble in the Medical Staff: A Practical Guide to Hospital Initiated Quality Assurance," *American Journal of Law and Medicine*, 7 (1981), 301–20.

FULTON, KATE, "Drug Abuse among Nurses: What Nursing Management Can Do," *Supervisor Nurse*, 12, 1 (January 1981), 18–20.

GREENLAW, JANE, "Communication Failure: Some Case Examples," *Law, Medicine & Health Care* (April 1982), 77–79.

———, "Malpractice Screening Panel: Do Nurses Have a Role?" *Nursing Law and Ethics*, 1, 7 (August/September 1980), 4–5.

———, "On Concealing Mistakes," *Nursing Law and Ethics*, 1, 8 (October 1980), 5–6.

———, "Reporting Incompetent Colleagues," Part 1, *Nursing Law and Ethics*, 1, 4 (February 1980); "Will I Be Sued for Defamation," Part 2, *Nursing Law and Ethics*, 1, 5 (May 1980).

GRISSUM, MARLENE, "How You Can Become a Risk-Taker and a Role-Breaker," *Nursing '76*, 6, 11 (November 1976), 89–98.

GUARRIELLO, DONNA LEE, "Nurses Don't Get Mad. They Get Even," *Medical Economics* (May 2, 1983), 67–70.

HULL, RICHARD T., "Blowing the Whistle While You Work," *Kansas Nurse*, 55, 11 (December 1980), 7.

ISLER, CHARLOTTE, "Six Mistakes That Could Land You in Jail," *R.N.*, 42, 2 (February 1979), 64–71.

LEWIS, RICHARD, "LPN Uncovers Medicaid Scheme," *American Medical News* (August 29, 1977), 13–14.

LIPMAN, MICHEL, "When Should a Nurse Blow the Whistle?" *R.N.*, 34, 10 (October 1971), 50–54.

"Nurses' Reports of MD's Sex Offenses Ignored," *American Operating Room Nursing Journal*, 30, 2 (August 1979), 307.

ORME, JUNE Y., AND ROSEMARY S. LINDBECK, "Nurse Participation in Medical Peer Review," *Nursing Outlook*, 22, 1 (January 1974), 27–30.

OWENS, ARTHUR, "Can a Hospital Sue You for a Nurse's Mistake?" *Medical Economics* (July 5, 1982), 66–69.

RAVEN-HANSEN, PETER, "Dos and Don'ts for Whistleblowers: Planning for Trouble," *Technology Review* (May 1980), 34–44.

REGAN, WILLIAM ANDREW, "How Do You Expose an Errant M.D.?—Very, Very Carefully!" *R.N.* (September 1978), 39–40.

REGARDIE, ARNOLD G., "If Unprofessional Conduct Is Charged by the California Board of Medical Quality Assurance," *Western Journal of Medicine*, 127 (1977), 438–41.

SCHWARTZ, WILLIAM B., AND NEIL K. KOMESAR, "Doctors, Damages and Deterrence: An Economic View of Medical Malpractice," *The New England Journal of Medicine*, 298 (1978), 1282–89.

SHOEMAKER, N. EUGENE, "My Battle with the Nursing Home That Barred Me," *Medical Economics* (September 14, 1981) 73–76.

WALTERS, KENNETH D., "Your Employee's Right to Blow the Whistle," in *Moral Issues in Business*, ed. Vincent Barry, pp. 166–75. Belmont, Calif.: Wadsworth Publishing Co., Inc. 1979.

WILEY, LOY, "Liability for Patient Death: Nine Nurses' Legal Ordeals," *Nursing 81*, 11, 9 (September 1981), 34.

WILLIAMS, K.J., "The Quandary of the Hospital Administrator in Dealing with the Medical Malpractice Problem," *Nebraska Law Review*, 55, 3 (1976), 401–16.

Nursing Power

AMERICAN NURSES' ASSOCIATION, *Power: Nursing's Challenge for Change*. Kansas City, Mo.: American Nurses' Association, 1979.

ASHLEY, JO ANN, "About Power in Nursing," *Nursing Outlook*, 21 (1973), 637–41.

BROOTEN, DOROTHY A., LAURA LUCIA HAYMAN, AND MARY DUFFIN NAYLOR, EDS., *Leadership for Change: A Guide for the Frustrated Nurse*. Philadelphia: J.B. Lippincott Company, 1978.

BULLOUGH, BONNIE, "The New Militancy in Nursing," *Nursing Forum*, 10 (1971), 273–88.

CANNINGS, KATHLEEN, AND WILLIAM LAZONICK, "The Development of the Nursing Labor Force in the United States: A Basic Analysis," *International Journal of Health Services*, 5 (1975), 185–215.

COHEN, HELEN A., *The Nurse's Quest for a Professional Identity*. Menlo Park, Calif.: Addison-Wesley Publishing Co., Inc., 1981.

DELOUGHERY, GRACE L., AND KRISTINE M. GEBBIE, *Political Dynamics: Impact on Nurses and Nursing*. St. Louis: The C.V. Mosby Company, 1975.

JACOX, ADA, "Collective Action and Control of Practice by Professionals," *Nursing Forum*, 10 (1971), 239–57.

KALISCH, BEATRICE J., AND PHILIP A. KALISCH, "A Discourse on the Politics of Nursing," *Journal of Nursing Administration*, 6, 3 (March/April 1976), 29–34.

KALISCH, BEATRICE J., "The Promise of Power," *Nursing Outlook*, 26, 1 (January 1978), 42–46.

LEMANN, NICHOLAS, "Let the Nurses Do It," in *The Nation's Health*, eds. Philip R. Lee, Nancy Brown, and Ida V.S.W. Red, pp. 218–23. San Francisco: Boyd & Fraser Publishing Co., 1981.

MAUKSCH, INGEBORG G., ED., "Control over Conditions of Practice," *Nursing Forum*, 10, 3 (1971), 229–332.

NATIONAL LEAGUE FOR NURSING, ED., *The Emergence of Nursing as a Political Force*. New York: National League for Nursing, 1979.

SEXTON, PATRICIA CAYO, *The New Nightingales: Hospital Workers, Unions, New Women's Issues*. New York: Enquiry Press, 1982.

SIDEL, VICTOR W., "Medical Ethics and Socio-Political Change," in *The Teaching of Medical Ethics*, eds., Robert M. Veatch, Willard Gaylin, and Councilman Morgan, pp. 29–37. Hastings-on-Hudson, N.Y.: Institute of Society, Ethics and the Life Sciences, 1973.

STORLIE, FRANCES J., "Power—Getting a Piece of the Action," *Nursing Management*, 13, 10 (October 1982), 15–18.

Strikes and Collective Actions

BADGLEY, ROBIN F., AND SAMUEL WOLFE, *Doctor's Strike*. New York: Lieber-Atherton Inc., 1967.

BELLIN, L.E., *The Nursing Home Strike: November 5–12, 1973, Mortality in Seven Struck Free-Standing Nursing Homes*. New York: New York City Department of Health, 1976.

BELMAR, R. AND VICTOR SIDEL, "An International Perspective on Strikes and Threatened Strikes by Physicians: The Case of Chile," in *Organization of Health Workers and Labor Conflict*, ed. Samuel Wolfe, Chap. 7. Farmingdale, N.Y.: Baywood Publishing Co., Inc., 1978.

CHANEY, PATRICIA S., "Protest," *Nursing '77*, 7, 2 (February 1977), 19–33.

COULTON, MARY R., "Labor Disputes: A Challenge to Nurse Staffing," *Journal of Nursing Administration*, 6, 4 (May 1976), 15–20.

CROSS, YVONNE, "Rogue Nurses: Striking," *Nursing Mirror*, 134, 9 (March 3, 1972), 12–13.

GAYNOR, DAVID, ET AL., "RN's Strike: Between the Lines," *Health/PAC Bulletin*, no. 60 (September/October 1974), 1–6, 10–14.

JARVIS, PETER, "Nursing Ethics of Withdrawing," *Nursing Mirror* (February 16, 1978), 30–31.

MILLER, MICHAEL H., "Nurse's Right to Strike," *Journal of Nursing Administration,* 5, 2 (February 1975), 35–39.

PHILLIPS, D., "San Francisco Nurses Strike," *Hospital Medical Staff* (October 1974), 13–20.

WERTHER, WILLIAM B., JR., AND CAROL A. LOCKHART, "Collective Action and Cooperation in the Health Professions," *Journal of Nursing Administration,* 7, 6 (July/August 1977), 13–19.

WOLFE, SAMUEL, ED., *Organization of Health Workers and Labor Conflict,* Chaps. 3 and 5. Farmingdale, N.Y.: Baywood Publishing Co., Inc., 1978.

Appendix:
Selected Documents

International Council of Nurses: Code for Nurses, 1973*

The fundamental responsibility of the nurse is fourfold: to promote health, to prevent illness, to restore health and to alleviate suffering.

The need for nursing is universal. Inherent in nursing is respect for life, dignity and rights of man. It is unrestricted by considerations of nationality, race, creed, colour, age, sex, politics or social status.

Nurses render health services to the individual, the family and the community and coordinate their services with those of related groups.

Nurses and People

The nurse's primary responsibility is to those people who require nursing care.

The nurse, in providing care, respects the beliefs, values and customs of the individual.

The nurse holds in confidence personal information and uses judgment in sharing this information.

Nurses and Practice

The nurse carries personal responsibility for nursing practice and for maintaining competence by continual learning.

The nurse maintains the highest standards of nursing care possible within the reality of a specific situation.

The nurse uses judgment in relation to individual competence when accepting and delegating responsibilities.

The nurse when acting in a professional capacity should at all times maintain standards of personal conduct that would reflect credit upon the profession.

*Reprinted with permission of the International Council of Nurses.

299

Nurses and Society

The nurse shares with other citizens the responsibility for initiating and supporting action to meet the health and social needs of the public.

Nurses and Co-Workers

The nurse sustains a cooperative relationship with co-workers in nursing and other fields.

The nurse takes appropriate action to safeguard the individual when his care is endangered by a co-worker or any other person.

Nurses and the Profession

The nurse plays the major role in determining and implementing desirable standards of nursing practice and nursing education.

The nurse is active in developing a core of professional knowledge.

The nurse, acting through the professional organization, participates in establishing and maintaining equitable social and economic working conditions in nursing.

American Nurses' Association: Code for Nurses, 1976*

Preamble

The *Code for Nurses* is based on belief about the nature of individuals, nursing, health, and society. Recipients and providers of nursing services are viewed as individuals and groups who possess basic rights and responsibilities, and whose values and circumstances command respect at all times. Nursing encompasses the promotion and restoration of health, the prevention of illness, and the alleviation of suffering. The statements of the *Code* and their interpretation provide guidance for conduct and relationships in carrying out nursing responsibilities consistent with the ethical obligations of the profession and quality in nursing care.

Point 1

The nurse provides services with respect for human dignity and the uniqueness of the client unrestricted by considerations of social or economic status, personal attributes, or the nature of health problems.

1.1 SELF-DETERMINATION OF CLIENTS. Whenever possible, clients should be fully involved in the planning and implementation of their own health care. Each client has the moral right to determine what will be done with his/her person; to be given the information

---

*Reprinted with the permission of the American Nurses' Association from *Code for Nurses with Interpretive Statements*, Kansas City: American Nurses' Association, 1976.

necessary for making informed judgments; to be told the possible effects of care; and to accept, refuse, or terminate treatment. These same rights apply to minors and others not legally qualified and must be respected to the fullest degree permissible under the law. The law in these areas may differ from state to state; each nurse has an obligation to be knowledgeable about and to protect and support the moral and legal rights to all clients under state laws and applicable federal laws, such as the 1974 Privacy Act.

The nurse must also recognize those situations in which individual rights to self-determination in health care may temporarily be altered for the common good. The many variables involved make it imperative that each case be considered with full awareness of the need to provide for informed judgments while preserving the rights of clients.

1.2 Social and Economic Status of Clients. The need for nursing care is universal, cutting across all national, ethnic, religious, cultural, political, and economic differences, as does nursing's responses to this fundamental need. Nursing care should be determined solely by human need, irrespective of background, circumstances, or other indices of individual social and economic status.

1.3 Personal Attributes of Clients. Age, sex, race, color, personality, or other personal attributes, as well as individual differences in background, customs, attitudes, and beliefs, influence nursing practice only insofar as they represent factors the nurse must understand, consider, and respect in tailoring care to personal needs and in maintaining the individual's self-respect and dignity. Consideration of individual value systems and life-styles should be included in the planning of health care for each client.

1.4 The Nature of Health Problems. The nurse's respect for the worth and dignity of the individual human being applies irrespective of the nature of the health problem. It is reflected in the care given the person who is disabled as well as the normal; the patient with the long-term illness as well as the one with the acute illness, or the recovering patient as well as the one who is terminally ill or dying. It extends to all who require the services of the nurse for the promotion of health, the prevention of illness, the restoration of health, and the alleviation of suffering.

The nurse's concern for human dignity and the provision of quality nursing care is not limited by personal attitudes or beliefs. If personally opposed to the delivery of care in a particular case because of the nature of the health problem or the procedures to be used, the nurse is justified in refusing to participate. Such refusal should be made known in advance and in time for other appropriate arrangements to be made for the client's nursing care. If the nurse must knowingly enter such a case under emergency circumstances or enters unknowingly, the obligation to provide the best possible care is observed. The nurse withdraws from this type of situation only when assured that alternative sources of nursing care are available to the client. If a client requests information or counsel in an area that is legally sanctioned but contrary to the nurse's personal beliefs, the nurse may refuse to provide these services but must advise the client of sources where such service is available.

1.5 The Setting for Health Care. The nurse adheres to the principle of non-discriminatory, non-prejudicial care in every employment setting or situation and endeavors to promote its acceptance by others. The nurse's readiness to accord respect to clients and to render or obtain needed services should not be limited by the setting, whether nursing care is given in an acute care hospital, nursing home, drug or alcoholic treatment center, prison, patient's home, or other setting.

1.6 The Dying Person. As the concept of death and ways of dealing with it change, the basic human values remain. The ethical problems posed, however, and the decision-making responsibilities of the patient, family, and professional are increased.

The nurse seeks ways to protect these values while working with the client and others to arrive at the best decisions dictated by the circumstances, the client's rights and wishes, and the highest standards of care. The measures used to provide assistance should enable the client to live with as much comfort, dignity, and freedom from anxiety and pain as possible. The client's nursing care will determine to a great degree how this final human experience is lived and the peace and dignity with which death is approached.

Point 2

The nurse safeguards the client's right to privacy by judiciously protecting information of a confidential nature.

2.1 DISCLOSURE TO THE HEALTH TEAM.   It is an accepted standard of nursing practice that data about the health status of clients be accessible, communicated, and recorded. Provision of quality health services requires that such data be available to all members of the health team. When knowledge gained in confidence is relevant or essential to others involved in planning or implementing the client's care, professional judgment is used in sharing it. Only information pertinent to a client's treatment and welfare is disclosed and only to those directly concerned with the client's care. The rights, well-being, and safety of the individual client should be the determining factors in arriving at this decision.

2.2 DISCLOSURE FOR QUALITY ASSURANCE PURPOSES.   Patient information required to document the appropriateness, necessity, and quality of care that is required for peer review, third party payment, and other quality assurance mechanisms must be disclosed only under rigidly defined policies, mandates, or protocols. These written guidelines must assure that the confidentiality of client information is maintained.

2.3 DISCLOSURE TO OTHERS NOT INVOLVED IN THE CLIENT'S CARE.   The right of privacy is an inalienable right of all persons, and the nurse has a clear obligation to safeguard any confidential information about the client acquired from any source. The nurse-client relationship is built on trust. This relationship could be destroyed and the clients' welfare and reputation jeopardized by injudicious disclosure of information provided in confidence. Since the concept of confidentiality has legal as well as ethical implications, an inappropriate breach of confidentiality may also expose the nurse to liability.

2.4 DISCLOSURE IN A COURT OF LAW.   Occasionally, the nurse may be obligated to give testimony in a court of law in relation to confidential information about a client. This should be done only under proper authorization or legal compulsion. Privilege in relation to the disclosure of such information is a legal right that only the patient or his representative may claim or waive. The statutes governing privilege and the exceptions to them vary from state to state, and the nurse may wish to consult legal counsel before testifying in court to be fully informed about professional rights and responsibilities.

2.5 ACCESS TO RECORDS.   If, in the course of providing care, there is need for access to the records of persons not under the nurse's care, as may be the case in relation to the records of the mother of a newborn, the person should be notified and permission first obtained whenever possible. Although records belong to the agency where collected, the individual maintains the right of control over the information provided by him, his family, and his environment. Similarly, professionals may exercise the right of control over information generated by them in the course of health care.

If the nurse wishes to use a client's treatment record for research or non-clinical purposes in which confidential information may be identified, the client's consent must first be obtained. Ethically, this insures the client's right to privacy; legally, it serves to protect the client against unlawful invasion of privacy and the nurse against liability for such action.

Point 3

The nurse acts to safeguard the client and the public when health care and safety are affected by incompetent, unethical, or illegal practice of any person.

3.1 ROLE OF ADVOCATE.   The nurse's primary commitment is to the client's care and safety. Hence, in the role of client advocate, the nurse must be alert to and take appropriate action regarding any instances of incompetent, unethical, or illegal practice(s) by any member of the health care team or the health care system itself, or any action on the part of others that is prejudicial to the client's best interests. To function effectively in the role, the nurse should be fully aware of the state laws governing practice in the health care field and the employing institution's policies and procedures in relation to incompetent, unethical, or illegal practice.

3.2 INITIAL ACTION. When the nurse is aware of inappropriate or questionable conduct in the provision of health care, concern should be expressed to the person carrying out the questionable practice and attention called to the possible detrimental effect upon the client's welfare. When factors in the health care delivery system threaten the welfare of the client, similar action should be directed to the responsible administrative person. If indicated, the practice should then be reported to the appropriate authority within the institution, agency, or larger system. There should be an established mechanism for the reporting and handling of incompetent, unethical, or illegal practice within the employment setting so that such reporting can go through official channels and be done without fear of reprisal. The nurse should be knowledgeable about the mechanism and be prepared to utilize it if necessary. When questions are raised about the appropriateness of behaviors of individual practitioners or practices of health care systems, documentation of the observed behavior or practice must be provided in writing to the appropriate authorities. Local units of the professional association should be prepared to provide assistance and support in reporting procedures.

3.3 FOLLOW-UP ACTION. When incompetent, unethical, or illegal practice on the part of anyone concerned with the client's care is not corrected within the employment setting and continues to jeopardize the client's care and safety, additional steps need to be taken. The problem should be reported to other appropriate authorities such as the practice committees of the appropriate professional organizations or the legally constituted bodies concerned with licensing of specific categories of health workers or professional practitioners. Some situations may warrant the concern and involvement of all these groups. Reporting should be both factual and objective.

3.4 PEER REVIEW. In addition to the role of advocate, the nurse should participate in the planning, establishment, and implementation of other activities or procedures which serve to safeguard clients. Duly constituted peer review activities in employment agencies directed toward the improvement of practice are one example. This ongoing method of review is based on objective criteria, it includes a mechanism for making recommendations to administrators for correction of deficiencies, it facilitates the improvement of delivery services, and it promotes the health, welfare, and safety of clients.

Point 4

The nurse assumes responsibility and accountability for individual nursing judgments and actions.

4.1 ACCEPTANCE OF RESPONSIBILITY AND ACCOUNTABILITY. The recipients of professional nursing services are entitled to high quality nursing care. Individual professional licensure is the protective mechanism legislated by the public to ensure basic and minimum competencies of the professional nurse. Beyond that, society has accorded to the nursing profession the right to regulate its own practice. The regulation and control of nursing practice by nurses demands that individual professional practitioners of nursing bear primary responsibility for the nursing care clients receive and be individually accountable for their practice.

4.2 RESPONSIBILITY. Responsibility refers to the scope of functions and duties associated with a particular role assumed by the nurse. As nursing assumes functions, these functions become part of the responsibilities or expectations of performance of nurses. Areas of responsibilities expected of nurses include: data collection and assessment of the health status of the client; determination of the nursing care plan directed toward designated goals; evaluation of the effectiveness of nursing care in achieving the goals of care; and subsequent reassessment and revision of the nursing care plan as defined in the ANA Standards of Nursing Practice. By assuming these responsibilities, the nurse is held accountable for them.

4.3 ACCOUNTABILITY. Accountability refers to being answerable to someone for something one has done. It means providing an explanation to self, to the client, to the employing agency, and to the nursing profession. Over and above the obligations such accountability imposes on the individual nurse, there is also a liability dimension to accountability. The nurse may be called to account to be held legally responsible for judgments exercised and actions taken in the course of nursing practice. Neither physician's prescriptions nor the employing agency's policies relieve the nurse of ethical or legal accountability for actions taken and judgments made. Accountability, therefore, requires evaluation of the effectiveness of one's performance of nursing responsibilities.

4.4 EVALUATION OF PERFORMANCE. *Self-evaluation.* The nurse engages in ongoing evaluation of individual clinical competence, decision-making abilities, and professional judgments. The nurse also engages in activities that will improve current practice. Self-evaluation carries with it the responsibility for the continuous improvement of one's nursing practice.

Evaluation by peers. Evaluation of one's performance by peers is a hallmark of professionalism, and it is primarily through this mechanism that the profession is held accountable to society. The nurse must be willing to have practice reviewed and evaluated by peers. Guidelines for evaluating the appropriateness, effectiveness, and efficiency of nursing practice are emerging in the form of revised and updated nurse practice acts, ANA's Standards of Nursing Practice, and other quality assurance mechanisms. Participation in the development of objective criteria for evaluation that provide valid and reliable data is the responsibility of each nurse.

Point 5

The nurse maintains competence in nursing.

5.1 PERSONAL RESPONSIBILITIES FOR COMPETENCE. Nursing is concerned with the welfare of human beings, and the nature of nursing is such that inadequate or incompetent practice may jeopardize the client. Therefore, it is the personal responsibility and must be the personal commitment of each individual nurse to maintain competence in practice throughout a professional career. This represents one way in which the nurse fulfills accountability to clients.

5.2 MEASUREMENT OF COMPETENCE IN NURSING PRACTICE. Competence is a relative term, and an individual's competence in any field may be diminished or otherwise affected by the passage of time and the emergence of new knowledge. This means that for the client's optimum well-being and for the nurse's own professional development, nursing care should reflect and incorporate new techniques and knowledge in health care as these develop and especially as they relate to the nurse's particular field of practice.

Measures of competence are developing; they include peer review criteria, outcome criteria, and ANA's program for certification.

5.3 CONTINUING EDUCATION FOR CONTINUING COMPETENCE. Nursing knowledge, like that in the other health disciplines, is rendered rapidly obsolete by mounting technological advances and scientific discoveries, changing concepts and patterns in the provision of health services, and the increasing complexity of nursing responsibilities. The nurse, therefore, should be aware of the need for continuous updating and expansion of the body of knowledge on which practice is based and should keep knowledge and skills current. The nurse should assess personal learning needs, should be active in finding appropriate resources, and should be skilled in self-directed learning. Such continuing education is the key to maintenance of individual competence.

5.4 INTRAPROFESSIONAL RESPONSIBILITY FOR COMPETENCE IN NURSING CARE. All nurses, be they practitioners, educators, administrators, or researchers, share responsibility for quality nursing care. Therefore all nurses need thorough knowledge of the current scope of professional nursing practice. Advances in theory and practice made by one professional must be disseminated to colleagues. Since individual competencies vary in relation to educational preparation, experience, client population and setting, when necessary, nurses should refer clients to and/or consult with other nurses with expertise and recognized competencies, e.g. certified nurses and clinical specialists.

Point 6

The nurse exercises informed judgment and uses individual competence and qualifications as criteria in seeking consultation, accepting responsibilities, and delegating nursing activities to others.

6.1 CHANGING FUNCTIONS. Because of the increased complexity of health care, changing patterns in the delivery of health services, continuing shortages in skilled health manpower, and the development and acceptance of evolving nursing roles, nurses are being requested or expected to carry out functions that have formerly been performed by physicians. In turn, nurses are assigning some nursing functions to variously prepared ancillary personnel. In this gradual shift of functions, as the scope of practice of each profession changes, the nurse must exercise judgment in seeking consultation, accepting responsibilities, and assigning responsibilities to others to ensure that clients receive quality care at all times.

6.2 JOINT POLICY STATEMENTS. Nurse practice acts are usually expressed in broad and general language in order to provide the necessary freedom for interpretation of the law so that future developments, new knowledge, and changing roles will not necessitate constant revision of the law. The nurse must not engage in practice prohibited by law or delegate to others activities prohibited by practice acts of other health care personnel or by other laws. Recognition by nurses of the need for a more definitive delineation of roles and responsibilities, however, has resulted in collaborative efforts to develop joint policy statements. These statements may involve other health care providers or associations and usually specify the functions that are agreed upon as appropriate and proper for the nurse to perform. Such statements represent a body of expert judgment that can be used as authority where responsibilities are not definitively outlined by legal statute.

6.3 SEEKING CONSULTATION. The provision of health and illness care to clients is a complex process that requires a wide range of knowledge and skills. Interdisciplinary team effort with shared responsibility is the most effective approach to provision of total health services. Nurses, whether practicing in clearly defined or new and emerging roles, must be aware of their own individual competencies. When the needs of the client are beyond the qualifications and competencies of the nurse, consultation must be sought from qualified nurses or other appropriate sources.

Discretion must be exercised by the nurse before intervening in diagnostic or therapeutic matters that are not recognized by the nursing profession as established nursing practice. Such discretion should be based on education, experience, legal parameters, and professional guidelines and policies.

6.4 ACCEPTING RESPONSIBILITIES OR DELEGATING ACTIVITIES. The nurse should look to mutually agreed upon policy statements for guidance and direction; but even where such statements exist, personal competence should be carefully assessed before accepting responsibility or delegating activities. Decisions in this area call for knowledge of and adherence to joint policy statements and the laws regulating medical and nursing practice as well as for the exercise of informed nursing judgments.

6.5 ACCEPTING RESPONSIBILITY. If the nurse does not feel personally competent or adequately prepared to carry out a specific function, the nurse has the right and responsibility to refuse. In so doing, both the client and the nurse are protected. The reverse is also true. The nurse should not accept delegated responsibilities that do not utilize nursing skill or competencies or that prevent the provision of needed nursing care to clients. Inasmuch as the nurse is responsible for the client's total nursing care, the nurse must also assess individual competence in assigning selected components of that care to other nursing service personnel. The nurse should not delegate to any member of the nursing team a function for which that person is not prepared or qualified to perform.

Point 7

The nurse participates in activities that contribute to the ongoing development of the profession's body of knowledge.

7.1 THE NURSE AND RESEARCH. Every profession must engage in systematic inquiry to identify, verify, and continually enlarge the body of knowledge which forms the foundations for its practice. A unique body of verified knowledge provides both framework and direction for the profession in all of its activities and for the practitioner in the provision of nursing care. The accrual of knowledge promotes the advancement of practice and with it the well-being of the profession's clients. Ongoing research is thus indispensable to the full discharge of a profession's obligations to society. Each nurse has a role in this area of professional activity, whether involved as an investigator in the furthering of knowledge, as a participant in research, or as a user of research results.

7.2 GENERAL GUIDELINES FOR PARTICIPATING IN RESEARCH. Before participating in research the nurse has an obligation:

1. To ascertain that the study design has been approved by an appropriate body.
2. To obtain information about the intent and the nature of the research.
3. To determine whether the research is consistent with professional goals.

Research involving human subjects should be conducted only by scientifically qualified persons or under such supervision. The nurse who participates in research in any capacity should be fully informed about both nurse and client rights and responsibilities as set forth in the publication *Human Rights Guidelines for Nurses in Clinical and Other Research* prepared by the ANA Commission on Nursing Research.

7.3 THE PROTECTION OF HUMAN RIGHTS IN RESEARCH. The individual rights valued by society and by the nursing profession have been fully outlined and discussed in *Human Rights Guidelines for Nurses in Clinical and Other Research;* namely, the right to freedom from intrinsic risks of injury and the rights of privacy and dignity. Inherent in these rights is respect for each individual to exercise self-determination, to choose to participate, to have full information, to terminate participation without penalty.

It is the duty of both the investigator and the nurse participating in research to maintain vigilance in protecting the life, health, and privacy of human subjects from unanticipated as well as anticipated risks. The subjects' integrity, privacy, and rights must be especially safeguarded if they are unable to protect themselves because of incapacity or because they are in a dependent relationship to the investigator. The investigation should be discontinued if its continuance might be harmful to the subject.

7.4 THE PRACTITIONER'S RIGHTS AND RESPONSIBILITIES IN RESEARCH. Practitioners of nursing providing care to clients who serve as human subjects for research have a special need to clearly understand in advance how the research can be expected to affect treatment and their own moral and legal responsibilities to clients. Here, as in other problematic situations, the practitioner has the right not to participate or to withdraw under the circumstances described in paragraph 1.4 of this document. More detailed guidance about the rights and responsibilities of nurses in relation to research activities may be found in *Human Rights Guidelines for Nurses in Clinical and Other Research.*

Point 8

The nurse participates in the profession's efforts to implement and improve standards of nursing.

8.1 RESPONSIBILITY TO THE PUBLIC. Nursing has the responsibility to admit to the profession only those who have demonstrated a capacity for those competencies believed essential to the practice of nursing. Areas of concern for nursing competence should include adequate performance of nursing skills, academic achievement, humanitarian concern for others, acceptance of responsibility for individual actions, and the desire to improve nursing practice. Nurses involved in the evaluation of student attainment carry a primary responsibility for ensuring that the profession's obligation to the public relative to entry qualifications for practice are met.

The nursing profession exists to give assistance to those persons needing nursing care. Standards of nursing practice provide guidance for the delivery of quality nursing care and are a means for evaluating that care received by clients. The nurse has a responsibility to the public for personally implementing and maintaining optimal standards.

8.2 RESPONSIBILITY TO THE DISCIPLINE.   The professional practice of nursing is founded on an understanding and application of a body of knowledge reflected in its standards. As the profession's organization for nurses, ANA has adopted standards for nursing practice, nursing service, and nursing education. The nurse has the responsibility to monitor these standards in everyday practice and through voluntary participation in the profession's ongoing efforts to implement and improve standards at the national, state, and local levels.

8.3 RESPONSIBILITY TO NURSING STUDENTS.   The future of nursing rests with new recruits to the profession. Nursing has a responsibility to maintain optimal standards of nursing practice and education in schools of nursing and/or wherever students engage in learning activity. This places a particular responsibility on all nurses whose services are concerned with the educational process.

Point 9

The nurse participates in the profession's efforts to establish and maintain conditions of employment conducive to high quality nursing care.

9.1 RESPONSIBILITY FOR CONDITIONS OF EMPLOYMENT.   The nurse must be concerned with conditions of economic and general welfare within the profession. These are important determinants in the recruitment and retention of well-qualified personnel and in assuring that each practitioner has the opportunity to function optimally.

The provision of high quality nursing care is the responsibility of both the individual nurse and the nursing profession. Professional autonomy and self-regulation in the control of conditions of practice are necessary to implement standards of practice as established by organized nursing.

9.2 COLLECTIVE ACTION.   Defining and controlling the quality of nursing care provided to the client is most effectively accomplished through collective action. Collective action may include assistance and representation from the professional association in negotiations with employers to achieve employment conditions in which the professional standards of practice can be implemented and which are commensurate with the qualifications, functions, and responsibilities of the nurse. The Economic and General Welfare program of the professional association is the appropriate channel through which the nurse can work constructively, ethically, and with professional dignity. This program, encompassing commitment to the principle of collective bargaining, promotes the right and responsibility of the individual nurse to participate in determining the terms and conditions of employment conducive to high quality nursing practice.

9.3 INDIVIDUAL ACTION.   A nurse may enter into an agreement with individuals or organizations to provide health care, provided that the agreement is in accordance with the Standards of Nursing Practice of the American Nurses' Association and the nurse practice law of the state and provided that the agreement does not permit or compel practices which are in violation of this Code.

Point 10

The nurse participates in the profession's effort to protect the public from misinformation and misrepresentation and to maintain the integrity of nursing.

10.1 ADVERTISING SERVICES. A nurse may make factual statements that indicate availability of services through means that are in dignified form, such as:

A professional card identifying the nurse by name and title, giving address, telephone number, and other pertinent data.

Listing name, title, and brief biography in reputable directories and reputable professional publications. Such published data may include the following: Name, address, phone, field of practice or concentrates; date and place of birth; schools attended, with dates of graduation, degrees, and other scholastic distinctions; offices held; public or professional honors; teaching positions; publications; memberships and activities in professional societies; licenses; names and addresses of references.

A nurse shall not use any form of public or professional communication to make self-laudatory statements or claims that are false, fraudulent, misleading, deceptive, or unfair.

10.2 USE OF TITLES AND SYMBOLS. The right to use the title "Registered Nurse" is granted by state governments through licensure by examination for the protection of the public. Use of that title carries with it the responsibility to act in the public interest. The nurse may use the title "R.N." and symbols of academic degrees or other earned or honorary professional symbols of recognition in all ways that are legal and appropriate. The title and other symbols of the profession should not be used, however, for personal benefit by the nurse or by those who may seek to exploit them for other purposes.

10.3 ENDORSEMENT OF COMMERCIAL PRODUCTS OR SERVICES. The nurse does not give or imply endorsement to advertising, promotion, or sale of commercial products or services because this may be interpreted as reflecting the opinion or judgment of the profession as a whole. Since it is a nursing responsibility to engage in health teaching and to advise clients on matters relating to their health, it is not unethical for the nurse to utilize knowledge of specific services and/or products in advising individual clients. In the course of providing information or education to clients or other practitioners about commercial products or services, however, a variety of similar products or services should be offered or described so that the client or practitioner can make an informed choice.

10.4 PROTECTING THE CLIENT FROM HARMFUL PRODUCTS. It is the responsibility of the nurse to advise clients against the use of dangerous products. This is seen as discharge of nursing functions when undertaken in the best interest of the client.

10.5 REPORTING INFRACTIONS. Not only should the nurse personally adhere to the above principles, but alertness to any instances of their violation by others should be maintained. The nurse should report promptly, through appropriate channels, any advertisement or commercial which involves a nurse, implies involvement, or in any way suggests nursing endorsement of a commercial product, service, or enterprise. The nurse who knowingly becomes involved in such unethical activities negates professional responsibility for personal gain, and jeopardizes the public confidence and trust in the nursing profession that have been created by generations of nurses working together in the public interest.

Point 11

The nurse collaborates with members of the health professions and other citizens in promoting community and national efforts to meet the health needs of the public.

11.1 QUALITY HEALTH CARE AS A RIGHT. Quality health care is mandated as a right to all citizens. Availability and accessibility to quality health services for all citizens require collaborative planning by health providers and consumers at both the local and national level. Nursing care is an integral part of quality health care, and nurses have a responsibility to help ensure that citizens' rights to health care are met.

11.2 RESPONSIBILITY TO THE CONSUMER OF HEALTH CARE. The nurse is a member of the largest group of health providers, and therefore the philosophies and goals of the nursing profession should have a significant impact on the consumer of health care. An effective way of ensuring that nurses' views regarding health care and nursing service are properly represented is by involvement of nurses in political decision making.

11.3 RELATIONSHIPS WITH OTHER DISCIPLINES. The complexity of the delivery of health care service demands an interdisciplinary approach to delivery of health services as well as strong support from allied health occupations. The nurse should actively seek to promote collaboration needed for ensuring the quality of health services to all persons.

11.4 RELATIONSHIP WITH MEDICINE. The interdependent relationship of the nursing and medical professions requires collaboration around the need of the client. The evolving role of the nurse in the health delivery system requires joint practice as colleagues, deliberations in determining functional relationships, and differentiating areas of practice between the two professions.

11.5 CONFLICT OF INTEREST. Nurses who provide public service and who have financial or other interests in health care facilities or services should avoid a conflict of interest by refraining from casting a vote on any deliberation affecting the public's health care needs in those areas.

The Code For Licensed Practical/Vocational Nurses*

The Code adopted by NFLPN in 1961 and revised in 1979 provided a motivation for establishing and elevating professional standards. Each LP/VN, upon entering the profession, inherits the responsibility to adhere to the standards of ethical practice and conduct as set forth in this Code.

1. Know the scope of maximum utilization of the LP/VN and function within this scope.
2. Recognize and respect cultural backgrounds, spiritual needs, and the religious beliefs of individual patients.
3. Safeguard the confidential information acquired from any source about the patient.
4. Refuse to give endorsement to the sale and promotion of commerical products or services.
5. Uphold the highest standards in personal appearance, language, dress, and demeanor.
6. Accept responsibility for membership in NFLPN and participate in its efforts to maintain the established standards of nursing practice and employment policies conducive to quality patient care.

CNA Code of Ethics: An Ethical Basis For Nursing In Canada†

Introduction

Nursing is a person-oriented health service. It is a service called forth by the experience of human pain and suffering, and directed to the promotion of health, the prevention and alleviation of suffering, and the provision of a caring presence for those for whom cure is not possible. The ethical norms that guide this service evolve from a belief system that perceives the human person to be of incalculable worth, and human life to have a sacred, precious and even mysterious character. Nursing is practiced in the context of human relationships, the dominant ethical determinant of which is the principle of respect for persons.

The concept which constitutes the unifying and ethical focus for nursing practice, education, administration and research is the concept caring. Caring, as a characteristic

*Used with permission of the National Federation of Licensed Practical Nurses.

†Originally prepared for the Canadian Nurses Association by M. Simone Roach, RN, PhD, csm, and approved by the Board of Directors, February 1980. The code has since been amended by the CNA and is reprinted here in its amended version with their permission.

descriptive of all authentic human action, is expressed within the discipline of nursing through the following attributes.

1. *Compassion*—the human response through which nurses participate in the pain and brokenness of humanity, by entering into the experience of another's suffering, misfortune or need in such a manner that the needs of that person are the primary basis for the use of the nurse's personal and professional skills.
2. *Competence*—the state of having the knowledge, skills, energy and experience adequate to provide the required service.
3. *Conscience*—the sense of what is right or wrong in one's conduct, and the awareness of, and the will to apply relevant ethical principles.
4. *Confidence*—the quality which fosters the development and maintenance of trusting relationships.
5. *Commitment*—a pledge, based on free choice, to devote oneself to meeting one's professional obligations.

In nursing, the human capacity to care is developed and professionalized through the acquisition of those intellectual, affective and technical skills required to carry out the responsibilities of specific nursing roles. The ethical obligations arising from caring as required by these roles are met at different levels of practice and within varying contexts. . . .

Caring and the Profession

The nursing profession as a whole has ethical obligations to society as well as to its own membership. The profession has an obligation to examine its own goals and the service it offers in the light of existing health problems, and to design its programs in collaboration with other professions which also provide health services within the society. Nursing, in keeping with its mandate as a service profession, is bound to see itself, not as an end to be promoted and served by society, but as a professional body, constituted and legitimized by society's approval, to offer a prescribed service required for the improvement of the health status of people.

In meeting its obligations to society, nursing has responsibility for monitoring the quantity and quality of persons entering the profession, and for identifying and implementing standards that promote the type and quality of nursing service dictated by society's needs. Nursing has a related responsibility to work for those conditions which will enable its members to provide the quantity and quality of service deemed necessary and desirable.

The nursing profession also has responsibilities to the international community. Since health is a basic condition for human development, and as no one nation or country can develop its potential in isolation, the interests of the profession transcend national boundaries. In fact, our credibility as a profession is called into question if we do not collaborate on an international level to promote the health of all peoples, and to work toward the relief of human suffering wherever it is experienced.

These broad obligations constitute the grounds for the ethical responsibilities of nursing's organized professional body, and include the following commitments:

1. In the context of existing health needs and problems, to identify Canada's need for nursing activities and services.
2. To establish relevant and realistic goals for the profession of nursing within Canadian society.
3. To foster collaboration with other health professions, political bodies, and other agencies in responding to the health needs of Canadians.
4. To collaborate with professional groups, institutions and agencies in promoting the welfare of peoples in other countries of the world.
5. To provide measures which will ensure that only those with the potential, motivation and

discipline required to function as caring persons are accepted into, and endorsed by the nursing profession.

6. To work for the realization of working conditions which enable nurses to function as caring persons with the required degree of autonomy.
7. To promote conditions for nurses which provide for legitimate personal, professional and economic rewards.
8. To demonstrate, in its own transactions, accountability for the use of internal and external resources.

Caring and the Individual Nurse

The final test of the credibility of ethical standards in nursing lies in the behavior of the individual nurse—educator, practitioner, administrator and researcher. Many of the responsibilities arising out of obligations of the profession as a whole, and the ethical demands of the caring community itself, are fulfilled only in the actions of the individual nurse. While the profession has the obligation to identify, promote and monitor ethical standards, the execution of such standards is a personal responsibility, the final guarantee of which is in the conscience and commitment of the individual nurse.

Guidelines

The following guidelines include general principles, with statements of ethical responsibility which flow from these principles. They are intended to provide a guide for reflection and for the articulation of more specific ethical rules and standards applicable to concrete experiences. With the increasing complexity of ethical conflicts in nursing, and the potential for greater ethical concerns in the future, ethical discernment in nursing is an exciting challenge, requiring knowledge, skill and great moral sensitivity. We have the capacity to meet this challenge—one which could be the greatest in the history of our profession.

GENERAL PRINCIPLES

1. The human person, regardless of race, creed, color, social class or health status, is of incalculable worth, and commands reverence and respect.
2. Human life has a sacred and even mysterious character and its worth is determined not merely by utilitarian concerns.
3. Caring, the central and fundamental focus of nursing, is the basis for nursing ethics. It is expressed in compassion, competence, conscience, confidence and commitment. It qualifies all the relationships in nursing practice, education, administration and research including those between nurse-client; nurse-nurse; nurse-other helping professionals; educator-colleague; faculty-student; researcher-subject.

STATEMENTS OF ETHICAL RESPONSIBILITY

1. Caring demands the provision of helping services that are appropriate to the needs of the client and significant others.
2. Caring recognizes the client's membership in a family and a community, and provides for the participation of significant others in his or her care.
3. Caring acknowledges the reality of death in the life of every person, and demands that appropriate support be provided for the dying person and family to enable them to prepare for, and to cope with death when it is inevitable.
4. Caring acknowledges that the human person has the capacity to face up to health needs and problems in his or her own unique way, and directs nursing action in a manner that will assist the client to develop, maintain or gain personal autonomy, self-respect and self-determination.

5. Caring, as a response to a health need, requires the consent and the participation of the person who is experiencing that need.
6. Caring dictates that the client and significant others have the knowledge and information adequate for free and informed decisions concerning care requirements, alternatives and preferences.
7. Caring demands that the needs of the client supersede those of the nurse, and that the nurse must not compromise the integrity of the client by personal behavior that is self-serving.
8. Caring acknowledges the vulnerability of a client in certain situations, and dictates restraint in actions which might compromise the client's rights and privileges.
9. Caring, involving a relationship which is, in itself, therapeutic, demands mutual respect and trust.
10. Caring acknowledges that information obtained in the course of the nursing relationship is privileged, and that it requires the full protection of confidentiality unless such information provides evidence of serious impending harm to the client or to a third party, or is legally required by the courts.
11. Caring requires that the nurse represent the needs of the client, and that the nurse take appropriate measures when the fulfillment of these needs is jeopardized by the actions of other persons.
12. Caring acknowledges the dignity of all persons in the practice or educational setting.
13. Caring acknowledges, respects and draws upon the competencies of others.
14. Caring establishes the conditions for the harmonization of efforts of different helping professionals in providing required services to clients.
15. Caring seeks to establish and maintain a climate of respect for the honest dialogue needed for effective collaboration.
16. Caring establishes the legitimacy of respectful challenge and/or confrontation when the service required by the client is compromised by incompetency, incapacity or negligence, or when the competencies of the nurse are not acknowledged or appropriately utilized.
17. Caring demands the provision of working conditions which enable nurses to carry out their legitimate responsibilities.
18. Caring demands resourcefulness and restraint—accountability *for* the use of time, resources, equipment, and funds, and requires accountability *to* appropriate individuals and/or bodies.
19. Caring requires that the nurse bring to the work situation in education, practice, administration or research, the knowledge, affective and technical skills required, and that competency in these areas be maintained and updated.
20. Caring commands fidelity to oneself, and guards the right and privilege of the nurse to act in keeping with an informed moral conscience.

College of Nurses of Ontario, *Guidelines for Ethical Behaviour in Nursing* (1980)*

Assumptions

1. The purpose of nursing is to promote human well-being. In this paper nursing is considered to include:
   a. Caring for individuals, families, and communities;
   b. Teaching those who are entering the profession or continuing their preparation within it;
   c. Advancing the theoretical aspects of nursing through research involving individuals or groups.

*Used with permission of College of Nurses of Ontario. (Abridged.)

2. Nursing is a form of intervention in the lives of others. As such, all nursing has an ethical component. Choices based on values must be made. The values upon which the choices must be based may vary from one individual to another: between two nurses, between nurse and client, and between a nurse and others who share the care of a single client. Since nurses have a particular responsibility to help others meet particularly sensitive human needs, a nurse needs skill in making ethical decisions.

3. The ethical decisions made in nursing—the decisions based on values—arise first from recognizing that each individual involved in the nursing interaction has a "human dimension," i.e., a unique set of biological, spiritual, psychological, and social characteristics. This is true of nurse, client, other people caring for the client, family members, etc. This "human dimension" commands respect, even as it entails rights and responsibilities.

4. The nurse's ability to fulfil ethical responsibilities is commensurate with the professional context within which the nurse works: i.e., appropriate professional preparation, suitable conditions for exercising nursing activity, social respect for the nurse as a responsible decision-maker, and social recognition of professional expertise.

5. Each nurse's ethical judgments flow from personal conscience. They include a weighing of alternatives (what *could* be done) and the resulting decision as to what *should* be done. Informed ethical decision-making rests on a theoretical reasoning process in which the alternative modes of action are "matched" against the individual's personal value-system. The result of this "matching" process is applied in a particular situation to determine the best course of action in that situation. The "matching" takes into account past experience, possible consequences, and personal strengths and weaknesses. Once the ethical decision is made, personal inventiveness in the situation and strength of will are important in carrying out the decision.

6. Help in clarifying personal ethical values is often available to the nurse from associates and colleagues in nursing, from members of other health disciplines, and from employers, family, and friends. The particular social, cultural, and religious value-systems which form the individual conscience are often helpful in resolving ethical dilemmas. Important in finding the best solution is a continuing recognition of the values of other persons and consideration for these values.

No set of guidelines can resolve the ethical dilemmas which a nurse may be called upon to face. As noted, this is a personal matter, unique to each individual and situation. Nevertheless, given the nature of nursing and the ethical responsibilities associated with it, and given the requests from nurses for "sign-posts" in this area, some statement of desirable ethical behaviour in selected nursing situations seems required.

Fulfilment of these criteria is only a beginning: the actual resolution of the continuing ethical problems presented to each individual nurse remains a continuing personal challenge.

Guidelines

1. *Role of the Nurse:* The nurse, as one of the providers of health care, has a unique and responsible role in health promotion, in preventing illness, and in helping individuals attain and maintain the highest level of health possible.

   Fulfilment of this role within the nurse-client relationship requires mutual recognition of responsibility for self and respect for human dignity.

2. *Competence:* The nurse is responsible for achieving and maintaining professional competence.

3. *Expanding Knowledge:* The nurse has a responsibility to contribute to expanding the body of nursing theory and its application.

4. *Quality of Care:* The nurse has a responsibility to improve the quality of care being given.

5. *Accountability:* As a member of the profession, the individual nurse accepts responsibility for certain acts and functions.

   The nurse is responsible and accountable for the consequences of nursing actions.

6. *Truth:* The nurse respects the role of truthfulness in health care.

7. *Consent:* The nurse respects the client's right to an informed and voluntary consent regarding care, treatment, and participation in research. As a responsible decision maker, the client has the right:
   a. To be advised of the probable and potential consequences of nursing and medical actions and of research activities;
   b. To decide whether or not to accept treatment or participate in research, without coercion or duress;
   c. To be involved in developing the plan of care.
8. *Confidentiality:* The nurse respects the client's right to confidentiality within the nurse-client relationship.
9. *The Health Team:* The nurse as a member of the health team has a responsibility to collaborate, to share information, and to participate in joint planning for the benefit of the client and to maintain the standard of the team.

   The client, being the reason the team exists, is included in discussions when advisable and feasible.
10. *Professional Goals:* The nurse has a responsibility to further the goals of the profession.
11. *Nurse as Citizen:* The nurse as citizen has a responsibility to serve the community by trying to improve the level of health care.

Royal College of Nursing (Rcn) Code of Professional Conduct: A Discussion Document*

I. Introduction

The profession of nursing has a commitment which is shared with other health care professions to promote optimal standards of health, combat disease and disability and alleviate suffering. A code of professional conduct is required in order to make explicit those moral standards which should guide professional decisions in these matters, and in order to encourage responsible moral decision making throughout the profession. It is recognized that no code can do justice to every individual case and therefore that any set of principles must remain constantly open to discussion both within the nursing profession and outside it.

II. Responsibility to Patients or Clients

The primary responsibility of nurses is to protect and enhance the wellbeing and dignity of each individual person in their care. As members of professional teams nurses should recognize and accept responsibility for the total effects of nursing and medical care on individuals. This responsibility is in no way affected by the type of origin of the person's need or illness or by his age, sex, mental status, social class, ethnic origins, nationality or personal beliefs. Therefore it follows that:

1. Nursing care should be directed towards the preservation, or restoration, as far as is possible, of a person's ability to function normally and independently within his own chosen environment.
2. Discrimination against particular individuals, for whatever reason, should never be tolerated.
3. During episodes of illness the autonomy of patients should be maintained throughout

*Reprinted with the permission of the Royal College of Nursing. The code is available from the Rcn, Henrietta Place, London W1M 0AB.

treatment, restrictions being imposed only when these are demonstrably necessary for their own wellbeing, or for the safety of others; and the active participation of patients in their own treatment should be facilitated by means of open and sensitive communication.

4. Measures which jeopardise the safety of patients, such as unnecessary treatments, hazardous experimental procedures and the withdrawal of professional services during employment disputes, should be actively opposed by the profession as a whole.

5. Information about patients or clients should be treated with the utmost confidence and respect, and should not be divulged to persons outside the primary care or treatment team without the person's consent, except in exceptional circumstances.

III. Responsibility for Professional Standards

The professional authority of nurses is based upon their training and experience in day-to-day care of ill persons at home or in hospital; and in the enhancement of positive health in the community at large. All members of the nursing profession have a responsibility to continue to develop their knowledge and skill in these matters.

IV. Responsibility to Colleagues

In general, relationships with colleagues in nursing and in other health care professions should be determined according to what will maximize the benefit of those in their care.

1. Professional relationships between nurses should be regulated according to the level of knowledge, experience and skill of each nurse. Clear chains of command should be established to deal with emergency situations, but except in such situations, free discussion of the reasons for established procedures should be encouraged at all levels.

2. Professional relationships between nurses and doctors should be regulated according to the particular expertise of each profession. In the case of medical treatments nurses are under an obligation to carry out a doctor's instructions except where they have a good reason to believe that harm will be caused to the patient by so doing. In cases in which nurses' continuous contact with the patient has given them a different insight into the patient's medical needs, they are under moral obligation to communicate this to the doctor in charge of the case. Nurses should support the multidisciplinary case-conference approach to treatment decisions, and should improve their ability to participate actively in such conferences.

3. Professional relationships between nurses and members of other health care professions should be based upon respect for each other's area of expertise and on the desire to gain a fuller understanding of the patient's or client's needs. Procedures should be established for regular inter-professional consultations.

V. Professional Responsibility and Personal Responsibility

As citizens of a state and as private individuals nurses should defend and actively pursue those moral values to which their profession is committed, namely, individual autonomy, parity of treatment and the pursuit of health. In some circumstances this may require protest against, and opposition to, social and political conditions which are detrimental to human wellbeing; and in others, the altering of personal habits which set a poor example in health care. In all other respects nurses have the right to regulate their private lives according to their own standards of morality, provided their style of life does not cast doubts on the integrity and trustworthiness of their profession.

Florence Nightingale Pledge For Nurses

I solemnly pledge myself before God and in the presence of this assembly to pass my life in purity and to practise my profession faithfully.

I will abstain from whatever is deleterious and mischievous, and will not take or knowingly administer any harmful drug.

I will do all in my power to elevate the standard of my profession, and will hold in confidence all personal matters committed to my keeping, and all family affairs coming to my knowledge in the practice of my calling.

With loyalty will I endeavour to aid the physician in his work, and devote myself to the welfare of those committed to my care.

A Patient's Bill of Rights: American Hospital Association, 1973*

The American Hospital Association presents a Patient's Bill of Rights with the expectation that observance of these rights will contribute to more effective patient care and greater satisfaction for the patient, his physician and the hospital organization. Further, the Association presents these rights in the expectation that they will be supported by the hospital on behalf of its patients, as an integral part of the healing process. It is recognized that a personal relationship between the physician and the patient is essential for the provision of proper medical care. The traditional physician-patient relationship takes on a new dimension when care is rendered within an organizational structure. Legal precedent has established that the institution itself also has a responsibility to the patient. It is in recognition of these factors that these rights are affirmed.

1. The patient has the right to considerate and respectful care.
2. The patient has the right to obtain from his physician complete current information concerning his diagnosis, treatment, and prognosis in terms the patient can be reasonably expected to understand. When it is not medically advisable to give such information to the patient, the information should be made available to an appropriate person in his behalf. He has the right to know by name, the physician responsible for coordinating his care.
3. The patient has the right to receive from his physician information necessary to give informed consent prior to the start of any procedure and/or treatment. Except in emergencies, such information for informed consent, should include but not necessarily be limited to the specific procedure and/or treatment, the medically significant risks involved, and the probable duration of incapacitation. Where medically significant alternatives for care or treatment exist, or when the patient requests information concerning medical alternatives, the patient has the right to such information. The patient also has the right to know the name of the person responsible for the procedures and/or treatment.
4. The patient has the right to refuse treatment to the extent permitted by law, and to be informed of the medical consequences of his action.
5. The patient has the right to every consideration of his privacy concerning his own medical care program. Case discussion, consultation, examination, and treatment are confidential and should be conducted discreetly. Those not directly involved in his care must have the permission of the patient to be present.
6. The patient has the right to expect that all communications and records pertaining to his care should be treated as confidential.
7. The patient has the right to expect that within its capacity a hospital must make reasonable response to the request of a patient for services. The hospital must provide evalua-

*Reprinted with the permission of the American Hospital Association, Copyright 1972.

tion, service, and/or referral as indicated by the urgency of the case. When medically permissible a patient may be transferred to another facility only after he has received complete information and explanation concerning the needs for and alternatives to such a transfer. The institution to which the patient is to be transferred must first have accepted the patient for transfer.

8. The patient has the right to obtain information as to any relationship of his hospital to other health care and educational institutions insofar as his care is concerned. The patient has the right to obtain information as to the existence of any professional relationships among individuals, by name, who are treating him.

9. The patient has the right to be advised if the hospital proposes to engage in or perform human experimentation affecting his care or treatment. The patient has the right to refuse to participate in such research projects.

10. The patient has the right to expect reasonable continuity of care. He has the right to know in advance what appointment times and physicians are available and where. The patient has the right to expect that the hospital will provide a mechanism whereby he is informed by his physician or a delegate of the physician of the patient's continuing health care requirements following discharge.

11. The patient has the right to examine and receive an explanation of his bill regardless of source of payment.

12. The patient has the right to know what hospital rules and regulations apply to his conduct as a patient.

No catalogue of rights can guarantee for the patient the kind of treatment he has a right to expect. A hospital has many functions to perform, including the prevention and treatment of disease, the education of both health professionals and patients, and the conduct of clinical research. All these activities must be conducted with an overriding concern for the patient, and, above all, the recognition of his dignity as a human being. Success in achieving this recognition assures success in the defense of the rights of the patient.

Massachusetts Cancer Nurses' Group Statement of Beliefs Related to Giving Cancer Patients Information*

Giving Information to Any Patient:

The nurse helps the patient to understand the implications of the diagnosis and recommended treatment consistent with his readiness, and in collaboration with the physician. The nurse also helps the patient to utilize his capabilities and make the best possible adjustment to his limitations.

Giving Information to the Cancer Patient:

1. In support of the Patient's Bill of Rights, the patient has the right to know his diagnosis and treatment, also to request and receive clarification from whomever he wishes. The nurse's role is to respond to the patient's information needs, also to his readiness and response to information.

2. The doctor has the initial responsibility to inform the patient of the diagnosis and treatment. The content and patient's response to the information should be communicated to

*From Beatrice Kay Kastenbaum and Rachel E. Spector, "What Should a Nurse Tell a Cancer Patient?" Copyright © 1978, American Journal of Nursing Company. Reproduced with permission from *American Journal of Nursing*, 78, 4 (April 1978), 640–41.

the remainder of the health team. (In some settings, a nurse is present when the patient is given information.)

3. The nurse has the responsibility of being informed about the patient's diagnosis and planned treatment. This includes the specific diagnosis and plans for a particular patient, and knowledge about the disease and treatment in general.
4. The nurse ascertains from the patient his understanding of his disease and treatment, and is aware of his changing needs for information.
5. The nurse communicates to the health team the patient's perceptions and questions, and the information being given to the patient. She provides for continuity of care between patient settings.
6. The rights of the patient to have knowledge of his diagnosis and make decisions about his care supersede the rights of family members. The health team is aware of the problems that the patient's illness engenders for the family. The family is included in teaching and planning in order to understand and assist in the patient's care. Children should participate in decisions about their care when possible, but parents or the legal guardian retain legal decision making responsibility for minors.
7. The child's questions concerning the disease and treatment are answered truthfully and at his level of understanding.
8. When a patient, who is fully aware of the consequences of the alternatives, does not wish to be a part of or to continue a research protocol, the patient is assisted to continue appropriate medical and nursing care in his chosen setting.

The Special Problems of Research and Informed Consent:

Informed consent is a term used to signify that the patient has been given and understands enough information about his disease and treatment to allow him to judge whether he wishes to become part of a study in which the treatment effectiveness has not been proved. The patient should know the drugs and procedures involved in the research study. Because denial is a normal emotional response to information about cancer, it is often difficult for a patient and family to adequately and quickly understand a proposed treatment. Some problems which develop as a result of this vulnerability are:

1. Lack of understanding of the effect of the treatment on the patient's present quality of life. (Side effects of drugs often reduce the patient's ability to perform activities of daily living and to gain enjoyment of life, for instance.)
2. Categorization into a treatment schedule which is inappropriate for the patient's life-style and needs. (Timing of treatments and requirements for hospitalization may interfere with the patient's work schedule or pose difficulties with transportation.)
3. Lack of awareness of alternatives to the proposed treatment. When the effectiveness of the treatment is not proven, the patient needs to be fully aware of the choices open to him.

Clearly, it is not the nurse's role to inform the patient of his/her specific diagnosis, treatment plan, and prognosis, especially when research is being contemplated. Because the nurse is aware of the Patient's Bill of Rights, we believe that *advocacy* is the appropriate role if problems develop.

An advocate has knowledge of the situation from more than one point of view. The nurse as an advocate communicates on behalf of the patient. The nurse assists others involved in decisions about the patient to understand his perception of the situation. The patient is assisted to understand his situation accurately. When necessary, the nurse helps the patient negotiate regarding his chosen medical treatment.

If advocacy activities fail to alleviate the patient's perceived problem, the nurse has the responsibility to use further organizational procedures on the patient's behalf. If appropriate procedures for handling situations in which problems are occurring do not exist, the nurse becomes active in pointing to the need for and creating procedures.

Cognitive Capacity Screening Test*

Examiner _____ Date _____

Instructions: Check items answered correctly. Write incorrect or unusual answers in space provided. If necessary, urge patient once to complete task.

Introduction to patient: "I would like to ask you a few questions. Some you will find very easy and others may be very hard. Just do your best."

Addressograph Plate

1) What day of the week is this? _____

2) What month? _____

3) What day of month? _____

4) What year? _____

5) What place is this? _____

6) Repeat the numbers 8 7 2. _____

7) Say them backwards. _____

8) Repeat these numbers 6 3 7 1. _____

9) Listen to these numbers 6 9 4. Count 1 through 10 out loud, then repeat 6 9 4. (Help if needed. Then use numbers 5 7 3.) _____

10) Listen to these numbers 8 1 4 3. Count 1 through 10 out loud, then repeat 8 1 4 3. _____

11) Beginning with Sunday, say the days of the week backwards. _____

12) 9 + 3 is _____

13) Add 6 (to the previous answer or "to 12"). _____

14) Take away 5 ("from 18"). _____
Repeat these words after me and remember them, I will ask for them later: HAT, CAR, TREE, TWENTY-SIX.

15) The opposite of fast is slow. The opposite of up is _____

16) The opposite of large is _____

17) The opposite of hard is _____

18) An orange and a banana are both fruits. Red and blue are both _____

19) A penny and a dime are both _____

20) What were those words I asked you to remember? (HAT) _____

21) (CAR) _____

22) (TREE) _____

23) (TWENTY-SIX) _____

24) Take away 7 from 100, then take away 7 from what is left and keep going: 100 − 7 is _____

25) Minus 7 _____

26) Minus 7 (write down answers; check correct subtraction of 7) _____

27) Minus 7 _____

28) Minus 7 _____

29) Minus 7 _____

30) Minus 7 _____

TOTAL CORRECT (maximum score = 30) _____

Patient's occupation (previous, if not employed) _____ Education _____ Age _____

Estimated intelligence (based on education, occupation, and history, not on test score):

Below average, Average, Above average _____

Patient was: Cooperative _____ Uncooperative _____ Depressed _____ Lethargic _____ Other _____

Medical diagnosis: _____

IF PATIENT'S SCORE IS LESS THAN 20, THE EXISTENCE OF DIMINISHED COGNITIVE CAPACITY IS PRESENT. THEREFORE, AN ORGANIC MENTAL SYNDROME SHOULD BE SUSPECTED AND THE FOLLOWING INFORMATION OBTAINED.

Temp. _____ BUN _____ Endocrine dysfunction? _____
T_3, T_4, Ca, P, etc.

B.P. _____ Glu _____

Hct _____ Po_2 _____ History of previous psychiatric difficulty _____

Na _____ Pco_2 _____ Drugs: _____
Steroids? L-Dopa? Amphetamines? Tranquilizers? Digitalis?

K _____

Cl _____ Focal neurological signs: _____

CO_2 _____

EEG _____ DIAGNOSIS: _____

ECG _____

California Natural Death Act: Guidelines and Directive†

These guidelines have been drafted by an ad hoc committee convened at the request of Assemblyman Barry Keene, composed of the Los Angeles County Bar Association's Com-

*Reprinted from Jacobs et al., "Screening for Organic Mental Syndromes," *Annals of Internal Medicine*, 86 (1977), 45, with the permission of the publisher and the author.

†The Natural Death Act, California Health and Safety Code 7185–7195 (West. Supp. 1977).

mittee on Bioethics, California Hospital Association Legal Counsel, California Medical Association Legal Counsel and representatives of the Office of Assemblyman Keene.

Guidelines for Signers

The DIRECTIVE allows you to instruct your doctor not to use artificial methods to extend the natural process of dying.

Before signing the DIRECTIVE, you may ask advice from anyone you wish, but you do not have to see a lawyer or have the DIRECTIVE certified by a notary public.

If you sign the DIRECTIVE, talk it over with your doctor and ask that it be made part of your medical record.

The DIRECTIVE must be WITNESSED by two adults who (1) are not related to you by blood or marriage, (2) are not mentioned in your will, and (3) would have no claim on your estate.

The DIRECTIVE may NOT be witnessed by your doctor or by anyone working for your doctor. If you are in a HOSPITAL at the time you sign the DIRECTIVE, none of its employees may be a witness. If you are in a SKILLED NURSING FACILITY, one of your two witnesses MUST be a "patient advocate" or "ombudsman" designated by the State Department of Aging.

You may sign a DIRECTIVE TO PHYSICIANS if you are at least 18 years old and of sound mind, acting of your own free will in the presence of two qualified witnesses.

No one may force you to sign the DIRECTIVE. No one may deny you insurance or health care services because you have chosen **not** to sign it. If you **do** sign the DIRECTIVE, it will not affect your insurance or any other rights you may have to accept or reject medical treatment.

Your doctor is bound by the DIRECTIVE only (1) if he/she is satisfied that your DIRECTIVE is valid, (2) if another doctor has certified your condition as terminal, and (3) at least 14 days have gone by since you were informed of your condition.

If you sign a DIRECTIVE while in good health, your doctor may respect your wishes but is not bound by the DIRECTIVE.

The DIRECTIVE is valid for a period of five years, at which time you may sign a new one.

The DIRECTIVE is not valid during pregnancy.

You may revoke the DIRECTIVE at any time, even in the final stages of a terminal illness, by (1) destroying it, (2) signing and dating a written statement, or (3) by informing your doctor. No matter how you revoke the DIRECTIVE, be sure your doctor is told of your decision.

Directive to Physicians

Directive made this _____ day of _____ (month, year).

I _____ , being of sound mind, willfully, and voluntarily make known my desire that my life shall not be artificially prolonged under the circumstances set forth below, do hereby declare:

1. If at any time I should have an incurable injury, disease, or illness certified to be a terminal condition by two physicians, and where the application of life-sustaining procedures would serve only to artificially prolong the moment of my death and where my physician determines that my death is imminent whether or not life-sustaining procedures are utilized, I direct that such procedures be withheld or withdrawn, and that I be permitted to die naturally.

2. In the absence of my ability to give directions regarding the use of such life-sustaining procedures, it is my intention that this directive shall be honored by my family and physician(s) as the final expression of my legal right to refuse medical or surgical treatment and accept the consequences from such refusal.
3. If I have been diagnosed as pregnant and that diagnosis is known to my physician, this directive shall have no force or effect during the course of my pregnancy.
4. I have been diagnosed and notified at least 14 days ago as having a terminal condition by _____ , M.D., whose address is _____ _____ , and whose telephone number is _____ _____ I understand that if I have not filled in the physician's name and address, it shall be presumed that I did not have a terminal condition when I made out this directive.
5. This directive shall have no force or effect five years from the date filled in above.
6. I understand the full import of this directive and I am emotionally and mentally competent to make this directive.

Signed _____

City, County and State of Residence _____

_____

The declarant has been personally known to me and I believe him or her to be of sound mind.

Witness _____

Witness _____

This Directive complies in form with the "Natural Death Act" California Health and Safety Code, Section 7188, Assembly Bill 3060 (Keene).

Summary and Guidelines for Physicians

INTRODUCTION. A person who is at least 18 years of age and of sound mind may sign a DIRECTIVE TO PHYSICIANS as contained in the 1976 California "Natural Death Act." This Act permits a person who meets certain qualifications to give legal effect to his/her wishes to avoid artificial prolongation of the dying process. It also imposes certain obligations—and provides certain protections—for a physician dealing with a person presenting a DIRECTIVE.

SIGNATURE AND WITNESSES. To be effective, the DIRECTIVE must be signed by the patient and witnessed by two persons who are not related to the patient by blood or marriage, are not mentioned in his/her will, are not potential claimants to his/her estate, and are not involved in the patient's medical care. Thus, the DIRECTIVE cannot be witnessed by you or any of your employees. Likewise it should not be witnessed by any other physician or his/her employees, or the employees of any health facility. In addition, if the patient is in a skilled nursing facility at the time of signing, a "patient advocate" or "ombudsman" (designated by the State Department of Aging) **must** be a witness.

The DIRECTIVE is effective for five years after which a person may sign a new one. A person signing a DIRECTIVE should, if possible, present the document to his/her physician so that it can be made part of his/her current medical record.

EFFECT OF A DIRECTIVE. Upon receipt of a DIRECTIVE from any patient (qualified or unqualified) the attending physician must determine that the DIRECTIVE meets legal requirements. Under the Act a "qualified patient" is a person diagnosed and certified in writing to be afflicted with a terminal condition by two physicians, one of whom shall be the attending physician, who have personally examined the patient.

Whether or not a DIRECTIVE is binding depends upon the condition of the patient at the time the DIRECTIVE was signed.

In order for the DIRECTIVE **to be binding** the patient must be qualified and have signed or re-executed the DIRECTIVE at least 14 days after being notified of his/her terminal condition. If you do not wish to carry out the DIRECTIVE of such a patient, you are required to transfer care of the patient to a physician who is willing to comply with the DIRECTIVE. If you do not transfer such a patient, you may be found guilty of unprofessional conduct. If you do carry out the DIRECTIVE, you are protected from civil and criminal liability.

The DIRECTIVE **is not binding** if the patient executed the DIRECTIVE while in good health (in anticipation of a terminal illness or injury). However, should the patient be subsequently diagnosed and certified as terminal, you may carry out the DIRECTIVE if, in your judgment, all of the circumstances known to you justify doing so. If you carry out the DIRECTIVE you are protected from civil and criminal liability.

Regardless of the binding or nonbinding nature of the DIRECTIVE, *it is not to be given effect until you have determined that death is imminent, whether or not "life-sustaining procedures" are utilized. Such procedures include mechanical or other "artificial means" which sustain vital functions only to postpone the moment of death. These do not include medications or procedures deemed necessary to alleviate pain.*

The DIRECTIVE *is invalid and has* **no effect** *if the patient is pregnant at the time it is to be carried out.*

REVOCATION. A patient may revoke the DIRECTIVE at any time by (1) destroying it, (2) signing a written statement or (3) communicating to the attending physician his/her wish to revoke the DIRECTIVE. Should you receive such revocation from or on behalf of a patient who has previously signed a DIRECTIVE, enter that information promptly and prominently in the patient's current medical record.

OTHER RIGHTS. No person may be forced to sign a DIRECTIVE. A person who has signed a DIRECTIVE may not be denied health care or health insurance. The DIRECTIVE has no effect on any insurance policy and does not limit a person's right to accept or reject health care of any kind.

PRECAUTIONS. A person who knowingly conceals or destroys a valid DIRECTIVE is guilty of a misdemeanor. A person who forges or falsifies a DIRECTIVE, or who withholds knowledge of a revocation of a DIRECTIVE may be guilty of unlawful homicide.

SUMMARY. Withholding "life-sustaining procedures" in compliance with a DIRECTIVE is **not** euthanasia or "mercy killing." The DIRECTIVE is **not** a "Living Will." The DIRECTIVE is merely a method, recognized under California law, by which a physician may respect a patient's instruction to permit an imminent death to proceed naturally.

Policies and Procedures Governing Violations of the Code for Nurses, Approved by the Board of Directors of the New York State Nurses Association*

Introduction

The Code for Nurses adopted by the American Nurses' Association, is intended to serve the nursing practitioner as a guide to the ethical principles that govern individual practice, conduct and relationships. The Code and the accompanying interpretive statements clarify the areas in which definite standards of practice and conduct are essential to the full and ethical discharge of each practitioner's responsibility to the public, to associated groups, and to the profession. Each practitioner has an obligation to uphold and adhere to the Code in individual practice and to ensure that colleagues do likewise. The professional organization has the obligation to protect the public in general, to protect the individual patient in particu-

*Reprinted with permission from *Journal, New York State Nurses Association*, 4, 2 (August 1973), 43–44.

lar, and to demonstrate concern for the profession of nursing. Therefore, the organization will take all appropriate measures to ensure adherence to the Code by all nursing practitioners.

The Board of Directors of each constituency of the American Nurses' Association has the authority and the responsibility for handling all alleged violations of the Code by their respective members.

All practitioners holding membership in the New York State Nurses Association are subject to such disciplinary action under Article V of the Bylaws. The 1971 New York State Nurses Association House of Delegates established a Committee on Ethical Practice and charged it with the responsibility for investigating any complaints of alleged violation of the Code for Nurses, and has prepared the following policies and procedures governing such matters.

Policies

1. Complaints may be initiated by a colleague, constituent nurses association or any individual who has cause to believe a nursing practitioner is in violation of the Code.
2. All complaints must be submitted to the Committee on Ethical Practice in writing and signed by the complainant.
3. Investigations are to be carried out in a manner which will safeguard the rights of all parties:
    a. Confidentiality shall be strictly maintained;
    b. All information pertinent to the alleged violation shall be collected and thoroughly evaluated;
    c. The individual alleged to be in violation shall be notified in writing that a complaint has been lodged and an investigation of the charge is pending;
    d. Precautions shall be taken to prevent reprisals against the complainant;
    e. In all instances of reported alleged violations, provision shall be made for a full and fair formal hearing;
    f. The privilege of a formal hearing may be waived by the individual alleged to be in violation;
    g. In presentation of the defense, the individual alleged to be in violation shall have the right to be accompanied by or represented by legal counsel or another individual of his choice;
    h. The individual alleged to be in violation shall have the right to introduce evidence on his behalf; to examine any evidence introduced against him; to examine and cross-examine every witness against him.
4. The recommended disposition of the complaint by the Committee on Ethical Practice shall be appropriate to the nature and circumstances of the alleged violation. Such disposition may include, but not necessarily be limited to, dismissal of the charges, reprimand, censure, suspension or expulsion from the New York State Nurses Association. Where the violation appears to be of a criminal nature, the New York State Nurses Association will refer the matter to the appropriate legal authorities.
5. Provision shall be made for notifying all parties, including other levels of the professional association when applicable, of the Association's decision in this matter.
6. Provision shall be made for an individual alleged to be in violation against whom disciplinary action has been decided, to have the right to appeal said decision in accord with the provisions of Article V of the Bylaws of the New York State Nurses Association.

Procedure

I. The New York State Nurses Association Committee on Ethical Practice shall:
    1. Receive all written, signed complaints:
        a. Acknowledge receipt of complaint;
        b. Request additional information if necessary;

    c. Notify the individual alleged to be in violation of the complaint;

    d. Notify complainant that the individual alleged to be in violation has been advised of the nature of the complaint and the name of the complainant.

2. Proceed with an investigation of the complaint:

    a. Determine whether additional information is necessary;

    b. Conduct interviews with the complainant and the individual alleged to be in violation, if necessary.

3. Provide for a full and fair formal hearing if necessary, or requested:

    a. Determine within 30 days from receipt of complaint whether a hearing is to be held;

    b. Notify complainant and individual alleged to be in violation of the date of the hearing at least 10 days prior to the scheduled date;

    c. Conduct the hearing within 60 days from receipt of complaint.

4. Recommend disposition of charges:

    a. Submit to the New York State Nurses Association Board of Directors a written report including recommendations for specific action to be taken, within sixty (60) days from receipt of complaint.

    b. Make available to the Board all pertinent findings when a case is appealed;

    c. Provide for any follow-up to determine that the violation has been corrected.

II. The New York State Nurses Association Board of Directors shall:

1. Receive the report and recommendations from the Committee on Ethical Practice;

2. Determine the final disposition of the case;

3. Notify all involved parties of its decision in the matter;

4. Receive and process requests for appeal as provided for in Article V of the New York State Nurses Association's Bylaws.

Note

    The Board of Directors of a district nurses association may request the New York State Nurses Association's Committee on Ethical Practice to carry out the procedure governing violations of the Code for its members if the district lacks the necessary resources or if the particular circumstances of an alleged violation preclude an unbiased investigation.

Index

Principles:
  conventional, 71–75
  moral vs. medical, 74
  regulation of, and actual adherence to, 75–78
  roots of, 73–75
Professionalism, 18–27
  and autonomy, 21–22, 52–53
  vs. bureaucratic authority, 52
  characteristics of (vs. "calling"), 18–21
  claim to competence in, 19–20
  ethics of, 4–5, 22–30, 203
  hazards of, 31–33
  and monopoly of health care, 21
  social value of, 20
Profits, medical, 103–7

Quality of life, 229, 253
Quarantine, 265
Quinlan, Karen, 197

Racism, 270–73
Rationality, 147
Reality Shock (Kramer), 5
Reciprocity:
  re gifts and tips, 101–2
  in medical information exchange, 171
  and rights and responsibilities, 139
Reduction-of-suffering argument, 232
Reflection, ethical, 152–60
Registered nurses (RN), 7–9, 11
Registries, nurses, 47
Religion:
  nursing's roots in, 222–23
  views on suffering, 221–22
Research:
  exploitative, 107–11
  models of, 160–62
  therapeutic, in NICU, 252
Respect for persons, 125–30, 148
respondeat superior, 40–41
Responsibility, 141–45
  capacity and, 143–45
  causal, 142, 205
  coercion and, 143–44
  collective, 145, 290
  and liability, 143, 145, 205–6
  and rights, 139
  unofficial, 144
Review, professional, 22–23
Rewards (*see* Sanctions)
Right:
  to death with dignity, 141
  to health, 265–66
  to health care, 263–65, 266
  to self-protection (nurses), 212–16
Rights, 138–41
  absolute, 139–40

and entitlement (to medical information), 172–73
  fundamental, 140, 264
  history of, 138–39
  informed consent and, 184
  legal vs. moral, 139
  positive and negative, 139
  protection of vs. provision for, 141
  and responsibilities, 139
  surveyable and enforceable, 140
Risk-benefit analysis, 94–95, 148
Risk management, 144
Risks, 214–16
  of experimentation, 107–11
  and informed consent, 186–87
  of medical procedures, 93–95
  to nurses, 214–16
Robb, Isabel Hampton, 28, 37, 118–19
Rogers, Martha, 262
Roles:
  and competence, 82
  extended, 28
  private vs. professional, 28–30
  and responsibility, 142–43
Royal College of Nursing Code of Professional Conduct, 314–15
Rule utilitarianism, 146–47
Rules, (over-)stringent, 145

Sacrifices, personal, 214–15
Sainthood, 215
Salaries, medical, 103–7
Sanctions and rewards:
  bureaucratic, 41
  professional, 23, 75–76
Sanger, Margaret, 286
Sartre, Jean Paul, 288–89
Scandals, experimental, 108–9
Scapegoating, 145
Schorr, Thelma, 287–88
Sedation, 213–14
Self-examination, philosophical, 61
Self-protection, right to, of nurses, 212–16
Self-sacrifice, 215–16
Semi-profession, nursing as, 21–22
Settlement House movement, 98
Sex relations, exploitative, 114–16
Sexism:
  in language, 42
  and nurses, 38–39
  and patients, 47–50
Silver nitrate controversy, 287–88
Slow code, 233
Social conflict theorists, 154–55
Socialization, moral, 152–53
Socrates, 160
Standardized procedures, 9
Standing orders, 9
"Statement on a Patient's Bill of Rights," 112